A Special Issue of
Neuropsychological Rehabilitation

The Self and Identity in Rehabilitation

Guest Editors

Fergus Gracey
The Oliver Zangwill Centre, Cambridge, UK

and

Tamara Ownsworth
Griffith University, Nathan, Australia

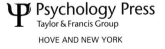

Ψ Psychology Press
Taylor & Francis Group

HOVE AND NEW YORK

First published 2009 by Psychology Press
27 Church Road, Hove, East Sussex BN3 2FA

www.psypress.com

Simultaneously published in the USA and Canada
by Psychology Press
270 Madison Avenue, New York NY 10016

Psychology Press is an imprint of the Taylor & Francis Group, an Informa business

British Library Cataloguing in Publication Data
A catalogue record for this book is available from the British Library

ISBN: 978-1-84169-863-2
ISSN: 0960-2011

Cover design by Hybert Design
Typeset in the UK by Techset Composition Limited, Salisbury
Printed in the UK by Henry Ling Limited at the Dorset Press, Dorchester
Bound in the UK by TJ International Ltd, Padstow, Cornwall

The publication has been produced with paper manufactured to strict
environmental standards and with pulp derived from sustainable forests.

Contents*

---

*This book is also a special issue of the journal *Neuropsychological Rehabilitation*, and forms issues 5 and 6 of Volume 18 (2008). The page numbers are taken from the journal and so begin with p. 513.

NEUROPSYCHOLOGICAL REHABILITATION
2008, 18 (5/6), 513–521

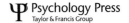

Foreword

Yehuda Ben-Yishay

Brain Injury Day Treatment Program, New York University Medical Center,
Rusk Institute of Rehabilitation, New York, NY, USA

The articles appearing in this issue examine, from different points of view, the fact that acquired brain injuries of varying aetiologies often result in damaged identity or self in the persons so afflicted. All the authors of these papers appear to take for granted that the readers will understand what, precisely, is being referred to by the construct of identity. But I believe that this assumption is questionable. For, we may ask, what is identity and why is it relevant in the context of the neuropsychological rehabilitation endeavour?

More than a century ago, William James in his *The Principles of Psychology* (1980) defined the self as "all that [a person calls] ME" (p. 291). James (1980) distinguished between the "social self [i.e.] the recognition which [the person] gets from his mates" (p. 293), and the "spiritual self [i.e.] a man's inner or subjective being, his psychic faculties or dispositions [which] are the most enduring intimate part of the self" (p. 296). This personal identity, James argued, is experienced by the individual as a "sense of sameness [of the] present self and [the] self of yesterday" (p. 332). But our perception of the "sameness" (i.e., the continuity) of the self is contributed only by those personal recollections of experiences from our childhood which, according to James, have "warm" and "intimate" feelings attached to them. Thus, stories we might be told by our parents, about some "clever" things we said or did as children, are not included in our sense of self, if we are unable personally to recall them (even though it may please us to hear such stories).

James (1980) emphasised that one of the major requirements for the persistence of our self is the continuum of those "intimate" personal

Correspondence should be sent to Yehuda Ben-Yishay, Brain Injury Day Treatment Program, New York University Medical Center, Rusk Institute of Rehabilitation, 550 First Avenue, New York, NY 10016, USA. E-mail: Yehuda.Ben-Yishay@nyumc.org

© 2008 Psychology Press, an imprint of the Taylor & Francis Group, an Informa business
http://www.psypress.com/neurorehab
DOI:10.1080/09602010802141525

recollections. For, "if a man wakes up some fine day unable to recall any of his past experiences, so that he has to learn his biography afresh ... he feels, and he says, that he is a changed person" (p. 336). Thus, the continuity of the sense of self cannot be taken for granted as (half a century later) Erik Erikson (1950) observed in war veterans who suffered, so-called, combat neuroses: "What impressed me most was the loss in these men of a sense of identity. They knew who they were; [but] it was as if subjectively their lives no longer hung together – and never would again" (p. 38). Similarly, some years later, Laing (1962) observed that – under certain pathological conditions – people manifested generalised feelings of unreality, a lack of a sense of temporal continuity, and a blurred sense of self.

We now turn our attention to some of Kurt Goldstein's ideas concerning the holistic neuropsychological rehabilitation of persons who sustained a traumatic brain injury (TBI). Goldstein (1959) asserted that when, following aTBI, it is impossible to restore the patient's cognitive and functional life-competencies to their pre-injury levels, others must structure and modify the patient's environment so that the patient will be able to cope with demands of the situations confronting him or her. Under those conditions the patient will feel "in a state of health" (p. 9) so to speak. Thus, despite the fact that the brain injury has resulted in permanent reductions in the patient's capacities, by making it possible for the patient to cope, we can foster a feeling of "health" (or well-being).

However, by structuring a patient's environment, we impose, by necessity, "restrictions" i.e., limitations on his or her freedoms. Hence, Goldstein (1959) taught us that to help the person with TBI to feel healthy, "demands the trans-formation of the individual's personality [to enable him or her] to bear restrictions [and that] it is our task in therapy to help the patient realise [and accept] the necessity [for bearing those] restrictions, to such a degree that life remains worth living in spite of [the] restrictions" (p. 10). The implications for neurop-sychological rehabilitation, according to Goldstein (1959) are obvious. Since, due to the impairments of cognitive functions and the presence of neurobehavioural and emotional disturbances, "a [significant aspect of the] therapy consists in making the patient understand [his or her] problems as much as possible in all [their] details" (p. 10); because, "therapy [can] be suc-cessful [only] if the patient participates in [his or her] treatments adequately [i.e., actively and voluntarily]" (p. 11).

Without a doubt, Goldstein's views on the neuropsychological rehabilita-tion endeavour, encompass the restoration of the impaired identity, or self, of the individual who suffered a TBI. His views have been the conceptual foun-dation of the New York University (NYU) holistic programme of neuropsy-chological rehabilitation, as it has been operationalised and programmatically implemented by us, in a "therapeutic community" setting, since its inception (Ben-Yishay, 1981, 1996, 2000; Ben-Yishay & Daniels-Zide, 2000; Ben-Yishay

& Diller, in press; Ben-Yishay et al., 1978, 1985; Daniels-Zide and Ben-Yishay, 2000).

Figure 1 illustrates the various overlapping stages in the process of remedial and therapeutic interventions (in the NYU Day Program) which (gradually) culminate in the reconstitution of the identity of patients following TBI.

Surrounded by their peers, their respective significant others, and the staff the patients are constantly encouraged, inspired, and exhorted to participate whole-heartedly in the programme activities; systematically made aware of and helped to understand the nature of their deficits, how they interact with each other, and their combined functional consequences; and are persuaded that to deal effectively with those deficits, it is necessary to undergo special-ised rehabilitative treatments. For, only by learning how to compensate for the deficits that resulted from the brain injury can patients hope to optimise their subsequent functional adjustment. The emphasis, thereafter, during each of the successive stages of the remedial process, is on ameliorating pro-blems due to disinhibition (e.g., difficulties controlling impulsive and poorly

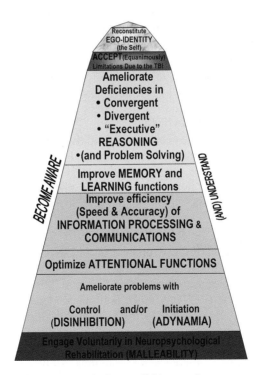

Figure 1. Stages in the remedial intervention process.

modulated behaviours) or problems due to adynamia (e.g., difficulties initiating and sustaining purposeful behaviours); optimising attentional functions; facilitating the speed and accuracy of information processing and interpersonal communications; improving memory functions (which includes teaching the patient effective mnemonic and review techniques); and on improving patients' convergent and divergent reasoning abilities, as well as their executive functions (e.g., organising, planning, prioritizing, problem-solving; and self-monitoring skills).

Supplemented by ongoing personal and conjoint family counselling, the preceding remedial efforts prepare many patients to accept their limitations with the degree of equanimity that is needed to find meaning in their attainments after rehabilitation; and finally, to reconstitute their shaken identity, or self.

Extensive clinical experiences, over the years, have shown that the construct of ego-identity, as it was articulated by Erik Erikson (1950, 1958, 1959), is particularly well suited in the context of neuropsychological rehabilitative programmes for persons who sustained TBI. The Eriksonian concept of ego-identity has a number of meanings. Although Erikson wrote about the subject extensively, it has been difficult to understand clearly the various nuances of his conception of ego-identity. Fortunately, Yankelowich and Barret (1970) provided a systematic and lucid description of Erikson's concept. According to Yankelowich and Barret (1970) we may distinguish between three components: (1) identity as the synthesis of all the imitations; (2) identity as the persistence of the sense of sameness within one's self through life; and (3) identity as self-definition. Each component is briefly described below.

Identity as imitation.   The roots of the imitative aspects are to be found in the psychological mechanism of the young child. For example, when the 2-year-old girl put on her mother's hat and shoes and declares, "I am a mommy", or when the young boy puts on a fireman's toy hat and says, "I am a fireman". As the child matures, the imitations become more complex; 4–5-year-old children "play" different roles using their own voices and mannerisms. As the child reaches early adolescence, the various imitations become fused "by the [process of the] "synthesizing ego [which] consolidates [the imitations] and forges them into a unity [which] transforms them into the unique sense of self [that Erikson called] the ego-identity" (Yankelowich & Barrett, 1970, p. 124). Following adolescence the imitation assumes increasingly more subtle forms, such as the special "dress codes" of teenagers, their mannerisms, and the special "vocabulary" they often affect. These also include the internalised beliefs, values and attitudes, that young adults "absorb" as they emulate parental figures or other adult role-models, which may also include literary or historical figures.

Identity as a sense of continuity and sameness.   The sense of a persistent sameness comes from the coherent memories which provide "a stable structure that endures in time" (Yankelowich & Barrett, 1970, p. 127). It is this enduring structure of sameness that the individual identifies as "Me" through the years, from childhood to adulthood (see James' earlier comments).

Identity as self-definition.   According to Yankelowich and Barret's (1970) rendition of the Eriksonian concept of ego-identity, as the person reaches early adulthood, the ego-identity metamorphoses into two complementary forms of self-definition. The first form of self-definition was described 2000 years ago by the Greek (stoic) philosopher Epictetus who said: "You should explicitly identify the kind of person you aspire to become. What are your personal ideas? Whom do you admire? What are their special traits that you would make your own?" (Lebell, 1994). An example of such a self-definition is the following, self-revealing, assertion that was made by a psychologist (as part of his "thank you" comments) when he received an award for his contributions to the field of neuropsychological rehabilitation: "I am an ambitious person who has striven since I have been a teenager to excel at what I have been doing. But, since I have always attempted to emulate my two role-models (my father and grandfather) who served their country (Israel) selflessly in war and peace in the spirit of the early pioneers, I have chosen this field; so that I may work toward realizing my ambition to excel, guilt-free and with the satisfaction of knowing that I am doing some good for others."

  The second form of self-definition, which is part of Erikson's ego-identity, was described by Yankelowich and Barret (1970) as "a form of transcendence, a way of reaching beyond one's own self and even beyond the limits of one's own times and culture" (p. 133). An excellent example of a "transcendental" type of self-definition can be found at the Holocaust Museum in Washington DC. Inscribed on a plaque is the following statement that is attributed to Albert Einstein: "A desire for knowledge for its own sake, a love of justice that borders on fanaticism, and a striving for personal independence – these are the aspects of the Jewish people's tradition that allow me to regard my belonging to it a gift of great fortune." Yankelowich and Barret (1970) thus present Erikson's construct of ego-identity as the culmination of the transformed imitations, internalized attitudes and values accumulated through childhood, adolescence, and adulthood, into a unified sense of selfhood, which "in later years, the person experiences [as the "me" which provides] a feeling of oneness with himself, with his environment, and his life" (p. 132). Figure 2 illustrates the evolution of the Eriksonian construct of ego-identity.

  The following case illustrations are typical of the patients who underwent intensive neuropsychological rehabilitation in the NYU Day Program (lasting

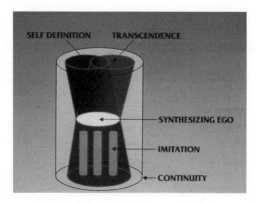

Figure 2. Evolution of ego identity.

in each case for at least one year). These individuals, following their discharge from rehabilitation, made excellent personal and occupational adjustments, found meaning in their lives, and have reconstituted their ego-identities.

CASE ILLUSTRATION 1

M was 46 years old when he suffered severe brain injuries as a result of encephalitis of unknown aetiology. He. was the chief of the gastroenterology service at a large urban hospital. After a long period of resistance to rehabilitation and depression, M made peace with his situation. M's self-definition after rehabilitation included the following: "I feel, in general, that I am a whole person. I don't look at myself as somebody who has a brain injury ... I don't look at myself as separate from the person I was in the past ... a result of my rehabilitation, there has been a synthesis ... I have learned enough to function at my best both cognitively and interpersonally ... I feel OK and am fortunate in having a loving supportive family ... being able to function with my wife and children, gives the ultimate meaning to my life ... the opportunity to function as a peer counsellor (at the NYU Day Program) supports my self-esteem."

CASE ILLUSTRATION 2

R was a successful 57-year-old engineer, attorney, and community leader. He suffered two strokes that left him with physical and cognitive disabilities. His self-definition contained the following: "To answer the question whom I am today, we have to go back to who I was before. In a way I am the same person. I still seek happiness, but in a different way. Before the stroke, I used to look for happiness in a material way ... I now realise that happiness does not come from things. It comes from the satisfaction of being a peer counsellor [which] serves my need to be of service [and it] makes me happy to be of service."

Initially, while he was still struggling to accept his limitations, R frequently expressed his wish to be able to emulate his "uncle Jimmy." Despite being severely incapacitated by polio, this uncle earned the admiration of all the members of his large extended family by his cheerfulness and dignified existence. When R, finally, managed to achieve his own acceptance, he defined himself as having become a role-model ("like my uncle Jimmy") to his children, his many nephews and nieces, and the younger members of his patient peer group at the NYU Day Program. He asserted: "I feel a bond with these young people, like with my own children, nieces and nephews ... By inspiring them, I also help myself ..."

CASE ILLUSTRATION 3

J was a 24-year-old student of economics when he sustained a moderately severe TBI in a motor vehicle accident. He was an athletic, ambitious, hard working, and practical man. Initially, J was hard to manage at the Day Program, because of his rebelliousness and insistence that rehabilitation following a brain injury was not different, in principle, from body-building (of the weight lifting variety, with the slogan "no pain – no gain"). He constantly demanded "challenging" tasks from the staff (e.g., "Ask each patient to summarise the news of the day") which were not part of the staff's remedial curriculum. But, aided by his religious faith and supported by his loving and wise parents, J finally accepted his situation. His self-definition was of the "transcendental" type, "The Lord intended that I become severely incapacitated so that I can be a role model to others for graceful acceptance." Following discharge from the Day Program, J became employed as a clerk at a health club. Three years later, he enrolled into slow and gradual academic studies towards a degree in rehabilitation counselling. After 10 years he finally graduated. As of this writing, J is employed at a rehabilitation centre.

CASE ILLUSTRATION 4

S, a 34-year-old bank executive who earned degrees in maths and statistics, was severely injured in a motor vehicle accident. Following intensive neuropsychological rehabilitation, S became employed (part-time) in a mid-level clerical capacity. S could work only 3–4 hours a day because longer hours would precipitate seizures. Yet she persisted at her work cheerfully and accepted calmly her need to be taken care of by a sister. S's self-definition statement was as follows, "I gave my 100% to everything I have ever done . . . I gave my rehabilitation 150%; this is my best . . . this is me."

CASE ILLUSTRATION 5

M was an academically outstanding college student and star athlete (on scholarship) at an "Ivy League" university, when she suffered severe TBI in a motor vehicle accident. M refused to accept (as she interpreted it) the "defeatist" message of rehabilitation ("they preach acceptance of a second-rate life of a cripple . . . !") She discharged herself against medical advice from two rehabilitation programmes in her State. For the next three years, M attempted to restore her cognitive abilities by spending many hours each day at the local library. To supplement her income, she attempted to work as a cashier at a local supermarket. However, she failed at both tasks. Then, at her mother's insistence, M. enrolled into the Day Program. At her "graduation" ceremony, M made the following self-defining statement: "The old me did strive to be successful in what I did. In my pre-injury life, I measured [success] on a scale geared for speed and agility . . . I have had to revise my pre-injury 'ruler' to a new, more appropriate measurement for success . . . I will be pleased [to be making progress] no matter how small [the steps may be] . . . I have the hardy strength and strong character of a cross-county runner."

Over the following 10 years (subsequent to her discharge from the NYU Day Program) M resumed her academic studies, obtained a BA (Cum Laude), enrolled into graduate studies in library sciences from which she graduated with an MA, secured a full-time position as a librarian at a college, was married (happily) to an airline pilot, and gave birth to her first child.

FINAL COMMENT

Experience has shown that only some of the individuals who attended the NYU Day Program over the years have attained a reconstituted ego-identity. Clinical observations suggested that those who did succeed in providing unambiguous self-definitions possessed some premorbid personality characteristics that helped them attain "examined" lives following rehabilitation after TBI. We are presently conducting several retrospective studies aimed at identifying those personality characteristics.

REFERENCES

Ben-Yishay, Y. (1981). Cognitive remediation: Toward a definition of its objectives, tasks and conditions. In Y. Ben-Yishay (Ed.), *New York University Medical Center, Rehabilitation Monograph No. 62* (pp. 14–42). New York: New York Medical Center.

Ben-Yishay, Y. (1996). Reflections on the evolution of the therapeutic milieu concept. *Neuropsychological Rehabilitation, 6,* 327–343.

Ben-Yishay, Y. (2000). Post-acute neuropsychological rehabilitation. In A. Christensen & B. Uzzell (Eds.), *International Handbook of Neuropsychological Rehabilitation* (pp. 131–139). New York: Kluwer Academic/Plenum Publishers.

Ben-Yishay, Y., Ben-Nachum, Z., Cohen, A., Gross, Y., Hoffien, D., Rattok, J., & Diller, L. (1978). Digest of a two-year comprehensive clinical research program for out-patient head injured Israeli veterans. In Y. Ben-Yishay (Ed.). *New York University Medical Center Rehabilitation Monograph No. 59* (pp. 1–61). New York: New York University Medical Center.

Ben-Yishay, Y., & Daniels-Zide, E. (2000). Examined lives: Outcomes after holistic rehabilitation. *Rehabilitation Psychology, 45* (2), 112–119.

Ben-Yishay, Y., & Diller, L. (in press). *Primer of Holistic Neuropsychological Rehabilitation* New York: Oxford University Press.

Ben-Yishay, Y., Rattok, J., Lakin, P., Piasetsky, E., Ross, B., Silver S.L., Zide, E., & Ezrachi, O. (1985). Neuropsychological rehabilitation: The quest for a holistic approach. *Seminars in Neurology, 5,* 252–259.

Daniels-Zide, E., & Ben-Yishay, Y. (2000). Therapeutic Milieu Day Program. In A. Christiansen & B. Uzzell (Eds.), *International Handbook of Neuropsychological Rehabilitation* (pp. 183–193). New York: Kluwer Academic/Plenum Publishers.

Erikson, E. H. (1950). *Childhood and Society.* New York: W.W. Norton.

Erikson, E. H. (1958). *Young Man Luther.* New York: W.W. Norton.

Erikson, E. H. (1959). Identity and the life cycle. *Psychological Issues, 1,* 102–110.

Goldstein, K. (1942). *After-Effects of Brain Injuries in War: Their Evaluation and Treatment.* New York: Grune and Straton.

Goldstein, K. (1952). *The Effects of Brain Damage on the Personality.* Presented at the Annual Meeting of the American Psychoanalytic Association, Atlantic City, NJ.

Goldstein, K. (1959). Notes on the development of my concepts. *Journal of Individual Psychology, 15,* 5–14.

James, W. (1980). *The Principles of Psychology* (Vol. 1). New York: Doer Publications.

Laing, R. O. (1962). *Ontological Insecurity in Psychoanalysis and Existential Philosophy.* New York: E.P. Dutton.

Lebell, S. (1994). *A Manual for Living. Epictetus – A New Interpretation.* San Francisco: Harper.

Yankelovich, D., & Barrett, W. (1970). *Ego and Instinct.* New York: Random House.

NEUROPSYCHOLOGICAL REHABILITATION
2008, 18 (5/6), 522–526

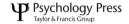

Editorial

Fergus Gracey[1] and Tamara Ownsworth[2]

[1]Oliver Zangwill Centre for Neuropsychological Rehabilitation, Princess of Wales Hospital, Ely, UK; [2]School of Psychology and Applied Cognitive Neuroscience Research Centre, Griffith University, Mt Gravatt, Australia

The importance of consideration of self and identity in neuropsychological rehabilitation following brain injury has historically been the preserve of the holistic approach (Ben-Yishay et al., 1985). However, there has been a recent growth of interest in the topic in three broad areas. Firstly, the development of the field of social neuroscience has brought functional neuroimaging and processes pertinent to self-awareness and systems of self-representation together. Secondly, critiques of the cognitive-behavioural model of emotional disorders in the early 1990s led to the development of more highly specified and rigorous theoretical models of cognition and emotion which include representation and processing of self-relevant information. Thirdly, there has been a growth in the extension of post-modern thinking to clinical psychology generally and neuropsychological rehabilitation particularly. This social-constructionist turn emphasises subjectivity, language, social processes and the importance of understanding individuals as actively constructing meaning in the context of interactions with others.

This special issue sets out to present examples of work drawn from these three areas that is of particular relevance to the development of understanding of the self and identity in rehabilitation. In the foreword to this Special Issue, Yehuda Ben-Yishay lays out the inception and development of a model for the integration of "ego-identity" change into the process of rehabilitation. This provides a historical and conceptual context for the papers that follow, which have been divided into three sections: conceptual and theoretical issues, research studies, and clinical interventions and service provision.

http://www.psypress.com/neurorehab   DOI:10.1080/09602010802141509

THEORETICAL AND CONCEPTUAL ISSUES

Wilson, Kopelman, and Kapur review their previous account of post-encephalitic patient CW's "denial of past consciousness" as a delusion in the context of a recent neurological model of consciousness and self. The potential applicability of this neurological account of self, incorporating a conceptualisation of systems of self-representation, self-regulation, memory and awareness, alongside the hypothesised neurological substrate for these processes, is highlighted, alongside other hypotheses for CW's denial of past consciousness.

Fotopoulou provides a contemporary account of confabulation which draws attention to the role of motivation as well as neuro-cognitive factors, contending that the self-related positive biases inherent in these false memories support self-enhancement and self-coherence. Fotopoulou suggests that understanding the identity formation function served by confabulations, in addition to underlying neuro-cognitive mechanisms, may lead to more successful clinical management and rehabilitation outcomes. Intriguing case material is used to illustrate the implications of a motivational approach in rehabilitation of confabulation.

Yeates, Gracey, and Collicutt-McGrath offer a social constructionist review of the use of the term "personality change" in brain injury rehabilitation. A biopsychosocial framework is employed to offer alternative accounts of what might lead to judgement or experience of "personality change". Clinical implications drawn from this highlight the need for sensitivity to the self-protective function an individual's language and behaviour may serve, and the need for integrated interventions that tackle the social contextual, neuro-cognitive, and self-representational systems that are implicated.

INVESTIGATIONS INTO SELF AND IDENTITY

Naylor and Clare investigate correlates of identity in their empirical study of the relationships between self-concept, awareness and autobiographical memory in early-stage dementia. Participants with a more positive and definite sense of self were found to display poorer awareness of their memory function and a greater impairment of autobiographical memory during the mid-life period. Consistent with the positions proposed by Fotopoulou and Yeates et al., these findings are interpreted using a biopsychosocial framework, whereby impaired awareness is proposed to have a protective function, namely, to maintain prior sense of self in the face of progressive functional decline.

Relationships between self-awareness, self-concept and cognitive function are also explored by Cooper-Evans and colleagues. This investigation of self-esteem and self-concept confirms that sense of self is negatively impacted by brain injury. In their long-term brain injury sample, self-esteem was found to be stable over a two-week interval. A higher level of self-esteem was related to reduced self-awareness and poorer cognitive function. Consistent with Gracey et al., the authors emphasise the need for subjective experiences to be a central focus in rehabilitation.

Using a group-based personal construct approach, Gracey et al. elicited bipolar constructs of self through structured small group discussions in a holistic rehabilitation setting. A key finding that emerged from the thematic analysis is that sense of self following acquired brain injury is primarily construed through subjective experiences associated with social and practical activities, thus highlighting how "meaning" and "doing" (in both tasks and social interactions) are intrinsically linked in reconstructing identity.

Extending the contextual dimension further, Cloute, Mitchell, and Yates take a social constructionist approach to understanding identity after traumatic brain injury (TBI) as experienced and constructed in the context of social interactions. A qualitative discourse analysis of interviews with participants with TBI and a significant other is presented. The authors find that people with brain injury can often be positioned as relatively passive in the context of a medical discourse about their injury, and may experience abandonment secondary to dependence on specialist services. A further theme of "progression and productivity" was also identified. The authors conclude that families require ongoing community support from brain injury services, and that such support needs to recognise the narratives and discourses used by clinicians, family members and the individual with TBI and "empower individuals with disabilities towards role engagement and participation in the community".

The social nature of identity is further emphasised in the study by Haslam et al. who look at social group membership after stroke. Since social identity theory suggests that participation in social contexts is the means by which we realise our identities, they hypothesise that social group membership may be related to well-being after stroke. They apply a new measure, the Exeter Identity Transitions Scale, and their findings suggest that those with membership of multiple social groups prior to stroke that are also maintained post-stroke rated higher levels of well-being.

CLINICAL INTERVENTIONS AND SERVICE PROVISION

With a similar focus to that of Naylor and Clare on both self-awareness and identity, Ownsworth, Turpin, Andrew, and Fleming describe the process of intervention with their patient CP who had poor self-awareness of deficits following thalamic stroke. They present a qualitative analysis of CP's rehabilitation designed to tackle metacognitive skills in a structured manner. The themes identified from interview with CP suggest that structured feedback in relation to tasks set in rehabilitation, in addition to allowing CP to "learn from experience" while having rehabilitation goals individually tailored, were significant to CP. The authors conclude that restructuring of self-knowledge may occur in rehabilitation through "a bi-directional feedback process between the client and therapist" rather than one way feedback to the client about deficits from the clinician.

This emphasis of a collaborative approach that includes a specific focus on identity by linking meaning, goals and tasks is also described and advocated by Ylvisaker, McPherson, Kayes, and Pellett. In this two-part paper, the authors discuss identity in the rehabilitation process following TBI drawing upon cognitive models of self-representation and goal-directed behaviour. First they outline the theoretical background to a clinical approach called "metaphoric identity mapping" aimed at integrating identity (and related motivational states) into goal setting and restructuring of self-knowledge in rehabilitation. The second part of the paper presents qualitative data from a pilot study of a related goal setting technique called "identity-oriented goal setting (IOG)". The qualitative analysis identified responses of both clients and clinicians emphasising the acceptability of this approach to clients, but some mixed responses from clinicians. A more negative response from one therapist was related to a perception of the approach being at odds with the skills and role of that professional.

Massimi, Berry, Browne, and Baecker present a descriptive treatment case study in which they describe the development and preliminary evaluation of "biography theatre", an innovative technology designed to preserve selfhood in Alzheimer's disease. The participant's use of an "in-home ambient computer display" to continuously play autobiographical information was associated with decreased apathy and more positive self-image. This exploratory study is part of an exciting frontier of technological advances to support or maintain sense of self in the context of progressive neurological conditions.

Holistic rehabilitation was developed with the aim of integrating issues such as cognitive rehabilitation and return to productive activity with attention to identity and awareness changes (Ben-Yishay et al., 1985). Coetzer provides a review of the background to how identity issues are addressed in intensive holistic rehabilitation, and then describes an alternative service configuration for such work based on longevity of input, rather than intensity. The argument here is that identity change is slow and many people have very long term, albeit varying, needs following brain injury. Furthermore, the need to tailor the service to the particular rural community was also a consideration. A case is presented illustrating the work undertaken by this service.

In our view, the papers presented in this special issue spell out the complex and interacting processes across biological, psychological and social domains that are required for a clinically relevant appreciation of the nature of changes to self and identity in the context of neuropsychological rehabilitation. At the biological level, emerging literature suggests a systematic deconstruction of broad notions such as "self" and "sense of self" into subsidiary processes based on neuroanatomical organisation. Certain types of injury or illness may differentially target neurological substrates of self-related processes, thus constraining access to the representations required to support a full and coherent experienced and enacted sense of self. Technological interventions, as well as innovative rehabilitation techniques, may seek to address such underpinning deficits so as to return access to self-representation or sense of self to those with such impairments. It appears that there is some variation in the way people make sense of changes in themselves after injury, such as retaining coherence in sense of self although described as having poor self-awareness, or experiencing a sense of discrepancy with prior self or "hoped for" self. However, the placing of experience and development of sense of self and identity in social context also emerges as an overwhelming theme across many of the papers presented. Discourses and experiences in the contexts of families, services, tasks and roles may disempower some individuals, provide experiential evidence for negative self-perceptions, and thus maintain poor clinical outcomes. On the other hand, engagement in a range of social groups, the use of bi-directional feedback between therapist and client on performance on specific tasks in rehabilitation, and the use of metaphor and other techniques to link goal setting and rehabilitative activity to more adaptive "possible selves" and identities appear to yield some positive gains for restructuring self-representations and experienced sense of self. The clinical outcomes described in the issue are tantalising in their tentativeness but together spell out a number of testable hypotheses regarding change processes in rehabilitation. The ideas represented across the issue are not inconsistent with the early ideas that contributed to the development of the holistic model as presented by Ben-Yishay, but provide interesting extensions of notions well established in holistic rehabilitation. In conclusion, a range of biological, psychological and social models is now contributing to significant developments in understanding self and identity in rehabilitation and these promise growth in research and clinical interventions.

REFERENCE

Ben-Yishay, Y., Rattok, J., Lakin, P., Piasetsky, E.D., Ross, B., Silver, S., Zide, E., & Ezrachi, O. (1985). Neuropsychologic rehabilitation: Quest for a holistic approach. *Seminars in Neurology*, 5, 252–259.

NEUROPSYCHOLOGICAL REHABILITATION
2008, 18 (5/6), 527–540

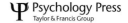

Prominent and persistent loss of past awareness in amnesia: Delusion, impaired consciousness or coping strategy?

Barbara A. Wilson[1], Michael Kopelman[2], and Narinder Kapur[3]

[1]Medical Research Council Cognition and Brain Sciences Unit, Cambridge and Oliver Zangwill Centre, Ely, UK; [2]King's College London, Institute of Psychiatry, London, UK; [3]Department of Neuropsychology, Addenbrooke's Hospital, Cambridge, UK

Profound loss of awareness for the past in amnesia has implications for our understanding of memory and belief systems, and how they may become disrupted in neurological conditions. We report the case of CW, a professional musician who became severely amnesic in 1985 following herpes simplex viral encephalitis (HSVE) at the age of 46 years. For many years CW stated several times a day that he had just woken up. He frequently wrote this in his diary too. When shown examples of his diary entries or videos of himself playing or conducting music, he recognised both his handwriting and himself on the video screen but stated vehemently that he "was not conscious then". In a previous paper (Wilson, Baddeley, & Kapur 1995), it was suggested that this lack of awareness for the past was a delusion, defined as a strongly held belief in the face of contradictory evidence (rather than implying any kind of psychiatric disorder per se). As a contribution to the academic debate regarding theories of "self", in the present paper we will review this explanation of CW's state as it had been in those early years, and we will also consider two other possibilities – namely, that CW had suffered from a loss of "autobiographical self" or "extended consciousness" (see Damasio, 2000, pp. 198–199), and that his verbal reports simply reflected a form of coping strategy to help him deal with the limited evidence he had available in "declarative" memory.

Correspondence should be sent to: Barbara A. Wilson, MRC Cognition and Brain Sciences Unit, Box 58, Addenbrooke's Hospital, Cambridge, CB2 2QQ, UK. E-mail: barbara.wilson@mrc-cbu.cam.ac.uk

Keywords: Amnesia; Awareness; Delusion; Impaired consciousness; Coping strategy.

INTRODUCTION

Severe memory loss, as in the amnesic syndrome, is often associated with differing degrees of lost orientation for person, age, time or place, and with varying degrees of memory distortion. Complete loss of self-knowledge, including loss of personal identity, is extremely rare in neurological disease, and is usually associated with psychogenic memory loss (Kopelman, 2002). Lack of awareness for one's age may occur in some neurological conditions, especially in the acute stages of a brain insult (Zangwill, 1953). Loss of awareness for time and place are usually associated with the acute phases of a brain injury (High, Levin, & Gary, 1990), with severe amnesia, or with the more advanced stages of a primary degenerative dementia. Distorted memories may take two broad forms – first, flawed "episodic memories", in which there is either distortion of events that have occurred, such that events that never occurred may be introduced or mislocation of a true event to a different time and place; and, secondly, flawed "semantic memories", where there are distortions in belief and knowledge structures. Delusions that accompany marked memory impairment could be seen to fall into the latter category (Schacter, 1995; Schacter & Scarry, 2000).

Delusions are notoriously hard to define. One definition is that a delusion is a belief that is clearly false and that indicates an abnormality in the affected person's content of thought (Hahn, 2003). Perhaps a tighter definition is that delusions are (1) false beliefs, held as (2) absolute convictions, (3) not amenable to argument, (4) not culturally explicable, and that (5) they are often bizarre, and (6) usually preoccupying (Clare, 1976; Mullen, 1979), but each component of this definition is debatable.

Delusions are not confined to psychiatric disorder but can be seen quite commonly in people with neurological conditions. The delusions most commonly reported in neuropsychological literature on people with brain damage are the (relatively rare) mono-thematic delusions, such as: (1) the Capgras syndrome, a belief that an acquaintance, usually a spouse or a close family member, has been replaced by an imposter (Ramachandran & Blakeslee, 1998); (2) the Fregoli delusion: the belief that one or several unfamiliar people are really someone very familiar (Ellis, Whitley, & Luaute, 1994; Markova & Berrios, 1994; Wright, Young, & Hellawell, 1993); (3) reduplicative paramnesia: a belief that a place or location has been duplicated (Sellal, Fontaine, van der Linden, Rainville, & Labrecque, 1996); and (4) Cotard's syndrome: a belief that one is dead or does not exist or is putrefying or has lost internal organs (Pearn & Gardner-Thorpe, 2002). The first three of these examples are delusional misidentifications, and all four are relatively rare. Much more common in neurological and neuropsychiatric practice are delusions of persecution and reference, delusions related to mood state (e.g., derogatory, grandiose), delusions of being burgled (especially in dementia), somatic and religiose delusions, or "first-rank" delusions of control and interference with thoughts (e.g., Cutting, 1997; Kopelman, in press; Lishman, 1998; Schneider, 1959).

In contrast to a delusion, a hallucination is a false perception occurring without any identifiable external stimulus (Hahn, 2003). More specifically, hallucinations involve: (1) false perceptions arising in the absence of an external stimulus, (2) occurring simultaneously with normal perceptions, and (3) having "substantiality" (i.e., they appear vivid, "real"). Furthermore, (4) they appear to be located in external space ("outside the head"), and (5) they arise independently (i.e., they cannot be conjured up or dismissed at will) (Kopelman, 1994; Mullen, 1979). One way of classifying hallucinations is according to sensory modality. Auditory hallucinations occur when people hear voices, sounds, noises or music in the absence of an external stimulus. The hearing of voices is the most common auditory hallucination, observed in many psychiatric patients but also in neurological and neuropsychiatric disorders.

Consciousness can be defined in several ways: Damasio (2000) offered a simple definition when he stated that it is "...an organism's awareness of its own self and surroundings" (p. 4). Cartlidge (2001) suggested that, in addition to awareness of self and one's surroundings, there should be an ability to respond to environmental factors. Gray (2004) suggested that, rather than trying to define consciousness, it may be more fruitful to consider the various distinctions that occur in discussions of conscious experience – he distinguished between conscious awareness of the outside world ("public cognitive space"), conscious awareness of one's thoughts and images ("private cognitive space"), and awareeness of inner bodily sensations, such as those of hunger or tiredness ("private bodily space"). In common with other authors (e.g., Zeman, 2002), he also argued that it is important to distinguish between the contents of conscious experience and states of consciousness – the latter usually referring to degrees of wakefulness.

We report on a very amnesic patient who, despite playing and conducting music and writing diary entries several times a day until approximately a year ago, consistently denied he was conscious at the time. Although this state persisted for many years, we have been unable to track down any reports of patients who have denied that they had ever been conscious since the onset of their illness, despite evidence to the contrary, for such long periods of time.

CASE REPORT

CW was born in 1938. He was an outstanding musician and gifted musical scholar, being one of the world's experts on Orlando Lassus, the Renaissance composer. He produced BBC Radio 3 programmes of Renaissance Royal wedding music to celebrate the wedding of Prince Charles and Lady Diana Spencer and was leader of the London Sinfonietta. In March 1985 at the age of 46 years, he developed an influenza type illness with headache and fever. He was admitted to hospital days later and the diagnosis of herpes simplex viral encephalitis (HSVE) was made. His level of consciousness fluctuated, and he was treated with acyclovir. This probably saved his life, but the virus destroyed large sections of his brain. (For a detailed account of the onset of his disorder, see Wearing, 2005, also Wilson & Wearing, 1995.)

An MRI scan was carried out in July 1991 (see Figure 1). Three independent raters agreed there were marked abnormalities bilaterally in the following areas: hippocampal formations, amygdalas, mamillary bodies, temporal poles, and substantia innominata. In addition there were marked abnormalities unilaterally (left) in the fornix, inferior temporal gyrus, anterior portion of middle temporal gyrus, anterior portion of superior temporal gyrus, and the insula. There were mild abnormalities in the posterior portion of left middle temporal gyrus, the left medial frontal cortex, the left striatum, the right insula, the right fornix and the anterior portion of right inferior temporal gyrus. In addition, the third ventricle and both lateral ventricles were significantly dilated. Both the left and the right thalami were considered to be intact and no other frontal abnormalities were seen other than the left medial frontal area mentioned above.

A second MRI (3-Tesla) was carried out in January 2006. As shown in Figure 2, there was very severe and extensive loss of left temporal lobe

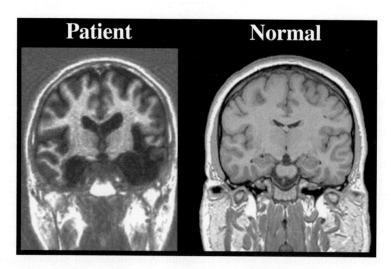

Figure 1. CW's MRI scan from 1991 compared with a non-brain damaged age-matched control.

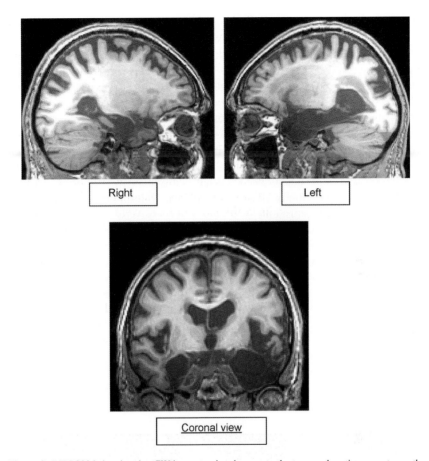

Figure 2. MRI 2006 showing that CW has extensive damage to the temporal cortices, greater on the left than on the right.

substance, and similarly severe loss of right medial temporal lobe tissue with some degree of generalised cortical atrophy throughout the brain. Comparing the 1991 and 2006 MRI scans, and allowing for improved imaging technology, there was very little change.

Neuropsychological assessment

CW was referred to one of us (BAW) in October 1985. A previous psychological report said there were extremely severe episodic memory deficits, some semantic memory impairments and CW's immediate memory span was normal.

A summary of the neuropsychological assessment of November 1985 can be seen in Table 1. In essence, CW's Verbal and Performance IQ scores were in the average range. This was, undoubtedly, a decline from his premorbid ability, which must have been in the superior or very superior range given his achievements. He showed evidence of executive dysfunction, particularly on a test of verbal fluency. As was the case in the earlier report (Wilson et al., 1995), his immediate memory, as measured by forward digit span (span of 7) and tapping a sequence of Corsi blocks (span of 5), was normal with delayed recall in the severely impaired range. Furthemore, CW, who had always been a city dweller, described a picture of a scarecrow as "a worshipping point for certain cultures" and, when asked, "What is a scarecrow?" he said, "A bird that flies and makes funny noises", which was interpreted as evidence of semantic memory impairment.

CW has been assessed on many occasions over the past 21 years. He has always scored zero on tests of delayed recall, and he has been unable to lay down new semantic information. In January 2006, on a test of new semantic knowledge, CW was given 50 words to define, which had come into the language over the past four decades (for example, e-mail, mad cow disease, and London Eye). The only word that CW defined accurately was "Eurotunnel", which could have been from guesswork. However, he has recently begun to show some evidence of new semantic learning, for

TABLE 1
Summary of CW's neuropsychological test scores

	1985	*1992*
•NART	122	111
•WAIS-R IQ	106	97
•WMS-R General index		<50
•Delayed index		<50
•RBMT	0/12	0/12
•Autobiog. Memory Interview	Severe impairment exc. childhood facts.	
•Graded Naming		2/30
•Semantic Battery Naming		
−Animate		30/60
−Inanimate		52/60
•Frontal/Executive:		
−Card sorting categories	4/6	6/6
−perseverations	8	0

Wilson et al., 1985, 1992.

example, the name and use of a mobile phone (for other examples, see Wearing, 2005).

CW has shown some evidence of residual learning capability, e.g., he could readily navigate to parts of the residential home in which he was living, such as the kitchen, even though it was difficult for him to give an explicit description of the route from memory if asked to do so. Furthermore, when CW took part in an errorless learning study (Baddeley & Wilson, 1994), he showed a major benefit for error-free over errorful learning, with a total of 12/36 correct in the errorful condition and 22/36 correct in the errorless condition. We argued that the superiority of errorless learning was due to implicit memory mechanisms, and Page, Wilson, Shiel, Carter, and Norris (2006) gave further support for this view. On a more formal test of implicit memory (Nannery, Sopena, Greenfield, & Wilson, 2007), CW showed some savings on a test of stem completion and on a perceptual priming (fragmented pictures) test. We have been unable to establish whether CW can learn new musical pieces, but he never learned pieces before he became ill as he always sight-read and he can still do this.

CW suffered an extensive retrograde amnesia, with markedly impaired recall on the Autobiographical Memory Interview (Kopelman, Wilson, & Baddeley, 1989) for all time-periods. He could recall very few facts from before the illness. Although he knew who he was and that he was a well-known musician, where he went to school, where he studied music, and that he married his wife, details were very patchy and he had lost most of his episodic memories for the 45 years prior to his illness. On a test of famous faces and names, CW was shown 18 well-known people. He recognised none of them and said only four were vaguely familiar (for example, he thought Margaret Thatcher was vaguely familiar and that she was a member of the Royal family and that Prince Philip was a member of CW's choir). When given their names, he gave identifying information for two, and four others were described as "vaguely familiar".

In summary, CW's memory functioning, as assessed by conventional neuropsychological tests, remained largely unchanged over 21 years, although Wearing (2005) noted some changes in everyday memory and conversation consistent with his being able to hold information in his memory longer than he used to (for example, he can now follow the plots of films more easily).

CW's auditory hallucination

In 1990 CW developed an auditory hallucination. He thought he could hear his music being played and said to is wife, "Listen, they're playing my music again." His wife believed he could genuinely hear it as he would start to hum the tune and pick it up mid-phrase. She indicated that if he were pretending to hear it then she thought he would start at the beginning of a phrase. This musical hallucination has remained and CW still "hears" his own music several times a week (described as "they're playing one of my tapes"), although he does not experience any other auditory hallucinations. Evers and Elger (2004) reviewed published cases of musical hallucinations associated with psychiatric and neurological aetiologies. They pointed out that, as in the case of CW, most patients with musical hallucinations perceive familiar songs, often the same one played repetitively (as in CW's case), implicating residual memory traces in the generation of the hallucinations. They also considered whether laterality of lesion was critical in generating musical hallucinations in neurological patients, and concluded that the small advantage for right-sided lesions "was not significant and supports the hypothesis that right-sided lesions play a role only marginally more important in the aetiology of musical hallucinations than left-sided lesions" (2004, p. 60). It thus remains possible that the origin of CW's musical hallucinations were from the more extensive left temporal lobe lesion that was characteristic of his lesion profile. It should also be noted that musical hallucinations are often associated with temporal lobe epilepsy (Lishman, 1998), and CW has indeed experienced complex partial seizures secondary to his extensive temporal lobe pathology, and he remains on anti-convulsant medication.

CW's belief that he was not previously conscious

For many years, CW did not appear to accept that he has a memory disorder, attributing his problems to the fact that he has not been conscious since he became ill. Indeed, one of CW's most often repeated phrases was that he had become conscious for the first time. In the early years, he reported this many times a day and added, "it is like being dead". A typical statement was: "I have just become conscious for the first time, this is the first sight I've had, the first taste I've had (sipping his coffee) it's like being dead. Does anyone know what it's like being dead? Answer, no". Sometimes he spoke as if he *were* dead. For example, on one occasion he was talking about millionaires and said, "When I was young there was only one millionaire, *but when I died* there were millions." If shown his diaries in which he had recorded his moments of just awakening, he accepted that the entries were in his handwriting but said, "But I wasn't conscious when I wrote that, I'm now conscious for the first time." If shown videotapes of himself playing the piano or conducting his choir (which he has done on occasion for television documentary programmes), he recognised himself in the video clips but, once again, said, "I wasn't conscious then". He did not accept that his problem was due to a memory impairment, but stated that it was due to a failure of consciousness since he became ill. Furthermore, if challenged about this belief he would become angry, because his subjective experience of amnesia was as awakening from total void – it could not be explained, because there was no vocabulary for CW's amnesic window on the world. Although it would have been interesting to discuss with CW what he actually meant when he said that he was now conscious for the first time, this was impossible because, as soon as one tried to engage in such a discussion, CW would interrupt to say that he had just woken up. In-depth conversations were impossible because of (1) his dense amnesia and (2) his preoccupation of having just regained consciousness.

In 1995 Wilson et al. suggested that this could perhaps be interpreted as a delusion, although without any psychiatric connotations. We reported that he must have been conscious when he wrote in his diary, played the piano and conducted his choir. We thought then that there were two aspects to consciousness – *being awake* and *being aware* and, as CW was both awake and aware, he must have had conscious experience.

Was CW suffering from a delusion?

At one level, it is obvious that CW was conscious in order to make the statement that he had not been conscious before. One cannot make such a statement if one is unconscious, asleep or in a coma. He also had experienced a recurrent auditory hallucination so he displayed two forms of misinterpretation about himself and the world about him. Was his belief about lack of past consciousness (i.e., loss of consciousness since his illness for he did not deny that he was *ever* conscious) due to the location of his brain damage or to the severity of his brain damage? Following Jaspers' (1913) distinction between the "form" of mental phenomena (or psychopathology) and their (specific) "content", Feinberg, Eaton, Roane, and Giacino (1999) have argued that memory and executive deficits are a necessary (although insufficient) condition for the occurrence of delusions in neurological disorders (and in psychiatric disorders), but that their content can be influenced by motivational and other factors. CW certainly had severe memory deficits and some executive deficits, although, of course, not all patients with combined executive and memory disorders experience delusions.

What about the specific content of CW's delusion? It may simply be an attempt to explain to himself *why* he cannot remember, and the content of the auditory hallucination may also have been influenced by fact that he is a musician. However, we know of no other reports in the literature where people have so persistently and predominantly denied past consciousness, although similar much more transient complaints do occasionally occur in amnesic patients. Ramachandran and Blakeslee (1998) suggest that Capgras syndrome is a result of a disconnection between temporal lobe and limbic system. There is no evidence that CW currently has any other delusions, either common ones, such as ideas of persecution or reference, or rare ones, such as the Capgras syndrome or Fregoli's syndrome.

Given the superficial resemblance between saying that one had not previously been conscious and saying that a body part or oneself is dead, it might appear pertinent to ask if CW had a variant of Cotard's syndrome. This does not seem to be the case, although he has occasionally spoken as if he had been dead (saying "after I died" instead of "after I became ill"), he was far more likely to say, "It is like being dead". In addition, he did not show other features of Cotard's syndrome such as suggesting that he did not exist or that he was putrefying or had lost his internal organs – moreover, unlike many Cotard patients, CW did not show any evidence of depression.

In brief, while the fixity of CW's belief is indeed consistent with its being *described* as "delusional", CW does not report other psychiatric features, which would suggest that an underlying "organic" psychosis is an *explanation* of his complaint of absent past consciousness. Thus, we have modified our original view and now no longer believe "a delusion" is a sufficient account of this phenomenon.

CW's belief as a form of impaired consciousness

Since our paper in 1995, much more has been written about consciousness. Zeman (2002), for example, in his excellent book reminded us of the complexity of consciousness and referred to scientific and philosophical theories of the phenomenon. In 2006, Zeman also wrote about self-consciousness in which he included self-perception, self-monitoring (metacognition), self-recognition (e.g., of body in mirror), awareness of awareness (possession of theory of mind) and self-knowledge (autonoetic awareness). Interesting though this topic is, it requires another paper to deal with it as it lies beyond the scope of this paper.

Damasio (2000) has argued that there are three types of consciousness or self. The most basic is proto self: "a coherent collection of neural patterns which map, moment by moment, the state of the physical structure of the organism in its many dimensions" (p. 154). Damasio (2000) went on to say that "we are not conscious of the proto self . . . [it] has no powers of perception and holds no knowledge" (p. 154). The next level is core self or core consciousness. This kind of self is condemned to endless and fruitless transiency. According to Damasio, all that core consciousness requires is a brief short-term memory, and we know that CW certainly had this. Then there is a higher form of consciousness that Damasio called autobiographical self, which is required for extended consciousness. Damasio wrote: "I use the term autobiographical memory to denote the organised record of the main aspects of an organism's biography." CW certainly had some knowledge of his autobiographical memory but this was impoverished for the period before he had become ill and, since his illness, he had laid down virtually no new autobiographical facts. According to Damasio, autobiographical self is constantly being refashioned as a result of experience. He also wrote that, "Extended consciousness depends on holding in mind, over substantial periods of time, the multiple neural patterns which describe the autobiographical self" (p. 200). We suggest that CW could not hold in mind these patterns over extended periods of time.

Autobiographical self then is the state when certain records of one's personal past are made explicit in reconstructed images as needed. This would appear to be the kind of deficit suffered by CW. He could not reconstruct images from his autobiographical memory. He had a very severe autobiographical memory impairment both for episodes prior to his illness and for the years since his illness. He could not lay down any new memories. Damasio argued that being conscious goes beyond being awake and attentive, it requires an inner sense of self in the act of knowing. The primary damage to CW's brain lies in the limbic areas which, Damasio argues, allow him to have core consciousness but not autobiographical consciousness. This leads to a life "being sensed but not really examined" (p. 217) and this, in turn, could explain why it was so difficult to have an in-depth, meaningful conversation with CW.

In support of this view, Damasio described a patient of his, David, who was similar to CW in the extent, severity and location of his brain lesions. Although David did not say he had just woken up or that he had not been conscious before, he did say that Damasio was his cousin, suggesting the presence of a form of Fregoli illusion. The amount of hippocampal damage seen in David was similar to that seen in HM (Scoville & Milner, 1957) but, unlike HM, David had damage to the cortices of the temporal lobes especially in the inferotemporal and polar regions. CW has similar damage to David, i.e., both in the hippocampal areas and in the temporal cortices (see CW's scan in Figure 2). Damage to the temporal cortices, then, should not impair core consciousness, since the structures required for this are intact, but it will impair the activation of autobiographical memory records and thus reduce the scope of extended consciousness. Presumably, the severity and extent of CW's temporal lobe damage relates to his failure to recognise the existence of his past consciousness.

Was CW's belief simply a form of coping strategy?

In her description of CW's "moments of awakening" in the early stages of his illness, Wearing (2005) noted, "As it seemed impossible to fix anything in his mind, it was as if every waking moment was the first waking moment. Clive was under the constant impression that he had just emerged from uncon-sciousness because he had no evidence in his own mind of ever being awake before." (p. 127). If this belief were challenged, he would become irri-table; and even if he were to be talked through the logic of what he was saying, he would rapidly return to this belief. Indeed, this irritability, in the absence of any overt depression or anxiety, was perhaps the most salient aspect of CW's mood state.

It would appear that CW had little or no declarative memory support when faced with situations which he had to explain, whether it was entries in his diary, meeting someone again a few minutes later, etc. His coping strategy for the absence of such declarative memory appeared to be to generate false memories, or to deny any previous experience with the items in ques-tion. It would appear that for CW, "consciousness" and "awareness" were interchangeable, and that if he had no "memory", and thus awareness, for immediately preceding events, he therefore believed that he was "aware" for the first time. He thus did not have the continual "stream of conscious-ness" or "stream of awareness" that Penfield eloquently referred to in his studies of patients with temporal lobe epilepsy (Penfield, 1959). CW's repeated denials could be seen to be a form of coping strategy to deal with this complete discontinuity in his stream of consiousness. As Bogousslavsky and Inglin (2007) have pointed out, beliefs can be seen to serve two functions – to represent a concept, and to form a justification for a viewpoint or for a course of action. In CW's case, his belief that he now had the impression of being conscious for the first time helped him to cope with his absent memory and also provided a justification for his subsequent statements and behaviours.

CONCLUSIONS

CW knew who was he but had limited knowledge about many aspects of his life. Klein, Rozendal, and Cosmides (2002) have argued that there are mul-tiple contributions to the concept of self, including episodic memories, rep-resentations of one's own personality traits, knowledge of the facts of one's own life, the sense of continuity of experience through time, a sense of per-sonal agency, and the ability to self-reflect on one's own mental states. Seen in this context, CW's sense of self had almost certainly been disrupted by his memory disorder. His persistent belief that he was "conscious for the first time" could be seen as a form of (isolated) delusion (without any psychiatric implication), or an impairment of consciousness, or a coping strategy to deal with the limited evidence that his cognitive deficits allowed him to have at his disposal. This belief no doubt fed into his disrupted sense of self, and com-bined to contribute to the personality and behaviour that he displayed in his interactions with others. We should perhaps add that, in recent years, there have been some changes in CW's semantic learning, his emotional disposition, and his insight (see Wearing, 2005), which we plan to investigate further in future publications.

REFERENCES

Baddeley, A. D., & Wilson, B. A. (1994). When implicit learning fails: Amnesia and the problem of error elimination. *Neuropsychologia, 32*, 53–68.

Bogousslavsky, J., & Inglin, M. (2007). Beliefs and the brain. *European Neurology, 58*, 129–132.

Cartlidge, N. (2001). States related to or confused with coma *Journal of Neurology, Neurosurgery, and Psychiatry, 71*(Suppl 1), i18–i19.

Clare, A. (1976). *Psychiatry in Dissent: Controversial Issues in Thought and Practice.* London: Tavistock.

Cutting, J. (1997). *Principles of Psychopathology.* Oxford: Oxford University Press.

Damasio, A. (2000). *The Feeling of What Happens: Body and Emotion in the Making of Consciousness.* New York: Harcourt Brace.

Ellis, H. D., Whitley, J., & Luaute, J.-P. (1994). Delusional misidentification: The three original papers on the Capgras, Frégoli and intermetamorphosis delusions. *History of Psychiatry, 5*, 117–118.

Evers, S., & Ellger, T. (2004). The clinical spectrum of musical hallucinations. *Journal of the Neurological Sciences, 227*, 55–65.

Feinberg, T. E., Eaton, L. A., Roane, D. M., & Giacino, J. T. (1999). Multiple Fregoli delusions after traumatic brain injury. *Cortex 35*, 383–387.

Gray, J. (2004). *Consciousness: Creeping up on the Hard Problem.* Oxford: Oxford University Press.

Hahn, J. (2003). Delusions. In *Gale Encyclopedia of Mental Disorders* Farmington Hills, MI: Thomson Gale Corporation.

High, W., Levin, H., & Gary, H. (1990). Recovery of orientation following closed head injury. *Journal of Clinical and Experimental Psychology, 12*, 703–714.

Jaspers, K. (1913). Casual and "meaningful" connections between life history and psychosis. *Zeitschrift Neurologie, 14*, 158–263. [Translated and republished in S. R. Hirsh & M. Shepherd (Eds.) (1974). *Themes and variations in European psychiatry.* Bristol, UK: John Wright & Sons.]

Klein, S. B., Rozendal, K., & Cosmides, L. (2002). A social-cognitive neuroscience analysis of the self. *Social Cognition, 20*, 105–135.

Kopelman, M. D. (1994). Structured psychiatric interview: Psychiatric history assessment of mental state. *British Journal of Hospital Medicine, 52*, 93–98.

Kopelman, M. D. (2002). Disorders of memory. *Brain, 125*, 2152–2190.

Kopelman, M. D. (in press) Varieties of confabulation and delusion. In R. Langdon & M. Coltheart (Eds.), *Confabulation and Delusion: Overlapping or Distinct Pathologies of Reality Distortion.* Macquarie Monographs in Cognitive Science.

Kopelman, M., Wilson, B. A., & Baddeley, A. D. (1989). *The Autobiographical Memory Interview.* Bury St Edmunds: Thames Valley Test Company.

Lishman, W. A. (1998). *Organic Psychiatry: The Psychological Consequences of Cerebral Disorders* (3rd ed.). Oxford: Blackwell.

Markova, I. S., & Berrios, G. E. (1994). Delusional misidentifications: Facts and fancies. *Psychopathology, 27*, 136–143.

Mullen, P. (1979). The phenomenology of disordered mental function. In P. Hill, R. Murray, & A. Thorley (Eds.), *Essentials of Postgraduate Psychiatry* (pp. 25–54). London: Academic Press.

Nannery, R. A, Greenfield, E., Wilson, B. A., Sopena, S., & Rous, R. (2007). Memory without memory: Accessing the integrity of implicit memory using the Implicit Memory Test. *Brain Impairment, 8*, 216.

Page, M., Wilson, B. A., Shiel, A., Carter, G., & Norris, D. (2006). What is the locus of the errorless-learning advantage? *Neuropsychologia, 44*, 90–100.

Pearn, J., & Gardner–Thorpe, C. (2002). Jules Cotard (1840–1889): His life and the unique syndrome which bears his name, *Neurology, 58*, 1400–1403.

Penfield, W. (1959). The interpretive cortex. The stream of consciousness in the human brain can be electrically reactivated. *Science, 129*, 1719–1725.

Ramachandran, V. S., & Blakeslee, S. (1998). *Phantoms in the Brain.* New York; William Morrow and Company.

Schacter, D. (Ed.) (1995). *Memory Distortion. How Minds, Brains and Societies Reconstruct the Past.* Cambridge: Harvard University Press.

Schacter, D., & Scarry, E. (Eds.) (2000). *Memory, Brain and Belief.* Cambridge: Harvard University Press.

Schneider, K. (1959). *Clinical Psychopathology* (5th ed., M. W. Hamilton, Trans.). New York: Grune & Stratton.

Scoville, W. B., & Milner, B. (1957). Loss of recent memory after bilateral lesions. *Journal of Neurology, Neurosurgery and Psychiatry, 20*, 11–21.

Sellal, F., Fontaine, S. F., van der Linden, M., Rainville, C., & Labrecque, R. (1996). To be or not to be at home? A neuropsychological approach to delusion for place. *Journal of Clinical and Experimental Neuropsychology, 18*(2), 234–248.

Wearing, D. (2005). *Forever Today: A Memoir of Love and Amnesia.* London; Doubleday.

Wilson, B. A., Baddeley, A. D., & Kapur, N. (1995). Dense amnesia in a professional musician following herpes simplex virus encephalitis. *Journal of Clinical and Experimental Psychology, 17*, 668–681.

Wilson, B. A., & Wearing, D. (1995). Prisoner of consciousness: A state of just awakening following herpes simplex encephalitis. In R. Campbell & M. Conway (Eds.), *Broken Memories: Case Studies in Memory Impairment* (pp. 14–30). Oxford: Blackwell.

Wright, S., Young, A. W., & Hellawell, D. J. (1993). Fregoli delusion and erotomania. *Journal of Neurology, Neurosurgery and Psychiatry, 56*, 322–323.

Zangwill, O. L. (1953). Disorientation for age. *Journal of Mental Science, 99*, 698–701.

Zeman, A. (2002). *Consciousness: A User's Guide.* Yale University Press.

Zeman, A. (2006). What do we mean by "conscious" and "aware"? *Neuropsychological Rehabilitation, 16*, 356–376.

NEUROPSYCHOLOGICAL REHABILITATION
2008, 18 (5/6), 541–565

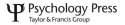

False selves in neuropsychological rehabilitation: The challenge of confabulation

Aikaterini Fotopoulou

Institute of Psychiatry, King's College London, UK

The presence of confabulation following brain damage can obstruct neuropsychological rehabilitation and management. A recent theoretical approach to confabulation emphasises that neurocognitive deficits are not sufficient to account for the content of confabulation. As a result, they are also insufficient to address the unique rehabilitation challenges that confabulation raises. Instead, confabulation could be best understood as the magnification of existing reconstructive memory processes, influenced by both neurocognitive and motivational factors. The paper reviews recent experimental findings showing that confabulations serve important functions of self-coherence and self-enhancement, despite their poor correspondence to reality. Case material is used to illustrate the meaningfulness of confabulation from the subjective perspective of the patient and to demonstrate that such a theoretical approach to confabulation can best inform management and rehabilitation efforts.

Keywords: Confabulation; Emotion; Memory; Rehabilitation; Self; Motivation.

INTRODUCTION

Brain damage may lead some patients to produce false memories without being aware of their falsehood. In severe cases, these false memories, termed confabulations, may completely dominate patients' speech and behaviour. Patients may narrate erroneous and even implausible stories about

Correspondence should be sent to Dr. Aikaterini Fotopoulou, Centre for Neuroimaging Sciences, Institute of Psychiatry De Crespigny Park, Box 089, London SE5 8AF, UK. E-mail: a.fotopoulou@iop.kcl.ac.uk

I am thankful to RM and his family. I am also particularly grateful to Stephen Tyrer and Philippa Griffiths for their valuable advice, collaboration and clinical insights.

DOI:10.1080/09602010802083545

themselves, misattribute their whereabouts, and confuse older recollections for recent ones and vice versa. Patients are typically unaware of their memory errors and may be so convinced of the truthfulness of their false claims that they act upon them (Schnider, von Däniken, & Gutbrod, 1996). Although confabulation occurs infrequently following brain damage, its presence and its related unawareness can obstruct neuropsychological management and rehabilitation (e.g., DeLuca, 1992; DeLuca & Locker, 1996). Patients may fail to see why they should comply with treatment requirements, and often direct feedback or efforts at distraction are ineffective as patients adhere more firmly to the truthfulness of their confabulations (Downes & Mayes, 1995; Talland, 1961). In chronic cases, the persistent presence of confabulation has been linked with increased need for supervision and hence reduced ability for independent living (Mills, Karas, & Alexander, 2006). Given the patients' poor insight into their condition, the presence of confabulation can increase caregivers' burden (Seltzer, Vasterling, Yoder, & Thompson, 1997). Moreover, to the extent that confabulating patients deny or distort common experiences and previously shared memories and facts, confabulation creates significant difficulties in patients' social environment (Weinstein, 1996).

Notwithstanding the unique clinical challenges that confabulation raises, most research on the topic has not hitherto been clinically pertinent. On the contrary, research has predominately approached confabulation as a useful neurocognitive symptom from which one can infer cognitive models of normal memory function (e.g., Dalla Barba, Cappelletti, Signorini, & Denes, 1997; Gilboa et al., 2006; Johnson, 1991). Thus, the exact prevalence, duration and taxonomy of confabulatory phenomena remain poorly investigated (Deluca, 2000; Johnson, Hayes, D'Esposito, & Raye, 2000). Most importantly, only a handful of studies present intervention programmes that focus on confabulation (Dayus & van den Broek, 2000), or even take it into account while attempting to address related deficits and rehabilitation targets (Deluca, 1992; DeLuca & Locker, 1996; Del Grosso Destreri et al., 2002).

The aim of this paper is not to provide a comprehensive review of the confabulation literature, nor to suggest a specific intervention approach. The paper will rather focus on a recent theoretical approach to confabulation that attempts to integrate previously opposing neurocognitive and motivational accounts. In this approach, the emphasis does not lie in describing the deficits that lead from perfect remembering to confabulation. Rather confabulations are seen as neurogenic exaggerations of the previously imperfect and dynamic functions serving personal memory and self-awareness. Moreover, despite their poor correspondence to reality, confabulations represent attempts to define one's self in time and in relation to the world. Thus, they are subject to motivational influences and they serve important identity formation functions. Recent evidence supporting this view will be reviewed.

Case material will be used to illustrate both the meaningfulness of confabulation from the subjective perspective of the patient and the neurocognitive deficits accompanying confabulation. It will be argued that such an approach can better address the clinical challenges posed by confabulation and can best inform management and rehabilitation efforts.

WHAT IS CONFABULATION?

Confabulations are false memories produced without conscious knowledge of their falsehood.

Amnesic confabulatory behaviour is considered pathognomonic of Wernicke-Korsakoff's syndrome, but confabulation has been observed in many other neuropathologies including anterior communicating artery (ACoA) aneurysms, Alzheimer's disease and traumatic brain injury (TBI) (see Johnson et al., 2000; Gilboa & Moscovitch, 2002 for extensive meta-analyses). Confabulation is frequently associated with lesions to the ventro-medial prefrontal cortex, as well as other surrounding areas, including the orbitofrontal cortex, the basal forebrain, the anterior cingulated cortex, and other "anterior limbic" areas (Johnson et al., 2000; Schnider, 2003).

Confabulation can take various forms, e.g., it can occur spontaneously or it can be provoked by questions; it may include the fabrication of new events or the misplacement of true experiences in time or space; it can include plausible recollections or completely implausible and non-realistic descriptions (e.g., Berlyne, 1972; Kopelman, 1987). Beginning with Korsakoff (1889/1996), some authors describe confabulatory manifestations on a continuum of severity (e.g., DeLuca & Cicerone, 1991). There is however some evidence suggesting that spontaneous confabulation is aetiologically different from other, less severe forms of provoked memory distortion or intrusion (Kopelman 1987; Schnider, 2003). Nevertheless, to date, the exact taxonomy of these characteristics and possible subtypes of confabulation remains unclear (for discussions see DeLuca, 2000; Metcalf, Langdon, & Coltheart, 2007).

NEUROCOGNITIVE MODELS OF CONFABULATION

Neuropsychological studies have focused on identifying the cognitive deficits causing the production of confabulation. Most studies seem to suggest that although impaired memory may be necessary for confabulation to occur, it is not sufficient to cause it (DeLuca, 2000; Gilboa et al., 2006; Johnson et al., 2000). Instead, most investigations suggest that some degree of executive function impairment seems also to be necessary for confabulation to occur (see DeLuca, 2000; Metcalf et al., 2007 for reviews). Nevertheless, the exact kind of this impairment and its role in memory processes remain debated. Two main classes of theories have been put forward; explanations that focus on impaired temporality or reality monitoring (Dalla Barba, 1993; Johnson et al., 2000; Schnider, 2003) and explanations that emphasise deficits in the control of memory retrieval (Burgess & Shallice, 1996; Gilboa et al., 2006; Moscovitch, 1989). These two theoretical approaches are discussed in turn below.

Confabulating patients often misattribute experiences of a given time to events that occurred at another time, or confuse the order of experienced events. This led a number of authors to suggest that confabulating patients have a disturbed ability to determine chronology (Dalla Barba, 1993; Talland, 1961; Schnider, 2003; Schnider et al., 1996). Support for this hypothesis came from a series of experiments that used a continuous recognition paradigm (reviewed by Schnider, 2003). Amnesic patients with spontaneous confabulation were distinguishable from amnesic patients with provoked confabulation based on their inability to differentiate between stimuli that were relevant to a previous run and stimuli that were relevant only to the current run. A more general version of this hypothesis suggests that confabulating patients are unable to distinguish the temporal or spatial source of different memories (source monitoring) or distinguish between real events and imagined ones (reality monitoring; Johnson, 1991; Johnson et al., 2000). For example, the patient who falsely claimed that he has just returned from a one-day trip to Tokyo may have confused his previous thoughts and wishes about travelling to Tokyo with real memories (Villiers, Zent, Eastman, & Swingler, 1996). Further, he may have misattributed to his recent past, the memory of a brief trip to a different destination he actually took a few years ago.

Alternatively, confabulation has been explained as a deficit in the control of memory retrieval. Confabulation can concern experiences encoded and stored before the onset of brain damage as much as it occurs for subsequent events. Thus, confabulation seems to be associated more with retrieval than encoding or storage difficulties. In the "strategic" or "generative" retrieval accounts confabulation is explained as a deficit in the strategic processes that are required during the organised and accurate retrieval of memories (Burgess and Shallice, 1996; Conway & Tacchi, 1996; Moscovitch, 1989; Moscovitch & Melo, 1997). According to these models, when memories are not elicited directly or automatically by a cue, a number of control processes, including memory search and monitoring processes, are called for to guide recollection. Confabulation represents a failure at one or more of these processes. For example, the aforementioned patient that claimed that he has just returned from a rather implausibly brief trip to Tokyo (Villiers et al., 1996), may have been unable to correctly perform a memory search and select the correct trip associations from a possible pool of alternative memories and thoughts. In addition, he may also have failed to monitor the selected memory for consistency and plausibility in the current and past context of his life.

IMPLICATIONS FOR NEUROPSYCHOLOGICAL REHABILITATION

In so much as confabulating patients suffer from some of the cognitive deficits described previously, namely amnesia, executive dysfunction, source monitoring impairments and strategic retrieval deficits, the management and rehabilitation of confabulation can focus on improving these cognitive abilities and related functional goals. Indeed, given the rarity of published rehabilitation studies on confabulating patients, it is assumed that these patients are treated alongside other patients with similar cognitive deficits. For example, confabulating patients may be managed alongside other non-confabulating amnesic patients suffering from ACoA "syndrome" (e.g., D'Esposito, Alexander, Fischer, McGlinchey-Berroth, & O'Connor, 1996; Mills et al., 2006). In these studies, confabulation may be assessed as an outcome measure, but little, if any, consideration is given to its initial presence and possible role in obstructing rehabilitation. As a result the persistent presence of confabulation has been found to correlate with poor rehabilitation results (Mills et al., 2006).

By contrast, a handful of cases have taken into account some of the specific rehabilitation challenges that confabulation may pose and they have designed interventions to address them (Dayus & van den Broek, 2000; Del Grosso Destreri et al., 2002; DeLuca, 1992; DeLuca & Locker, 1996). For example, Dayus and van den Broek (2000) predicted that enhanced self-monitoring through Self-Monitoring Training (Alderman, Fry, & Youngson, 1995), would result in confabulation reduction even in the absence of any other treatment. A patient showing highly aggressive confabulations that were specific in content and had persisted for over six years (see also Downes & Mayes, 1995) was trained to self-report his confabulation-related swearing using a hand-held clicker. Over a period of a few weeks, he exhibited a dramatic reduction in both swearing and confabulation frequency that was maintained at a three month follow-up.

This study demonstrates the importance of impaired self-monitoring in confabulation (e.g., Burgess & Shallice, 1996; Gilboa et al., 2006). However, the study does not report the effects of monitoring training to the patient's own perspective on his deficits, his mood and his own self-image. DeLuca (1992) reported that after initial training, patients may become more cautious at responding to questions for fear of embarrassment or feelings of inadequacy. In addition, several patients experience their confabulations with the same recollective quality as their true memories (Dalla Barba, 1993; Ciaramelli & Ghetti, 2007). Thus, one cannot exclude the possibility that the patient continued to form aggressive false memories and experienced the associated unpleasant emotions but learned not to express them. Self-monitoring training may prove to be important for controlling the utterance of false memories, but its role in the formation and subjective experience of memories is unclear.

In treating a patient with severe amnestic-confabulatory behaviour following herpes simplex encephalitis, Del Grosso Destreri and colleagues (2002) emphasised the need to manage confabulation at the acute stage following brain damage. Staff and the patient's relatives were asked to spend time contradicting the patient using written material and the patient's intact reasoning abilities. The authors claim that the treatment of confabulation was a prerequisite for the treatment of other cognitive functions and functional goals. However, as in the study reviewed previously, little consideration was given to the patient's subjective experience, her emotional state or her self-regard. Other studies show that confrontation may be met with resistance, may create anxiety and negative mood and may prove unsuccessful unless care is taken for the early establishment of working alliance between patient and therapist (e.g., DeLuca, 1992; DeLuca & Locker, 1996; Heinrichs et al., 1992).

Similar concerns have been raised in the rehabilitation of unawareness following acquired brain injury and dementia; the efficacy of confrontation and direct feedback has been questioned (Bieman-Copeland & Dywan, 2000; Lewis, 1991; Novack, Berquist, Bennett, & Gouvier, 1991; Prigatano, 1999; Toglia & Kirk, 2000; Ylvisaker & Szekeres, 1989). Confronting individuals with their deficits very early in the adjustment process may lead to heightened emotional distress and can be potentially harmful (Bieman-Copeland & Dywan, 2000; Langer & Padrone, 1992). It seems that when treating neurological patients who are unaware that their memories or perceptions are inaccurate, their subjective experience, associated emotions and several social factors need to be taken into account alongside neurocognitive deficits (Clare, 2004; Ownsworth & Clare, 2006; Ownsworth, Clare, & Morris, 2006; Prigatano, 1999). Unfortunately, there are no systematic studies assessing the role of patients' subjective experience, self-esteem, and mood in the rehabilitation of confabulation. Importantly, the relation between these factors and the unawareness that typically accompanies confabulation is far from clear. However, recent research provides preliminary indications that emotional and motivational factors have an important role in confabulation. Specifically, the next sections present an approach to confabulation that emphasises that neurocognitive deficits are not sufficient to account for the content of confabulation and the effects this has on patients' own self-regard. Subsequently, case material is used to highlight the implications of this approach to the rehabilitation of confabulating patients.

SELF-NARRATIVES FOLLOWING BRAIN DAMAGE

One factor that may influence the way people react to rehabilitation, and is of particular interest here, is patients' subjective experience of themselves following brain damage.

Recent studies highlight that the role of patients' own perspectives on their postmorbid "self" may influence functional outcome and psychosocial well-being in traumatic brain injury (Cantor et al., 2005; Nochi, 1998; Tyerman & Humphrey, 1984; Wright & Telford, 1996), in dementia (Clare, 2004; Finnema, Droes, Ribbe, & Van Tilburg, 2000) and in stroke (Ellis-Hill & Horn, 2000; Ellis-Hill, Payne, & Ward, 2000). Patients may feel severe anxiety and depression because they experience a loss of their premorbid self-identity (Cantor et al., 2005), or a significant and unbridgeable difference between their premorbid and postmorbid self-images (Dewar & Gracey, 2007; Wright & Telford, 1996).

For example, studies on stroke survivors suggested that stroke, similar to chronic illness, may represent a "biographical disruption" in the formation of people's narrative identity, i.e., an event that undermines people's sense of coherence with their past and thus renders the future uncertain and hard to predict (Ellis-Hill & Horn, 2000). Stroke survivors may settle for a restricted future self (Ellis-Hill et al., 2000), or they may cling onto unrealistic hopes of returning to their positive and perhaps even idealised premorbid self (Tyerman & Humphrey, 1984).

DAMAGED SELVES IN NEUROPSYCHOLOGICAL REHABILITATION

This sense of self-discrepancy or discontinuity is of special consideration in cases of significant memory impairment. There is a long philosophical tradition that argues that memory is the basis of personal identity (Locke, 1690, reprinted 1959; James, 1890/1950). Amnesia does not normally lead to a complete loss of identity (Schacter & Tulving, 1982). Nevertheless, the ability to appropriately encode, store and retrieve episodic and autobiographical memories is a necessary precondition for the construction of a coherent and continuous narrative self (Conway & Fthenaki, 2000; Gallagher, 2000; Schacter, 1996). Thus, lost or disrupted memories may lead to the experience of a discontinued and fragmented identity, over and above other postmorbid difficulties and concerns. For example, it has been shown that people with amnesia may be forced to draw upon immediate memories as the only remaining sources of self-identity (Bachna, Sieggreen, Cermak, Penk, & O'Conner, 1998). Alternatively, patients may escape into their preserved memories and begin to live in the past (Conway & Tacchi, 1996;

Fuchs, 1995). Loss of autobiographical memories may also lead to negative per-spectives on patients' current abilities and social roles (Dewar & Gracey, 2007).

FALSE SELVES IN NEUROPSYCHOLOGICAL REHABILITATION

Confabulation represents a different disruption of memory than amnesia, yet one that may have equally disruptive effects on identity formation. Amnesic errors are errors of omission. Patients seem unable to remember certain experi-ences or information. Typically, amnesic patients have lost the ability to encode or store information appropriately. On the contrary, confabulating patients are thought to be unable to remember their past, not because they fail to encode or store it, but because they have difficulty retrieving it in a systematic and reality-consistent manner (Gilboa et al., 2006; Moscovitch, 1989). Confabula-tions are by definition errors of commission. Patients remember something, even if that is highly distorted or completely fabricated. In this sense, confabu-lating patients do not simply have discontinued self-narratives. They instead construct false "selves", potentially insisting they are somewhere else, doing something else and having a different profession and family. Thus, confabula-tion could be seen as an extreme example of reconstructive memory (Bartlett, 1932). More generally, severe amnesia and confabulation can be seen as path-ologies that exemplify the two extremes of a long and debated history on the nature of personal identity; philosophers and psychologists have argued that a coherent sense of one's own past, present and future life is created through the remembering and narrating of personal memories. However, whether one's personal identity could be seen as pure fiction constructed in the narration or whether it is mostly anchored and constrained by reality is an issue of con-siderable debate (see Phillips, 2000 for review). Several recent philosophical approaches to the latter question seem to favour centrist positions in which nar-rative identity "must be seen as an unstable mixture of fabulation and actual experience" (Ricoeur, 1992; p. 192).

Similarly, psychologists have stressed that autobiographical memory is neither pure reproduction of past events, nor a pure present creation. Rather it is a relative reconstruction of the past in the light of the present (Conway & Pleydell-Pearce, 2000; McAdams, 2001; Neisser, 1988; Pillemer, 2001; Ross, 1989; Singer & Salovey, 1993). For example, Neisser (1988) proposed that remembering is both an act of "utility" (using the past in the service of the present) and "verity" (retracing what took place in the past). Conway (2005) suggested that autobiographical memory is faced with two opposing demands; memories may be altered and even fabricated in order to make the past consistent with current goals and self-images (the demand of "coherence"). Set against this tendency is the requirement of "reality corre-spondence". Memories should up to a degree correspond to past experience, irrespective of current concerns (see Langdon & Coltheart, 2000 for similar considerations in belief formation).

CONFABULATION AS EXAGGERATED MEMORY RECONSTRUCTION

Some recent studies have used the perspectives on memory and personal identity reviewed in the previous section to explain confabulation (Conway & Tacchi, 1996; Fotopoulou, Solms, & Turnbull, 2004). These studies propose that confabulation can be best understood as the magnification of existing "normal" misremembering instances. Specifically, they suggest that memory following brain damage may show similar patterns of omission, distortion, and fabrication as observed in normal memory reconstruction, albeit in a degree exaggerated by brain damage and its consequences. Furthermore, the content of confabulations will be determined by the exact combination of intact and damaged memory processes. For example, the relatives of the aforementioned patient (Villiers et al., 1996), who persistently confabulated about having recently returned from a trip to Tokyo, informed his doctors that for many years he was explicitly wishing to travel to Tokyo. It is thus possible that his confabulation represents a reality monitoring failure (an impaired memory function), leading him to confuse his memory of his longstanding wish (intact memory function) with a truly experienced event. A number of recent models of confabulation adhere to this approach (Burgess & Shallice, 1996; Conway & Fthenaki, 2000; Fotopoulou et al., 2004; Gilboa et al., 2006; Johnson et al., 1997; Metcalf et al., 2006). It is also of interest that similar suggestions have been made for the false and disorganised self-narratives produced by schizophrenic and deluded patients (Feinberg & Roane, 1997; Gallagher, 2000; McKay, Langdon, & Coltheart, 2007; Phillips, 2000). However, while some of these models have mainly emphasised the cognitive mechanisms leading to exaggerated reconstruction, others have focused on both cognitive and emotional factors (Conway & Fthenaki, 2000; Fotopoulou et al., 2004; Johnson et al, 2000; Solms, 2000).

Conway and colleagues (reviewed by Conway, 2005) have conceptualised autobiographical memory as a database of information in the service of the "working-self", which is conceived as a hierarchical template of currently active goals. The latter, in conjunction with input from the autobiographical memory base, sets goals, determines accessibility to autobiographical memory and supervises its output. According to this model, the dysfunctional executive control processes seen in confabulation compromise both the search in autobiographical memory and the evaluation of long-term memory output. Thus, patients are unable to distinguish between memory constructions created by the "current self", and the ones grounded in and constrained by autobiographical knowledge. As a consequence, the degree of involvement in memory construction of the wished-for-self (ungrounded goals and plans) is disproportionately larger than the "actual" self (Conway & Pleydell-Pearce, 2000). For example, the frontal patient OP, reported by Conway and Tacchi (1996) persistently maintained a set of plausible but confabulated memories. These rewrote the disappointments in familial inter-actions of her past into a history of successful and supportive intimacy with certain family members. From the patient's subjective point of view, these memories established a "coherence" with her own wished-for self-concept of a loved grandmother, irrespective of the fact that her memories had little "correspondence" to reality.

THE MOTIVATED CONTENT OF CONFABULATION

To investigate the validity of the above theoretical framework, a number of recent studies set out systematically to study the emotional content of confabu-lation (see Fotopoulou et al., in press-b, for review). The main hypothesis put forward by these investigations was that the false recollections of confabulating patients should show a self-serving bias that is greater than that typically encountered in studies on healthy volunteers (e.g., Walker, Skowronski, & Thompson, 2000). Of course, the vicissitudes of human motivation extend far beyond self-serving biases, but this reductionist definition of motivated confabulation was considered a useful first approach to the challenge of system-atically studying the complex role of motivation in confabulation. This exag-geration of self-serving biases was primarily expected due to the reported damage of the ventromedial frontal cortex in confabulation, which is more gen-erally thought to be responsible for affective regulation (Bechara, Damasio, & Damasio, 2000). In addition, given that exaggerated self-serving memory biases have been observed in amnesic patients with damage to the medial tem-poral lobes and without confabulation (e.g., Buchanan, Tranel, & Adolphs, 2005), in the studies reviewed below emotional bias was studied in the memory of amnesic patients with and without confabulation.

Consistent with the above hypothesis, the content of spontaneous confabu-lation has been found to contain mostly positive and wishful descriptions in a number of single-case and group studies (Fotopoulou et al., 2004, in press-a; Turnbull, Berry, & Evans, 2004). For example, patients described themselves as healthy and as being in familiar surroundings, in professional or leisure activities instead of the hospital (see also Turnbull et al., 2004). Some of these errors could of course be attributed to their amnesia for recent life periods. However, patients often accurately remembered neighbouring plea-sant events of the same time period (Fotopoulou, Conway, & Solms, 2007b). Patients also often minimised their current disabilities and attributed them to premorbid traits and attitudes. This can be seen as an extreme adherence to one's premorbid self-identity and a need to maintain a coherent self-narrative that is healthy, independent and competent. Given the neurocognitive deficits of these patients these needs for self-coherence were met with poor executive control and reality monitoring. Thus, their memory could not adequately respond to the demand for reality correspondence and patients maintained a continuous, yet false, self-identity.

Moreover, some confabulating patients persistently denied the death of close relatives and other unpleasant events of the remote or recent past and they were noted to inflate their abilities, exaggerate their previous professional skills and overstate their social and financial position (Fotopoulou et al., 2007a). Often these descriptions were accompanied by dramatisation of the circumstances or consequences of their injury and hospitalisation (see also Case Study presented in the next section). This can be seen as a form of idealisation of one's self-identity.

Social psychology has provided considerable evidence that people are motivated to view their current self favourably and engage in considerable memory distortion in order to maintain such a view (e.g., Walker et al., 2000; Wilson & Ross, 2003). This is particularly evident in older adults who show a strong self-serving positivity bias in their autobiographical recollections and this seems to have positive effects on their mood and well-being (for review see Mather & Carstensen, 2005). Older adults and confabulating patients show deterioration and dysfunction respectively in prefrontal brain regions (Braver & Barch 2002; Hedden & Gabrieli, 2004) and thus we have claimed that the exaggeration of self-enhancement through memory may be linked to the resulting deterioration of executive memory processes (Fotopoulou et al., in press-b).

The above observations on spontaneous confabulation were also supported by studies that experimentally manipulated the emotional content of memories. For example, a recent study showed that confabulating patients ($N = 4$) were more likely to misrecognise past self-referent events as currently true when these were of pleasant rather than unpleasant consequences (Fotopoulou et al., 2007b). Similar emotional biases were observed at the amnesic non-confabulating group ($N = 4$) but their overall errors were far less and thus the effect was of lesser importance in the construction of their self-representation. By contrast, the combination of poor memory monitoring and self-enhancement motivation led the confabulating patients to even accept as part of their autobiography a number of suggested pleasant events that had never taken place. These errors were only minimal in the case of unpleasant events. Thus, for example, a patient was significantly more likely to falsely claim that he actually remembered winning the lottery recently than to falsely claim that he remembered losing his job.

In a recent prose recall study, confabulating patients ($N = 15$) showed a selective bias in recalling negative self-referent stories, in that they recalled such information in a manner which portrayed a more positive image of them-selves (Fotopoulou et al., in press-b). This positive bias was not present in stories that were not encoded in a self-referent manner, nor in the amnesic control group. This study shows that confabulating patients do not have a dif-ficulty in processing negative emotions in general. Instead, they show a specific self-related motivational bias in their memory. This has implications for the provision of information to confabulating patients using "the third person" (see Case Study presented in the next section). More generally, this study shows that given the deficits of confabulating patients in the control and regulation of memory retrieval, their recall is highly susceptible to motivational distortions and their confabulations may reveal the influence of their self-related wishes, concerns and preoccupations.

Finally, the results of a recent investigation into the mood of confabulating patients are of particular relevance to rehabilitation. The study showed that although all of the 10 tested patients showed a positive bias in their confabulations, the greater the patients' self-reported depression, the greater their tendency to produce self-enhancing and wishful confabulations (Fotopoulou et al., in press-a). No relation was observed between patients' self-reported anxiety and the emotional content of their confabulations. This association between depression and confabulation may suggest that the production of positive confabulations is most frequently associated with low mood, or with topics that diminish one's self-esteem (see also Bentall & Kaney, 1996; McKay, Langdon, & Coltheart, 2007 for similar find-ings in delusions). This raises the possibility that confabulations have a direct adaptive function (as originally proposed by psychodynamically-oriented authors, e.g., see Weinstein, 1996). On the other hand, this association highlights that even if confabulations have a mood-regulatory (or defensive) function, their effect must be temporary or incomplete for patients to remain depressed. It is thus hard to conclude reliably that correction or spontaneous recovery from confabulation may lead to increased sadness. Furthermore, given that patients are typically unaware of their symptoms it is unlikely that mood regulation occurs at a conscious level. More generally, the highly complicated and dynamic relation between motivated confabulation, mood and awareness requires further systematic investigation through rehabilitation studies (see DeLuca, 1992 for a relevant single-case study).

Thus, in summary, the above studies suggest that confabulating patients show an exaggerated self-serving bias in their false recollections in relation to healthy controls. This is comparable in degree to the self-serving positive biases observed in amnesic non-confabulatory patients. However, given the latter have a lesser propensity to confabulate (i.e., have greater cognitive control over their memory) the pragmatic and clinical significance of the biases observed in confabulating patients is greater. Confabulation may have a mood-regulatory effect but such a conclusion would be premature given the current lack of systematic study on the matter.

PSYCHOGENIC AND NEUROGENIC MOTIVATIONAL INFLUENCES ON CONFABULATION

It should be noted that similar motivational influences on confabulation have been proposed before (Berlyne, 1972; Talland, 1961 for review; Weinstein, 1996). However, in most of these approaches the emotional and social factors are thought to arise as a consequence of the brain injury as a whole (a secondary emotional reaction to the injury) and not as the specific consequence of a particular neurocognitive deficit. For example, Weinstein and colleagues (Weinstein, Kahn, & Malitz, 1956) argue that confabulations implicitly express current preoccupations and anxieties, which the patient is not capable of fully appreciating and explicitly expressing. These unconscious compensatory coping mechanisms are thought of as instigated by excessive anxiety and as appearing in a number of different neurological syndromes. Thus, in at least some of the papers published by Weinstein and colleagues, the content of confabulation is thought of as independent of the specific neuropathological features of the syndromes they aim to explain and are more related to patients' premorbid personality and social environment.

By contrast, the motivational account of confabulation proposed here attempts to escape the Cartesian dualism inherent in descriptions of a partition of direct (neurocognitive) and indirect (emotional and social) consequences of brain damage (Goldstein, 1942; Yeates, Henwood, Gracey, & Evans, 2006 for discussion). Given the trade-off between the influence of cognitive control and motivational influences on memory (Conway, 2005; Ochsner & Gross, 2005), impairment in one aspect may generate exaggeration in the other; when irrelevant memory representations are not inhibited and memories are not retrieved in appropriate manner, motivational factors may acquire a greater role in determining which memories are selected for retrieval and accepted as true (see also Fotopoulou et al., 2004, 2007b). In the next section, a case of severe confabulation is used to illustrate how the theoretical framework presented in this paper may be relevant for the clinical management and rehabilitation of patients with confabulation[1].

---

[1] The term confabulation has also been used to describe the unintentionally false statements of patients in many other memory-independent neurological syndromes, such as right-hemisphere unawareness syndromes (e.g., Feinberg & Roane, 1997; Fotopoulou & Conway, 2004; Tallberg, 2001). Some of the issues raised here in relation to confabulations about personal memory may be of relevance to the rehabilitation of other forms of false memories and beliefs. However, different neurocognitive deficits and motivational factors may need to be emphasised in each syndrome and these considerations go beyond the scope of the current paper.

BRIEF CASE REPORT

RM was a 19-year-old window fitter with 11 years of education, hospitalised following a severe road traffic accident. His GCS (Glasgow Coma Scale) score on admission was 4/15. He was found to have a subarachnoid haemorrhage, left frontal and bilateral temporal contusions and compressed ventricles. He required a bifrontal decompressure craniotomy and insertion of an external ventricular drain (EVD) five days post-admission following increased intracranial pressure. Subsequent computed tomography (CT) scans revealed bi-frontal damage with small contusions in the left frontal lobe and a larger single contusion in the right medial aspect of the frontal lobe. There was extensive low density in the left anterior frontal region.

He was transferred to a multidisciplinary neurorehabilitation in-patient ward six months following his injury. He had made a good physical recovery but his disorientation in time, his profound amnesia, and his spontaneous confabulation were immediately evident. He also had problems in initiating behaviour, planning ahead his activities and monitoring himself (see Fotopoulou et al., 2007b for formal neuropsychological testing). Relatives described substantial changes in RM's personality in that he kept talking about himself and he was often irritable and tearful. RM also appeared anosognosic (unaware of his deficits), in that he believed he had recovered fully from his accident, he could work, drive and live independently without any assistance.

RM participated in various individual and group sessions of a multidisciplinary rehabilitation programme, which aimed to address RM's cognitive difficulties and a number of functional and vocational goals. His engagement in rehabilitation activities was initially very poor as he was not motivated and required constant prompting and supervision. Attempts to contradict his anosognosia and increase his motivation were often ineffective as RM immediately provided a series of confabulations to support his alleged abilities and he was particularly sensitive to poor performance and negative feedback. Using written materials for reality orientation and confrontation had some effect, but it was extremely time-consuming as RM was quick to make up long and complicated stories. It was particularly difficult to prevent him from completing the story he had decided to convey.

RM was recruited to a study on confabulation using the framework outlined in the preceding sections. Previous findings on the motivated content of confabulation were communicated to the clinicians responsible for his care. This perspective was integrated in his rehabilitation programme; particularly in his individual sessions with the clinical neuropsychologist and the occupational therapist, and in staff members' decision to contradict his confabulations only in well-structured sessions and only in non-self-threatening ways (see below). Nine months following the completion of his in-patient rehabilitation programme RM had achieve his main goal of living alone with merely visiting carers and with a potential for paid employment in the near future. His executive functions and memory had improved and he confabulated only minimally. The next sections do not attempt to describe the full details of his rehabilitation. Rather emphasis is placed on the content of RM's confabulations, the challenges faced at the initial stages of his rehabilitation and the practical steps taken to address them.

The influence of the premorbid self

RM's relatives confirmed that several of his confabulations were false versions of real past experiences. These had typically been important to RM and may have served as sources of personal identity. For example, he often confabulated about important school events and prizes he had won. Interestingly, RM often remembered some events of his past with great vividness and emotion, although his relatives confirmed that at the time RM was rather unaffected by these experiences. For example, RM often referred to his grandfather's death and cried while he narrated how upset he was at his funeral. RM's family were bewildered by these confabulations as RM had not previously appeared particularly preoccupied by his grandfather's death and he had not been to his funeral. The examiner explained to his family that such memories may relate to RM's experience of current losses and his efforts to make sense of them in the context of his unawareness and in relation to his premorbid self-identity.

The idealised self

While many of RM's confabulations referred to true past events, these tended to be highly exaggerated in ways that enhanced RM's abilities and achievements. For example, while RM had indeed been a good soccer player at school and had been once named "player of the year", RM often referred to this event as having happened 4 or 5 years in a row. RM gave lengthy descriptions of such events that included significant praise by others of his physical and intellectual abilities and somewhat created a impression of a young man who feels the need to assert himself and "show-off" his abilities in his false and exaggerated recollections. RM also often rewrote unpleasant events of his past in ways that he would clearly have preferred them to be. For example, although he was generally aware of his parents' divorce that preceded his accident by a few months and had greatly upset him, he sometimes claimed that he had managed to convince his parents not to divorce.

The wishful self

Often RM's confabulations were directly related to his current needs. For example, almost every ring of the ward phone or doorbell would prompt a confabulation by RM about his relatives calling him or coming to see him. At times, it was very hard to distract him from his need to "go and check" whether his mother had come and was waiting for him. Staff and his relatives had agreed to a very consistent visiting schedule and RM had in time learned this. Nevertheless, he continued to confabulate such visits and a combination of cognitive training and non-confrontational discussions about his wishes were required to assist him to relax and reduce these confabulations.

Implications for rehabilitation

The above clinical examples of premorbid, idealised and wishful "false selves" highlight that rehabilitation staff and relatives need to understand these confabulations beyond their apparent contradiction with reality and their incorrect contextualisation in past self-defining and self-enhancing memories. Furthermore, clinicians could try to explore with patients and their relatives the subjective meaning of these confabulations for the continuity of patients' self-identity and the preservation of self-esteem. For example, for as long as RM's confabulations did not directly impede his everyday activities, responsibilities and social interactions, rehabilitation staff were encouraged to refrain from directly confirming or contradicting RM's confabulations. Instead, they were asked (1) to respond to his statements at face value with natural interest and curiosity, (2) to discreetly suggest and add correct background information to his stories, when possible, (3) to pace the conversation and help RM to stay within a given conversational topic, and (4) to explore memories and current facts in ways that take into account both his emotions and also the emotions of others and their need for a shared reality. More specific examples of the application of this approach to RM's rehabilitation are given below.

Dramatisation of injury and related feelings

RM remembered his car accident accurately but in almost every description of the event he somewhat dramatised his initial post-injury state. He described a complete loss of personal identity, no recollection of semantic or episodic memories, weakness, and a series of somatic symptoms. He then immediately went on to narrate how much he had improved since and how he was "back to [his] own-self". In order to "prove [his] point" he kept repeating personal semantic information (e.g., he cited his address and listed the names of several of his relatives correctly) and proposing to the examiner to perform tasks that would demonstrate his strength. These confabulations bear some resemblance to a tendency shown by healthy individuals to derogate their past in order to enhance the current self-image (Wilson & Ross, 2003).

Interestingly, RM's confabulations often involved different road traffic accidents. Usually he was a passenger in the car (as in his real road traffic accident) but he was often required to drive the car and "save the day". Typically, his narrations involved some driving-related complication which endangered the people in the car and which forced RM to drive and take the situation under his control. This would soon lead to a positive resolution and RM would be praised and thanked by the car's passengers. These confabulations suggested a preoccupation with the circumstances of his injury and its resulting difficulties. When possible, staff were asked not to contradict RM. The subjective meaning of these confabulations and his potential need to mentally revisit and "undo" the accident were suggested to his relatives. Crucially, these concerns were explored in individual sessions with RM by asking him questions about how he felt about these experiences and by exploring the emotional consequences of alternative scenarios, e.g., what he feared would have happened if he had not "taken control". These confabulations seemed to decrease in time.

Violent content: Beyond monitoring

One of the aspects of RM's management that care staff found particularly challenging was the content of his confabulations, which typically concerned violent events and often included swearing. These descriptions were indeed very frequent and they seemed to be remarkably similar in narrative unravelling. In the alleged events RM and important others were threatened, or mistreated by some stranger. However, RM managed to protect them by using significant force and violence, or extraordinary speed. Frequently, the police arrived at the scene and they praised RM for his accomplishment. Finally, his relatives explicitly thank him for his protection.

Without confronting the veracity of his stories, the rehabilitation team decided to ask RM to refrain from narrating stories with violent content. RM understood that his stories maybe upsetting others and agreed to monitor himself. With prompting, RM gradually learned the demand made upon him. However, it soon became evident that staff members' requests found their way into the content of RM's confabulations. He now narrated stories in which he was challenged and invited by others to perform violent acts (which he described to his examiner in detail) but he refrained from doing so because he knew "that smashing someone's head with a baseball bat may upset some people". The following example is characteristic of a confabulation with "reduced" violence:

> "One day I was at home, and I had a mobile, and it was ringing and it was late and I thought ah yes, it's my dad, 'cause he was coming to see me and he was late and I picked it up and went, 'Hello dad I love you' and he went, 'Hello son, I love you too, do you know the mobile shop on the corner?'. 'Yeah, you stuck there?' 'No, I'm not stuck there, me and

a police officer was chasing Fred', the lad who did the murder, that was his name, and I can't remember the second name, but I knew what he looked like. I said to dad, I said, 'Dad, I'll be there in 5 minutes, I'll sprint there'. 'Will you?' I said, 'Yeah' 'Will you be knackered?' I said, 'Don't worry dad', so I just drained the rest of me tab and stuck it out and just ran all he way up, which was one and a half mile away, and then, I said to him, the policeman, 'Look mate, us three split up and see if we can find him', and then I ran into sort of like a school site, 'cause that's where he hangs around, that's where he hung around, and when I saw him he tried to hit me and get away but I sort of rugby tackled him, and the policeman had three handcuffs sets and we had one each. So I got him to hit the floor and funnily enough, he span round, so I knelt on his back, not knelt, sorry, I just got hold of his arms, put them close together, put the hand cuffs on them, picked up and put him on my shoulder, opened the police back door, put him in, there you go, and then, I just waited there in case he tried to escape, and then the police ... and then the police come, and they said 'Bloody hell, he was just round corner, he was hiding, bloody hell, did you have to, fight him?', I said, 'No, I just rugby tackled him.' I said 'Look mate, I was helping the police and if you try to arrest us mate, I'll flip, I will I'll flip.' My dad said, 'He isn't going to arrest you, you just rugby tackled him.' And the policeman said, 'Well, you did good because he's got some strength to fight you off, and you put the handcuffs on as well, well done. Thank you.'"

Weinstein and colleagues (1956) claimed confabulations of violence were common in patients with head injury, and they may contain symbolic representations of their current preoccupations and disabilities. RM's violent narratives clearly showed a preoccupation with his physical strength and speed, danger, regaining control, and being safe from harm. This was suggested to RM in individual non-confrontational sessions and the subjective meaning of these narratives was progressively explored in the following ways: RM was encouraged to think how he would feel if he had not managed to avoid danger and protect others, what he expected others will feel about him in this case and finally he was asked whether he thought these stories may have some relation to his accident. RM initially spoke of the constant and great danger his close relatives are in and of how much they need his protection. However, after a few sessions he reflected on his fears of residual weakness, lack of control and independence and his related social embarrassment. He also expressed anger over what had happened to him and the inability of others to prevent it, or "make it right". These insightful instances did not automatically lead to cessation of his related confabulations but RM appeared relaxed, less distracted and irritable during these sessions and even admitted his tendency to "think of things that may have never happened". In a session following a particularly insightful previous session, RM greeted the examiner by saying, "You are here to make some stories up again, aren't you?". More importantly, RM started to narrate confabulations in which he used "his father's name", or his "wit" to convince others to leave or to apologise and thus to defuse the dangerous situation. Moreover, it was progressively possible to start discussing and planning with RM his future activities and social role in a more realistic manner. This example highlights that memory monitoring is not sufficient to address confabulations that may be accompanied by subjectively important emotions and thoughts.

Discussions in the third person

In a study reviewed in previous sections, we showed that confabulating patients were able to remember accurately the unpleasantness of certain stories when these concerned someone else, while they "confabulated away" negative self-referent information (Fotopoulou et al., 2008b). Marcel, Tegner, and Nimmo-Smith (2004) observed that unaware patients are more likely to acknowledge their stroke-induced paralysis if asked in third- as opposed to first-person questions, and at times if asked in a less serious emotional tone.

RM also appeared to confabulate less when he was prompted to discuss his injury and associated difficulties in the "third person" (see also McGlynn & Kaszniak, 1991; Reisberg, Gordon, McCarthy, & Ferris, 1985). The examiner mentioned "a man she knew who had suffered a brain injury after a car accident" and RM immediately contributed highly insightful comments into the discussion. He said the man must feel very scared and upset about his condition and he must think that everybody else sees him as a fool. He said he was unsure whether that man could ever find a girlfriend again and it seemed like he may never be able to "go back to his own self". In this context, the examiner asked whether the man in question could still find a way to lead a satisfactory life, different than before but still happy. RM stood uncharacteristically silent for a while and then said, "The man will need help, the problem is he does not know how to ask for it." Discussions about the "abilities" and the future of this man became progressively more optimistic and in one session RM spontaneously concluded, "I like that man, he is a bit like me and the rest of the lads here." This example suggests that "third-person" conversations with patients may be a powerful tool for exploring and ameliorating patients' concerns, and for building a therapeutic rapport between patient and therapist. Crucially, these conversations seem not to be obstructed by patients' unawareness to the same degree as first-person perspectives on patients' deficits.

The social context of confabulation and others' needs

It should be evident from the preceding sections that RM's confabulations were not stable but changed over time and were modified by the team's interventions. RM's confabulations were also noted to be somewhat different from one social occasion to another. Indeed, patients have been observed who confabulate in everyday life but not during formal testing, or in certain social occasions (Papagno & Muggia, 1996; Villiers et al., 1996). This of course highlights that patients' social environment may have an influence over the content and occurrence of confabulations (Weinstein et al., 1956). These influences include the wider socio-cultural context (Gainotti, 1975), as well as family and everyday environmental influences (Prigatano, 1999; Weinstein et al., 1956). The importance of these psychosocial factors has been raised in the literature on acquired brain injury and disease and it has been particularly emphasised in recent theoretical reviews on unawareness (Clare, 2004; Ownsworth et al., 2006; Toglia & Kirk, 2000).

One social dimension that seems to be of particular importance in confabulation is the sudden lack of shared reality between a patient and his significant others. As revealed by many of the examples given in previous sections, RM distorted many important family events. At times, his confabulations clearly revealed wishes and criticisms about his parents' divorce or included descriptions of violent fighting and abuse between his family members. These caused significant concern and embarrassment to his family. More generally, Weinstein (1996) has shown that a significantly higher incidence of separation or divorce was observed in patients who persistently confabulated about family members than in those who did not.

In addition, patients and carers may have different perspectives on current reality following acquired brain injury (Yeates, Henwood, Gracey, & Evans, 2007). Relatives and friends may need to emphasise how patients have changed in order to define their loss and the change in social roles. On the contrary, patients may need to highlight their continuity and coherence with their past self and may not be able to understand or deal with the loss of their previous family and social role. In the case of confabulation, carers may also feel particularly motivated not to allow patients to disrupt their previously shared reality (e.g., RM's aforementioned confabulations about family matters). This attitude may in turn lead patients to further entrench their confabulations and even produce secondary false memories to support them (Moscovitch, 1989). Explaining these different emotional needs to relatives is of crucial importance, as it is informing them about the cognitive deficits that allow patients to misremember reality in the face of these needs and without consciously understanding their errors (e.g., reality and temporality monitoring deficits).

SUMMARY

Psychologists have long proposed that individuals' recollections reconstruct the past in ways that serve a coherent self-narrative. Through autobiographical memory one weaves together diverse experiences and creates a sense of unity over time and a defined purpose for future action. Loss of access to memories following brain damage may lead to a sense of self-discontinuity and lack of self-coherence. Conversely, loss of the ability to remember experiences in an organised way may lead to exaggerated reconstruction and poor correspondence of the self to reality. The latter disruption is seen in confabulating patients. Given their poor executive control over memory and their defective sense of temporality, patients' recollections are dominated by premorbid self-values, previous coping strategies and current inner drives. This paper presented a theoretical approach to confabulation that places emphasis on these motivational factors and the ways they shape confabulatory content. Finally, the paper argued that rehabilitation interventions need to take into account, alongside neurocognitive deficits, the motivated content of confabulation and the functions of self-coherence and self-enhancement it serves. Specific recommendations for clinicians include liaising with significant others to understand and explain how confabulations are cognitively and motivationally constructed and influenced by social context; discouraging rehabilitation staff from confirming or contradicting patients' confabulations; using individual sessions to progressively explore the subjective meaning of confabulations and provide non-theatening feedback, and finally building a rapport with the patient by initially discussing negative experiences, vulnerability and disability within the third person.

REFERENCES

Alderman, N., Fry, R. K., & Youngson, H. A. (1995). Improvement of self-monitoring skills, reduction of behaviour disturbances and the dysexecutive syndrome: Comparison of response cost and a new programme of self-monitoring training. *Neuropsychological Rehabilitation*, 5, 193–221.

Bachna, K., Sieggreen, M. A., Cermak, L., Penk, W., & O'Conner, M. (1998). MMPI/MMPI-2: comparisons of amnesic patients. *Archives of Clinical Neuropsychology*, 13(6), 535–542.

Bartlett, F. C. (1932). *Remembering*. Cambridge: Cambridge University Press.

Bechara, A., Damasio, H., & Damasio, A. R. (2000). Emotion, decision making and the orbito-frontal cortex. *Cerebral Cortex*, 10, 295–307.

Bentall, R. P., & Kaney, S. (1996). Abnormalities of self-representation and persecutory delusions: A test of a cognitive model of paranoia. *Psychological Medicine*, 26, 1231–1237.

Berlyne, N. (1972). Confabulation. *British Journal of Psychiatry*, 120, 31–39.

Bieman-Copeland, S., & Dywan, J. (2000). Achieving rehabilitative gains in anosognosia after TBI. *Brain & Cognition*, 44, 1–18.

Braver, T.S., & Barch, D. M. (2002). A theory of cognitive control, aging cognition, and neuro-modulation. *Neuroscience and Behaviour Review*, 26, 809–817.

Buchanan, T. W., Tranel, D., & Adolphs, R. (2005). Emotional autobiographical memories in amnesic patients with medial temporal lobe damage. *Journal of Neuroscience*, *25*, 3151–3160.

Burgess, P. W., & Shallice, T. (1996). Confabulation and the control of recollection. *Memory*, *4*, 359–411.

Cantor, J. B., Ashman, T. A., Schwartz, M. E., Gordon, W. A., Hibbard, M. R., Brown, M., Spielman, L., Charatz, H., & Cheng, Z. (2005). The role of self-discrepancy theory in understanding post-traumatic brain injury affective disorders: A pilot study. *Journal of Head Trauma Rehabilitation*, *20*(6), 527–543.

Ciaramelli, E., & Ghetti, S. (2007). What are confabulators' memories made of? A study of subjective and objective measures of recollection in confabulation. *Neuropsychologia 8*(7), 1489–1500.

Clare, L. (2004). The construction of awareness in early-stage Alzheimer's disease: A review of concepts and models. *British Journal of Clinical Psychology*, *43*(2), 155–175.

Conway, M. A. (2005). Memory and the self. *Journal of Memory and Language*, *53*, 594–628.

Conway, M. A., & Fthenaki, A. (2000). Disruption and loss of autobiographical memory. In F. Boller, & J. Grafman (Eds.), *Handbook of Neuropsychology* (Vol. 2, 2nd ed., pp. 281–312). Amsterdam: Elsevier Science.

Conway, M. A., & Pleydell-Pearce, C. W. (2000). The construction of autobiographical memories in the self-memory system. *Psychological Review*, *107*, 261–288.

Conway, M. A., & Tacchi, P. C. (1996). Motivated confabulation. *Neurocase*, *2*, 325–338.

Dalla Barba, G. (1993). Confabulation: Knowledge and recollective experience. *Cognitive Neuropsychology*, *10*, 1–20.

Dalla Barba, G., Cappelletti, Y. J., Signorini, M., & Denes, G. (1997). Confabulation: Remembering 'another' past, planning 'another' future. *Neurocase*, *3*, 425–436.

Dayus, B., & van den Broek, M. D. (2000). Treatment of stable delusional confabulations using self-monitoring training. *Neuropsychological Rehabilitation*, *10*(4), 1960–2011.

Del Grosso Destreri, N. D., Farina, E., Calabrese, E., Pinardi, G., Imbornone, E., & Mariani, C. (2002). Frontal impairment and confabulation after herpes simplex encephalitis: A case report. *Archives of Psychical Medicine and Rehabilitation*, *83*(3), 423–426.

DeLuca, J. (1992). Rehabilitation of confabulation: The issue of unawareness of deficit. *NeuroRehabilitation*, *2*(3), 23–30.

DeLuca, J. (2000). A cognitive perspective on confabulation. *Neuro-Psychoanalysis*, *2*(2), 119–132.

DeLuca, J., & Cicerone, K. D. (1991). Confabulation following aneurysm of the anterior communicating artery. *Cortex*, *27*, 417–423.

DeLuca, J., & Locker, R. (1996). Cognitive rehabilitation following anterior communicating artery aneurysm bleeding: A case report. *Disability Rehabilitation*, *18*(5), 265–272.

D'Esposito, M., Alexander, M. P., Fischer, R., McGlinchey-Berroth, R., & O'Connor, M. (1996). Recovery of memory and executive functioning following anterior communicating artery aneurysm rupture. *Journal of the International Neuropsychological Society*, *2*, 565–570.

Dewar, B., & Gracey, F. (2007). "Am not was": Cognitive-behavioural therapy for adjustment and identity change following herpes simplex encephalitis. *Neuropsychological Rehabilitation*, *17*(4), 602–620.

Downes, J. J., & Mayes, A. R. (1995). How bad memories can sometimes lead to fantastic beliefs and strange visions. In R. Campbell & M. A. Conway (Eds.), *Broken Memories: Case Studies in the Neuropsychology of Memory* (pp. 115–123). Oxford: Blackwell.

Ellis-Hill, C., & Horn, S. (2000). Change in identity and self-concept: A new theoretical approach to recovery following a stroke. *Clinical Rehabilitation 14*(3), 299–307.

Ellis-Hill, C., Payne, S., & Ward, C.D. (2000). Self-body split: Issues of identity in physical recovery following a stroke. *Disability and Rehabilitation 22*(16), 725–733.

Feinberg, T. E., & Roane, D. M. (1997). Anosognosia. In J. F. Feinberg & M. J. Farah (Eds.), *Behavioural Neurology and Neuropsychology* (2nd ed., pp. 324–362). New York: McGraw Hill.

Finnema, E., Droe, R., Ribbe, M., & Van Tilburg, W. (2000). The effects of emotion-oriented approaches in the care for persons suffering from dementia: A review of the literature. *International Journal of Geriatric Psychiatry*, *15*, 141–161.

Fotopoulou, A., & Conway, M. A. (2004). Confabulations pleasant and unpleasant. *Neuropsychoanalysis 6*(1), 26–33.

Fotopoulou, A., Solms, M., & Turnbull, O. (2004). Wishful reality distortions in confabulation: A case report. *Neuropsychologia*, *42*, 727–744.

Fotopoulou, A., Conway, M. A., Griffiths, P., Birchall, D., & Tyrer, S. (2007a). Self-enhancing confabulation: Revising the motivational hypothesis. *Neurocase*, *13*, 6–15.

Fotopoulou, A., Conway, M. A., & Solms, M. (2007b). Confabulation: Motivated reality monitoring. *Neuropsychologia*, *45*, 2180–2190.

Fotopoulou, A., Conway, M. A., Tyrer, S., Birchall, D., Griffiths, P., & Solms, M. (in press-a). Positive emotional biases in confabulation: An experimental study. *Cortex*.

Fotopoulou, A., Conway, M. A., Solms, M., Tyrer, S., & Kopelman, M. (in press-b). Self-serving confabulation in prose recall. *Neuropsychologia*.

Fuchs, T. (1995). In search of lost time-memory in dementia. *Fortschritte der Neurologie-Psychiatrie*, *63*(1), 38–43.

Gainotti, G. (1975). Confabulation of denial in senile dementia: An experimental study. *Psychiatria Clinica*, *8*, 99–108.

Gallagher, S. (2000). Self-narrative in schizophrenia. In T. Kircher & A. David (Eds.) *The Self in Psychiatry and Neuroscience*. Cambridge: Cambridge University Press.

Gilboa, A., Alain, C., Stuss, D.T., Melo, B., Miller, S., & Moscovitch, M. (2006). Mechanisms of spontaneous confabulations: A strategic retrieval account. *Brain*, *129*(6), 1399–1414.

Gilboa, A., & Moscovitch, M. (2002). The cognitive neuroscience of confabulation: A review and a model. In A. Baddeley, M. Kopelman, & B. Wilson (Eds.), *Handbook of Memory Disorders*. (2nd ed., pp. 315–342) Chichester: John Wiley.

Goldstein, K. (1942). *After Effects of Brain Injuries in War*. New York, Grune & Stratton.

Hedden, T., & Gabrieli, J. D. E. (2004). Insights into the ageing mind: A view from cognitive neuroscience. *Nature Reviews, Neuroscience 5*, 87–96.

Heinrichs, R., Levitt, H., Arthurs, A., Gallardo, K., Hirsheimer, K., MacNeil, M., Olshansky, E., & Richards, K. (1992). Learning and retention of a daily activity schedule in a patient with alcoholic Korsakoff's syndrome. *Neuropsychological Rehabilitation*, *2*(1), 43–58.

James, W. (1890). *The Principles of Psychology*. New York: Dover Publications.

Johnson, M. K. (1991). Reality monitoring: Evidence from confabulation in organic brain disease patients. In G. P. Prigatano & D. L. Schacter (Eds.), *Awareness of Deficit After Brain Injury* (pp. 176–197). Oxford: Oxford University Press.

Johnson, M. K., Hayes, S. M., D'Esposito, M., & Raye, C. (2000). Confabulation. In F. Boller & J. Grafman (Eds.), *Handbook of Neuropsychology: Vol 2: Memory and its Disorders* (2nd ed., pp. 383–407). Amsterdam: Elsevier Science.

Kopelman, M. D. (1987). Two types of confabulation. *Journal of Neurology, Neurosurgery, and Psychiatry*, *50*, 1482–1487.

Korsakoff, S. S. (1889/1996). Medico-psychological study of a memory disorder. *Consciousness and Cognition*, *5*, 2–21.

Langdon, R., & Coltheart, M. (2000). The cognitive neuropsychology of delusions. In M. Davies & M. Coltheart (Eds.), *Pathologies of Belief* (pp. 183–216). London: Blackwell.

Lewis, L. (1991). Role of psychological factors in disordered awareness. In G. P. Prigatano & D. L. Schacter (Eds.), *Awareness of Deficit After Brain Injury: Clinical and Theoretical Issues* (pp. 223–239). New York: Oxford University Press.

Locke, J. (1959). *An Essay Concerning Human Understanding*. New York: Dover.

Marcel, A. J., Tegnér, R., & Nimmo-Smith, I. (2004). Anosognosia for plegia: Specificity, extension, partiality and disunity of bodily unawareness. *Cortex, 20,* 19–40.

Mather, M., & Carstensen, L. L. (2005). Aging and motivated cognition: The positivity effect in attention and memory. *Trends in Cognitive Sciences, 9*(10), 496–502.

McAdams, D. P. (2001). The psychology of life stories. *Review of General Psychology, 5*(2), 100–122.

McGlynn, S. M., & Kaszniak, A. W. (1991). Unawareness of deficits in dementia and schizophrenia. In G. P. Prigatano, & D. L. Schacter (eds.), *Awareness of Deficit After Brain Injury: Clinical and Theoretical Issues* (pp. 84–110). New York: Oxford University Press.

McKay, R., Langdon, R., & Coltheart, M. (2007). The defensive function of persecutory delusions: An investigation using the Implicit Association Test. *Cognitive Neuropsychiatry, 12*(1), 1–24.

Metcalf, K., Langdon, R., & Coltheart, M. (2007). Models of confabulation: A critical review and a new framework. *Cognitive Neuropsychology, 24*(1), 23–47.

Mills, V. M., Karas, A., & Alexander, M. P. (2006). Outpatient rehabilitation of patients with chronic cognitive impairments after ruptured anterior communicating artery aneurysms reduces the burden of care: A pilot study. *Brain Injury, 20*(11), 1183–1188.

Moscovitch, M. (1989). Confabulation and the frontal system: Strategic versus associative retrieval in neuropsychological theories of memory. In H. L. Roediger & F. I. M. Craik (Eds.), *Varieties of Memory and Consciousness: Essays in the Honour of Endel Tulving* (pp. 133–160). Hillsdale, NJ: Lawrence Erlbaum Associates.

Moscovitch, M., & Melo, B. (1997). Strategic retrieval and the frontal lobes: Evidence from confabulation and amnesia. *Neuropsychologia, 35,* 1017–1034.

Neisser, U. (1988). Five kinds of self-knowledge. *Philosophical Psychology, 1,* 35–59.

Nochi, M. (1998). Struggling with the labeled self: People with traumatic brain injuries in social settings. *Qualitative Health Research, 8*(5), 665–681.

Novack, T. A., Bergquist, T. F., Bennett, G., & Gouvier, W. D. (1991). Primary caregiver distress following severe head injury. *Journal of Head Trauma Rehabilitation, 6,* 69–77.

Ochsner, K. N., & Gross, J. J. (2005). The cognitive control of emotion. *Trends in Cognitive Sciences, 9,* 242–249.

Ownsworth, T. L., & Clare, L. (2006). The association between awareness deficits and rehabilitation outcome following acquired brain injury. *Clinical Psychology Review, 26,* 783–795.

Ownsworth, T. L., Clare, L., & Morris, R. (2006). An integrated biopsychosocial approach for understanding awareness disorder in Alzheimer's disease and brain injury. *Neuropsychological Rehabilitation, 16,* 415–438.

Papagno, C., & Muggia, S. (1996). Confabulation: Dissociation between everyday life and neuropsychological performance. *Neurocase, 2*(2), 111–118.

Phillips, J. (2000). Schizophrenia and the self-narrative. In T. Kircher & A. David (Eds.), *The Self in Psychiatry and Neuroscience*. Cambridge: Cambridge University Press.

Pillemer, D. B. (2001). Momentous events and the life story. *Review of General Psychology, 5,* 123–134.

Prigatano, G. P. (1999). *Principles of Neuropsychological Rehabilitation.* Oxford: Oxford University Press.

Reisberg, B., Gordon, B., McCarthy, M., & Ferris, S. H. (1985). Clinical symptoms accompanying progressive cognitive decline and Alzheimer's disease. In V. L. Melnick & N. N. Duber (Eds.), *Alzheimer's Dementia* (pp. 295–308). Clifton, NJ: Humana Press.

Ricoeur, P. (1992). *Oneself as Another.* Chicago: University of Chicago Press.

Ross, M. (1989). Relation of implicit theories to the construction of personal histories. *Psychological Review, 96,* 341–357.

Schacter, D. L. (1996). *Searching for Memory: The Brain, the Mind, and the Past.* New York: Basic Books.

Schacter, D. L., & Tulving, E. (1982). Memory, amnesia, and the episodic semantic distinction. In R. L. Isaacson & N. E. Spear (Eds.), *The Expression of Knowledge* (pp. 33–65). New York: Plenum.

Schnider, A. (2003). Spontaneous confabulation and the adaptation of thought to ongoing reality. *Nature Reviews Neuroscience, 4*, 662–671.

Schnider, A., von Däniken, C., & Gutbrod, K. (1996). The mechanisms of spontaneous and provoked confabulations. *Brain, 119*, 1365–1375.

Seltzer, B., Vasterling, J. J., Yoder, J. A., & Thompson, K. A. (1997). Awareness of deficit in Alzheimer's disease: Relation to caregiver burden. *Gerontologist, 37*(1), 20–24.

Singer, J. A., & Salovey, P. (1993). *The Remembered Self: Emotion and Memory in Personality*. New York: Free Press.

Solms, M. (2000). A psychoanalytic perspective on confabulation. *Neuro-psychoanalysis, 2*, 133–143.

Talland, G. A. (1961). Confabulation in the Wernicke-Korsakoff syndrome. *Journal of Nervous and Mental Disease, 132*, 361–381.

Tallberg, I. M. (2001). Deictic disturbances after right hemisphere stroke. *Journal of Pragmatics, 33*(8), 1309–1327.

Toglia, J., & Kirk, U. (2000). Understanding awareness deficits following brain injury. *Neuro-Rehabilitation, 15*, 57–70.

Turnbull, O. H., Berry, H., & Evans, C. E. (2004). A positive emotional bias in confabulatory false beliefs about place. *Brain and Cognition, 55*(3), 490–494.

Tyerman, A., & Humphrey, M. (1984). Changes in self-concept following severe head injury. *International Journal of Rehabilitation Research, 7*, 11–23.

Villiers, C. D., Zent, R., Eastman, R. W., & Swingler, D. (1996). A flight of fantasy: False memories in frontal lobe disease. *Journal of Neurology, Neurosurgery and Psychiatry, 61*, 652–653.

Walker, W. R., Skowronski, J. J., & Thompson, C. P. (2000). Life is pleasant and memory helps to keep it that way. *Review of General Psychology, 7*(2), 203–210.

Weinstein, E. A. (1996). Symbolic aspects of confabulation following brain injury: Influence of premorbid personality. *Bulletin of the Menninger Clinic, 60*, 331–350.

Weinstein, E. A., Kahn, R. L., & Malitz, S. (1956). Confabulation as a social-process. *Psychiatry, 19*(4), 383–396.

Wilson, A. E., & Ross, M. (2003). The identity function of autobiographical memory: Time is on our side. *Memory, 11*, 137–149.

Wright, J., & Telford, R. (1996). Psychological problems following minor head injury: A prospective study. *British Journal of Clinical Psychology, 35*, 399–412.

Yeates, G., Henwood, K., Gracey, F., & Evans, J. (2006). Awareness of disability after acquired brain injury: Subjectivity within the psychosocial context. *Neuro-Psychoanalysis, 8*, 175–189

Yeates, G., Henwood, K., Gracey, F., & Evans, J. (2007). Awareness of disability after acquired brain injury and the family context. *Neuropsychological Rehabilitation, 17*(2), 1960–2011

Ylvisaker, M., & Szekeres, S. F. (1989). Metacognitive and executive impairments in head-injured children and adults. *Topics in Language Disorders, 9*, 34–49.

NEUROPSYCHOLOGICAL REHABILITATION
2008, 18 (5/6), 566–589

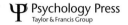

Psychology Press
Taylor & Francis Group

A biopsychosocial deconstruction of "personality change" following acquired brain injury

Giles Noel Yeates[1,2], Fergus Gracey[2], and
Joanna Collicutt McGrath[3]

[1]*Community Head Injury Service, Aylesbury, UK;* [2]*Oliver Zangwill Centre for Neuropsychological Rehabilitation, Ely, UK;* [3]*Heythrop College, University of London, UK*

The judgement of personality change following acquired brain injury (ABI) is a powerful subjective and social action, and has been shown to be associated with a range of serious psychosocial consequences. Traditional conceptualisations of personality change (e.g., Lishman, 1998) have largely derived from individualist concepts of personality (e.g., Eysenck, 1967). These assume a direct link between neurological damage and altered personhood, accounting predominantly for their judgements of change. This assumption is found as commonly in family accounts of change as in professional discourse.

Recent studies and perspectives from the overlapping fields of social neuroscience, cognitive approaches to self and identity and psychosocial processes following ABI mount a serious challenge to this assumption. These collectively identify a range of direct and indirect factors that may influence the judgement or felt sense of change in personhood by survivors of ABI and their significant others. These perspectives are reviewed within a biopsychosocial framework: neurological and neuropsychological deficits, psychological mechanisms and psychosocial processes. Importantly, these perspectives are applied to generate a range of clinical interventions that were not identifiable within traditional conceptualisations of personality changes following ABI.

Keywords: Brain injury; Personality change; Biopsychosocial; Deconstruction.

Correspondence should be sent to: Dr Giles Yeates, Clinical Psychologist, Community Head Injury Service, Buckinghamshire PCT, Camborne Centre, Jansel Square, Aylesbury, Bucks, UK. E-mail: Giles.Yeates@buckspct.nhs.uk

THE LANGUAGE OF PERSONALITY CHANGE

The concept of "personality change" following acquired brain injury (ABI) refers to an alteration or discontinuity in personhood post-injury. When considering many survivors of ABI, this alteration is undisputed by most professionals and families involved in the lives of these individuals. For many survivors themselves, there is a subjective discontinuity in their felt, embodied or social experience of who they are now in comparison with who they were. For others around them, there is an obvious change in "something" about them. The term "personality change" features prominently in professional discourse (literature, clinical documentation) and in the narratives and conversations of families (Oddy, 1995; Weddell & Leggett, 2006).

When personality change is defined by significant others, a number of serious clinical outcomes are more likely to ensue. Relatives' ratings of personality change following ABI have been identified in both cross-sectional and longitudinal outcome studies to be greater predictors of relatives' burden or stress in comparison with (traditionally-defined) cognitive or physical changes (e.g., Brooks, Campsie, Symington, Beattie, & McKinlay, 1987; Oddy, Humphrey, & Uttley, 1978; Weddell & Leggett, 2006). For the survivor of ABI, threats to self, identity and adjustment have been discussed in relation to psychological coping (Cantor et al., 2005; Jackson & Manchester, 2001; Nochi, 1997; 1998; 2000) and anxiety (Dewar & Gracey, 2007; Gracey, Oldham, & Kritzinger, 2006; McMillan, Williams, & Bryant, 2003). So the clinical prioritisation of the discontinuities referred to under the umbrella term of "personality change" is not controversial.

The critical theory practice of deconstruction (Derrida, 1977) is used across many contemporary disciplines to highlight the relative value and limitations of differing professional and everyday languages. This can be usefully applied to the use of the term "personality change", along with the assumptions supporting this usage. The professional use of this term in the ABI literature (e.g., Lishman, 1998; Tate, 2003) can be seen to be founded upon an individualist conceptualisation of personality. Typified by the work of Hans Eysenck (1967), stable personality traits are conceptualised to be located within the individual's cranium, to be fairly stable given non-pathological conditions (McCrae & Costa, 1996), and directly representing tendencies or biases within neurological process. It follows within this perspective that damage to this underlying neurological substrate results in a direct alteration of personality. This brain–mind alteration is considered to predominantly account for the "noticing" of personality change clearly evident in many families and wider social networks around a survivor of ABI.

While this shared reality of survivors, families and others is not disputed here, the assumption of a direct brain–mind alteration predominantly accounting for these experiences may be problematic. The aforementioned concepts of personality have been criticised by social psychologists emphasising the variable, heterogeneous aspects of personhood, dependent on the wider social context and the intersubjective, social actions of others (e.g., Antaki & Widdicombe, 1998; Potter & Wetherell, 1987; Tajfel & Turner, 1979). In addition to these ontological and epistemological challenges, the Eysenckian notion of a biologically determined, stable personality, directly altered through damage to neurological substrate leads to a clinical dead end. Clinicians have no options other than to stand by and try to help individuals and families cope with these permanent changes.

This limited potential for clinical application is disproportionate to the widespread use of the term personality change and associated assumptions. In contrast, a selective but broader literature is reviewed below within a biopsychosocial organisation, justified by two principles. Firstly, the reviewed concepts open up a more diverse and specific set of hypothesised deficits and processes that may contribute to alteration in personhood, extending beyond a damaged neurological substrate to psychological and psychosocial domains. Secondly, this specificity can be directly translated to multiple avenues for intervention that may be useful to survivors of ABI and their families, unidentifiable within a biologically-deterministic account of personality change. These interventions are reviewed alongside the theoretical and experimental literature.

A BIOPSYCHOSOCIAL REVIEW

The position that personality simply amounts to a set of immutable biologically endowed traits is challenged by the fields of social neuroscience, cognitive approaches to affect regulation, self and identity, and investigations of family communication after ABI. This conflicting evidence and its clinical implications is reviewed below within a biopsychosocial organising framework.

Biology: Altered neurological and neuropsychological function

Brain injury often results in physical changes that make the individual seem different to themselves and others (Collicutt McGrath, 2007). These changes may be morphological (e.g., limb shortening, or weight gain), or motor (e.g., weakness, nystagmus or ataxia). Change in voice, gait, fluidity of facial expression, or body shape render the individual less recognisable. Even more significant is the impact of neuropsychological deficits in socio-affective and neuro-cognitive mechanisms (Obonsawin et al., 2007).

Socio-affective neuropsychological processes. Neuroscientists have for some time described personality change and altered social relationships following damage to orbitofrontal and ventromesial frontal cortical areas (e.g., Stuss, Gow, & Hetherington, 1992). However, contemporary studies have introduced greater specificity in conceptualising associated neuropsychological impairments (Obonsawin et al., 2007). A number of neuroscientists now focus on the process of interoception as a core foundation of continuity in sense of personhood (e.g., Damasio, 1994; Panksepp, 1999; Dunn, Dalgleish, & Lawrence, 2006). Damasio (1999) describes cumulative, successively founding levels of personhood: the proto-self, core-self and auto-biographical self. The proto-self is the organism's non-conscious neural patterns regulating vital life functions. The core self is generated from moment to moment interactions with both internal and external objects/representations, and is consciously experienced as a shifting but undisrupted personal continuity. Finally, the autobiographical self makes use of more sophisticated linguistic, memory and executive cognitive systems together with extra-personal socially constructive processes. This is subjectively experienced as an "I" to be thought about, elaborated and located within a historical biography and narrative, extending forwards within a structure of aspirations and intentions.

Damasio evidently describes a trend towards increasing sophistication across these levels, with progressively greater involvement of numerous cortical areas and a wider range of cognitive operations. However, all levels are founded upon, and characterised by moment-to-moment interoception of homeostatic changes in internal milieu visceral states and proprioceptive feedback. This anchoring dimension of experience is subserved predominantly by brainstem, basal forebrain, paralimbic cortices and parietal cortical structures, and is characterised by a "felt" sense of background emotion (Damasio, 1999) and subjective continuity. It follows that damage to these neural structures will produce corresponding shifts in core subjective experience, perhaps accounting for some ABI survivors' descriptions of "just 'feeling' different now" post-injury. For a similar account with a more cognitive emphasis see Turk, Heaherton, Macrae, Kelley, and Gazzaniga (2003).

When taking survivors of ABI in their social interactional context, these somatic/affective considerations become even more significant. Frith (2003; Frith & Wolpert, 2003) outlines three concurrent phases of social neuropsychological activity within a dyadic encounter: (1) predicting the intentions of others, (2) aligning to other's subjectivity, and (3) influencing the subjectivity and behaviour of the other. Interoceptive, visceral and imitative processes mediated through inferior parietal and anterior cingulate networks have been identified as core to the aligning phase, which involve an internal simulation (Frith, 2003; Frith & Wolpert, 2003; Gallese, 1999) of others' emotional states. This simulation is now largely accepted to involve the personal experiencing of those emotional states (Gallese, 1999) as the individual perceives the social cues commensurate with a particular emotion displayed by others. Some would argue this alignment also involves a more immediate, automatic, "contagion" of affect passing between people (Hatfield, Cicioppa, & Rapson, 1994; Watt, 2007).

Selective difficulties have been reported in the perception of basic emotions such as fear and anger following amygdala damage (Adolphs, Tranel, Damasio, & Damasio, 1994; Park et al., 2001), disgust following damage to the insula (Calder, Keane, Manes, Antoun, & Young, 2000), and sadness following frontal injury (Blair & Cipolotti, 2000). Sequelae from both strokes and focal lesions have been shown to include an empathic failure regarding others' complex emotional states (Adophs et al., 2000; Eslinger et al., 2002; Shamay-Tsoory et al., 2003). In support of the internal simulation–emotion recognition hypothesis, some authors have identified a simultaneous disruption to the individual's subjective experience of those particular emotions (Blair & Cipolotti, 2000; Hornak, Rolls, & Wade, 1996). These data suggest that social experience can serve to highlight altered embodied experience, where feelings of other and self are difficult to access, distorted or misrepresented. Some authors have integrated these ideas to suggest alteration of self–other representations and forms of relating in various types of brain injury (Fotopoulou, Solms, & Turnbull, 2003; Turnbull, 2002; Turnbull, Evans, & Owen, 2005).

A failure to align with another may result from these core neuro-affective deficits following ABI, and/or other difficulties in the comprehension or production of social, pragmatic and prosodic aspects of verbal communication and social inference of sarcasm and irony (Cicerone & Tenenbaum, 1997; Martin & McDonald, 2003; Milders, Fuchs, & Crawford, 2003). Reciprocally, the failure to align with another will alter others' experience of the survivor of ABI. This may be in addition to the survivor's earlier failure to predict others' intentions via a deficit in mentalising, often found following damage to anterior cortices, temporal poles and superior-temporal sulcus (e.g., Baird, Dewar, Critchley, Dolan, Shallice, & Cipolotti, 2006; Channon, 2004; Channon & Crawford, 1999, 2000). It has recently been suggested that mentalising and imitation–emotional simulation abilities are mediated through an interconnected fronto-parietal network (Schulte-Ruther, Markowitsch, fink, & Piefke, 2007).

Similarly, adaptive predictive encoding and aligning stages may be undermined by neuropsychological pathologies in social behaviour, social judgements, or decision-making to appropriately influence the behaviour of the other. Following damage to anterior and temporal regions, difficulties have been reported in affect regulation and frustration tolerance within social situations (Burgess & Wood, 1990), detecting social norms (Blair & Cipolotti, 2001), accessing social knowledge (Channon, 2004; Channon & Crawford, 1999), and social problem-solving (perhaps also secondary to general executive dysfunction, Dimitrov, Grafman, & Hollnagel, 1996; Grafman, 1994; Grafman et al., 1996). In the case of ventral medial frontal damage, Damasio and colleagues argue that there may be intact access to social knowledge but a problem in using somatic, interoceptive information to guide decision-making in ambiguous situations, typically social in nature (Bechara, Damasio, Damasio, & Anderson, 1994; Damasio, 1994; Saver & Damasio, 1991).

Using these constructs, it is possible to specify how both subjective experience and social interactions can be differentially altered through neuro-anatomical damage. Furthermore, some of these constructs may have been approached in the operationalisation of "personality changes" and "behaviour problems" in early studies finding an association between these variables and caregiver strain and burden (Brooks et al., 1987; Weddell, Oddy, & Jenkins, 1980). Weddell and Leggett (2006) have recently returned to study these associations, while employing contemporary social neuropsychological concepts. They have found indirect measures of impaired orbito-frontal and social neuropsychological function to be one set of predictors for relatives' judgements of personality change and by association increased levels of relatives' psychological distress.

Cognitive neuropsychological functioning.   The early family outcome studies also included in the categories of personality and behavioural problems descriptors such as "aspontaneity", "stubbornness", "difficulties responding to changes in routine", and "disinhibition" (Brooks et al., 1987). Following the subsequent accounts of Baddeley (1986) or Shallice and Burgess (1996), these would now be recognised as dysexecutive problems. More recently, executive difficulties demonstrated through neuropsychological assessment have indeed been shown to be associated with significant other's judgements of personality change (Melamed, Stern, Rahmani, Groswasser, & Najenson, 1985), strained social relationships (Mazaux et al., 1997; Yeates et al., 2008) and other psychosocial outcomes (Tate, 1999; Villki et al., 1994).

In addition to problems with executive function, memory impairment may also contribute to the experience or judgement of "personality change" (empirically demonstrated by Weddell & Leggett, 2006). Sense of self is to some extent dependent on the construction of a set of reasonably coherent narratives based on past events (Conway, 2005; McAdams, 1990, 1993). These are punctuated by "self-defining memories" (Singer & Salovey, 1993). Events may be linked into coherent wholes through their relationship to enduring personal concerns and intentions (Dennett, 2004). A loss of auto-biographical memory as part of retrograde amnesia removes large portions of personal history and can thus devastate narratives about the self, while ante-rograde amnesia can also interfere with personal narratives by interrupting their construction.

Neuropsychological interventions. The specificity of relevant neuropsychological impairments identified above result in an increased array of rehabilitation options in response to the direct consequences of a damaged biological substrate. Training to identify emotional expression from facial, bodily and conversational cues (Von Cramon & Mattes-von Cramon, 1994) is now a common component in neuro-rehabilitation. In addition to these skills, social skills training can provide additional teaching on social responses and adhering to social norms (e.g., Boake, 1996). Other training packages developed within the field of autistic spectrum disorders, also include components on recognising and accessing emotional states in self (using external scaling procedures) and others, practising emotional expression and eye contact, perspective taking and mentalising (Solomon, Goodlin-Jones, & Anders, 2004). Social problem solving frameworks, addressing executive problems, emotional regulation and related social processes have been proven efficacious within ABI samples (Rath, Simon, Langenbahn, Sherr, & Diller, 2003).

Within experimental studies, Anderson and Phelps (2000) and Park and colleagues (2001) report an ability of ABI survivors with bilateral amygdala damage to produce explicit information relating to negative emotions when overtly cued to do so, despite their inability to process such information automatically. This suggests that external cues may have a role as an intervention to facilitate socially-congruent experience and discourse.

The recent work on interoception in social decision-making has not been formally applied to treatment approaches. However, the problem of subjective access to affective-somatic experience has been reconceptualised from an absence of such signals to a continuum of dampened to intense signal post-injury. As such, experimental procedures to increase the intensity of these signals in healthy subjects have been described by Damasio and colleagues (2000). In the assessment of interoception during decision-making by survivors of ABI, scaling and biofeedback paradigms are used to gather more detailed information (Dunn et al., 2006; Turnbull, 2004, personal communication). Future studies are required to see if intensity modulation, scaling and feedback protocols can be used as interventions to improve ABI survivors' access to interoceptive signals in emotional experience and social decision making, thereby effecting resultant social responses comparative with that pre-injury.

Finally, given the role of memory, language and executive processes in subjective continuity, notably autobiographical and representational aspects, compensatory interventions targeting these functions (e.g., Collicutt McGrath, 2008; Robertson, 1996; Wilson, Emslie, Quirk, & Evans, 2001) can be considered to be helpful in also re-establishing subjective continuity. Dewar and Gracey (2007) describe interventions developed with an

individual (VO) with post-encephalitic syndrome and related significant retrograde amnesia and prosopagnosia. These interventions were used to both
compensate for autobiographical memory loss and simultaneously to reaffirm
felt sense of social identity and belonging (see section on psychosocial processes below).

Psychological cognitive processes in affect regulation

As in the biological/organic literature, the use of the term "personality" and
the application of specific theories of personality appear superseded by the
cognitive approach. Here, "personality" is replaced with ideas about representation of "self", for example as a cognitive structure (Markus, 1977),
including goals (e.g., Conway, 2005) or as a "discourse" or narrative
(Antaki & Widdicombe, 1998). The literature on emotional and behavioural
changes post-injury as briefly summarised by Williams (2003) also provides
an alternative language to that of "personality change" (namely application of
cognitive models of coping style and related ideas about adjustment, grief and
trauma). We suggest that perception or experience of changed "personality"
following ABI can be considered in terms of alterations to the representational content and output (perceived as, for example, coping style or
emotional disorder) of systems governing experience or perception of self
in specific contexts.

Coping after brain injury.   The literature on coping has been concerned
with identifying categories of coping "style", based on cognitive models
(e.g., Godfrey, Knight & Partridge, 1996; Lazarus & Folkman, 1989)
which predict good and poor emotional outcome. Curran, Ponsford, and
Crowe (2000) found worry, wishful thinking, and self-blame to be predictive
of anxiety and depression, whereas problem solving and having a positive
outlook correlated with lower levels of anxiety. Locus of control beliefs
(Moore & Stambrook, 1992) and external causal attribution (Williams,
Williams, & Ghadiali, 1998) have also been found to correlate with poorer
emotional outcome. Thus cognitive-behavioural techniques to support
coping style change have been advocated (e.g., Ponsford, Sloane, & Snow,
1995, in brain injury rehabilitation; Moorey, 1996, in the context of terminal
illness). However, Lazarus and Folkman's coping model has been criticised
for failing adequately to recognise the nature, severity, and complexity of
the external stressor, a criticism especially relevant to the range of stressors
arising after ABI. As we describe below, clinical application of a cognitive
coping approach may fail to address the relationship between coping style
and underpinning self-representations, and thus the acceptability to the individual of suggested changes in coping style.

Adjustment and trauma. In understanding the emotional reaction to sudden onset, extreme life events such as an acquired brain injury, models of post-traumatic stress disorder (PTSD) may be helpful. Early accounts suggested the traumatic event might "shatter" the assumptions of an individual (Janoff-Bulman, 1989). Horowitz (1986) described the processing by the individual of a traumatic event until full integration or "completion" is reached. These ideas have been developed and integrated with contemporary cognitive, behavioural and neuroscientific ideas about trauma in Ehlers and Clark's (2000) cognitive model of PTSD. This describes the attempted integration of new trauma-derived information discrepant to, or activating of, enduring schema or representations of self, others and the world, together with cognitive coping and memory processes. It carries as a central motif the notion that it is psychological "threat to self" that underpins the traumatic response and subsequent development and maintenance of PTSD symptoms. Coping responses (e.g., avoidance, worry, rumination) aiming to reduce threat to self are suggested to impact upon processes that allow integration of trauma-related representations into prior, enduring representations of self, others and the world. Thus the need to consider the individual's personal values and expectations, and how these might be of particular relevance to the trauma incident and subsequent reactions, becomes critical in uncovering the underlying traumatic meanings to be addressed in therapy. Such notions may be of particular utility following brain injury in reconceptualising what may appear to be "personality change" in terms of the combined output of organic and cognitive changes and the process of psychological adjustment or adaptation (McGrath, 1997). In the brain injury literature, evidence in support of the notion of threat to self comes from Nochi (1998) describing "loss of self", and Cantor et al. (2005) reporting pre–post injury self-discrepancy to be associated with distress following brain injury.

Using PTSD as a vehicle for considering cognitive processes and representations relevant to affective disorders, Dalgleish argues for the application of cognitive models with multiple systems of representation. These include Dual Representation Theory (DRT; Brewin, 2001); Interacting Cognitive Subsystems (ICS; Teasdale & Barnard, 1993); and the Schematic, Propositional, Analogue and Associative Representational Systems model (SPAARS, Power, & Dalgleish, 1999). These models propose a range of representational and processing systems such as lower level sensory responses or body state, propositional information (thoughts and images), and higher level, abstract schematic representations including goals.

Perhaps the most relevant of these models, with a range of clinical applications derived from it in the field of psychological therapies for emotional disorders, is the ICS model (Teasdale & Barnard, 1993). This conceptualises information underpinning the "self" (including "felt sense" of self) as being stored in the "implicational" subsystem, abstracted over time from massed representations of ongoing autobiographical experiences. Depending on the mode of processing one may be more or less able to reflect on this "felt sense". Consistent with the social neurosciences literature described above, interventions to improve internal self-monitoring and to accept thoughts and feelings (mindfulness-based cognitive therapy) have been described (Segal, Williams, & Teasdale, 2003).

Goal processing and autobiographical memory.   Another particularly helpful way of construing "personality" at the intrapsychic level is in relation to personal goals (Emmons, 1999). An apparently random collection of unrelated habitual behaviours may achieve coherence if seen in the light of personal goals. These goals are variously described by researchers as "current concerns", "life tasks", "personal projects", and "personal strivings". Mundane habitual goals, such as getting the grocery shopping done, are thought to be connected to more fundamental goals, often expressed in terms of values related to personal identity, such as being a good mother (Carver & Scheier, 1990; Dewey, 1922; McGrath & Adams, 1999; Sheldon & Kasser, 1995). The changes that arise from brain injury constitute sudden major interruption to and thwarting of goal-directed activity. This is experienced as unpleasant affect, initially frustration as the individual attempts to continue with the same activity directed towards cherished goals, e.g., "being a good parent, competent student, physically fit and attractive mate"; then anxiety, confusion, or defensive aggression as problems in executing the required behaviours persist; then despair or depression as attempts at the behaviours cease and the cherished goals are relinquished. In addition to these affective responses, there is a profound change in the individual's sense of identity because previous habits, values, and ambitions are no longer in the picture.

Conway (2005; Conway & Pleydell-Pearce, 2000) presents an integrated account of memory, goal-directed behaviour and self-representation called the "self-memory system". Within this model, autobiographical memory processes provide a store of past experiences in which our possible "selves" are represented at an abstract level. At any given moment a particular "working self", may be active, carrying with it certain personally salient goals or sub-goals that direct and constrain action and cognition as required. Thus, self-representations abstracted from autobiographical experiences may significantly influence goal-directed behaviour in the here and now through the imposition of specific personally salient goals. In addition to the examples of the impact of ABI on personally salient goals described above, one can readily conceive how brain injury could lead to disruption of stores and processes that may impact upon the capacity to retrieve and maintain a context-specific "working self" in a given situation and for behaviour and emotion to be appropriately controlled.

An individual's coping response could then be seen as an emotionally potent (and thus resistant to change especially through verbal discussion) attempt to protect from conscious or non-consciously perceived threat to self. Any one of the resulting emotional reactions could be experienced (or denied) by the individual as personality change, and related behaviour changes could provide the basis for judgement of personality change by another. Over time, interactions between self and other would become represented within autobiographical memory systems, thus providing an increasingly rehearsed and therefore encoded representational substrate for altered sense of self in specific social contexts.

Psychological interventions.   The use of cognitive-behavioural techniques following ABI to address coping or learning of skills for managing emotional or behavioural changes (e.g., Ponsford, Sloane, & Snow, 1995), are not based on a specific cognitive model of emotional changes post-brain injury. In light of the above brief review the notions of loss of, threat to, and discrepant sense of self need to be taken into account when devising clinical intervention. One might argue that a goal for therapy is for the individual to integrate the meaning of the occurrence and the consequences of the injury, as well as any required adaptations such as strategies, into self-representations. For example, an individual may logically know and understand the potential usefulness of pacing oneself to reduce fatigue and irritability (for example), but this may clash with fundamental meanings associated with hard work and capacity for endurance. The suggested strategy would thus not be taken up, or experienced as one brain injured individual described potential use of a personal organiser as "bad, wrong and disloyal" to the pre-injury self.

Clinical approaches attempting to address such issues have drawn on contemporary cognition–emotion research and theory as described briefly above. For example, Ylvisaker and Feeney's (2000) use of "identity mapping", and the application of behavioural experiments in CBT, are thought to address what the ICS model describes as "implicational level meaning" (Bennett-Levy et al., 2004). Change at this level is described as in the "heart" rather than the "head", and may bring about more enduring change in mood and behaviour (Teasdale, 1999). Unhelpful patterns of processing, such as rumination, may present a barrier to such change (Teasdale & Barnard, 1993) and so there may be potential for application of approaches designed to disrupt such processing patterns (e.g., mindfulness-based cognitive therapy, Segal et al., 2003).

McGrath and King (2004) describe the specific application of behavioural experiments in cognitive-behavioural therapy following acquired brain injury. Cases noting how such experiments can be integrated into holistic rehabilitation are also offered by Gracey and others (2005; Gracey et al., 2006; and Dewar & Gracey, 2007). Some attention has been given to the potential of focusing on cherished goals as a means of addressing unpleasant affect in rehabilitation (Siegert, McPherson, & Taylor, 2004). Gracey (2005) and Ylvisaker and Feeney (2000) describe the development of diagrams with brain-injured individuals, which capture salient personal meanings associated with adaptive change after injury. Such "graphic organisers" or "positive formulations" provide a blueprint for individuals to accumulate further experiences that serve to develop or consolidate adaptive meanings post-injury. External support, cues or alerts may be helpful for maintaining gains. Thus, the systematic challenging of the notion of "personality change" post-injury using contemporary cognitive models of affect regulation and self-representation is allowing the development of theory-based rehabilitative and psychotherapeutic techniques that show initial promise (e.g., Ylvisaker et al., 2008 this issue).

Psychosocial processes

Many of the mechanisms described at the neuropsychological and psychological levels are realised at the psychosocial level. These are manifest in the socially-constructed subjectivities of the survivors of ABI and those around them, in the communicative processes in which they are related and organised, and in broader contextual dimensions in which they are situated. Prior to considering how the neuropsychological, cognitive and emotional is realised and influenced by the social, it is necessary to specify processes of influence unique to the psychosocial domain, independent of neuropsychological deficit.

In a series of qualitative studies Nochi (1997, 1998, 2000) has highlighted in the reliance of the ABI survivor on the broader social contextual dimension. Pre- and post-injury languages, social meanings and social roles have been described as necessary contextual parameters in survivors' post-injury sense-making and identity formation (Cloute, Mitchell, & Yates, 2008 this issue; Haslam, Holme, Haslam, Iyer, Jetten, & Williams, 2008 this issue; Nochi, 2000). Certain authors have drawn attention to altered roles within education, the workplace (Petrella, McColl, Krupa, & Johnston, 2005) and the family (e.g., parenting responses and responsibilities, Maitz & Sachs, 1995) post-injury as core limitations to both self and family identity.

Nochi (2000) has shown that the collaboration of significant others is necessary in this social identity reconstruction. However, Oddy (1995) has highlighted how some families are more able to preserve the continuity of the ABI survivor's pre-injury personhood (i.e., recognise the survivor as being essentially the same person) than others. Johnson and McCown (1997) have noted that within a given family, certain relatives who have had the majority of pre-injury contact with an individual at a particular developmental stage are going to identify differing quality or quantity of personality changes than those who are basing their comparison on a differing stage in life (e.g., parents versus a spouse). Yeates, Henwood, Gracey, and Evans (2006, 2007) have also highlighted breaks in continuity of personhood in family conversation. This was as part of a process of family negotiation and contestation where languages of pre-injury identity and the consequences of brain injury are often held in tension with one another.

Krefting (1990) has described both the investment and tensions of self-constructions and positions held by ABI survivors, relatives and clinicians as they communicate with one another. Mental distress in a social system seems to be a key precondition for judgements of personality change within that system, irrespective of the nature of cognitive impairment following ABI. In a case study of PTSD following ABI, McGrath (1997) noted that significant others had made a judgement of personality change as a result of the ABI survivor's anxiety and consequent withdrawal of social activity. Successful psychological treatment resulted in a corresponding witnessing by others of a "return of personality". The key point here is that no specific social neuropsychological deficit was identified or necessary.

In a multivariate analysis of a large sample of ABI survivors and relatives, Weddell and Leggett (2006) found that while traditional and social neuropsychological factors did predict relatives' judgements of personality change, it was in fact the level of psychological distress in both survivors and relatives that was most predictive (see also Obonsawin et al., 2007, for empirical modelling of interactions between these factors). An immediate clinical (and ethical) implication of these studies is that the presence of mental health problems in both survivors of ABI and their relatives may be related to a given judgement of personality change. These would be potentially treatable/reversible through psychological intervention (and so "reverse" personality change), but may be missed in the biologically-deterministic assumptions of the "personality change" label.

Some authors have attempted to highlight and conceptualise key nodal points of interconnection between social and neuropsychological influence on changes to identity or "personality". Several authors have pointed to the failure, following post-traumatic amnesia and any subsequent memory problems, to maintain socially-available continuous self-narratives (Nochi, 1997; Cloute, Mitchell, & Yates, 2008 this issue). Other investigators have focused on the relationship between altered embodied experience and socio-cultural parameters (e.g., Prigatano & Weinstein, 1996; Morin, Thibierge, Bruguière, Pradat-Diehl, & Mazevet, 2005). These authors have identified pre-injury socio-linguistic parameters of meaning that are used by ABI survivors in constructing an account of self, but also the distortion of this constructive process through neuro-linguistic and/or body representational deficits.

Others have focused on interpersonal interaction as a meeting point for neuropsychological and social process. Sabat and Harré (1992) have highlighted how continuity in a person's social self, already challenged by memory and language difficulties in neuro-disability, is further undermined by social processes driven by others, such as conversational repair, prohibited initiation of conversations, and conversational exclusion. The authors described the resultant loss of agency in the person's input and representation in conversation, and an associated progressive loss of social self. Similarly, in the case presented by Dewar and Gracey (2007), the clinical formulation describes ongoing threats and disruption of identity that are mediated by interactions between neuro-cognitive, psychological and family factors.

As described above, social neuropsychological deficits of various kinds can be hypothesised to stimulate and intensify an altered socio-emotional interaction with close others. The internal simulation models of emotion recognition and contagion (Gallese, 1999; Hatfield et al., 1994) discussed above in relation to survivors of ABI can also be applied to consider the subjectivities of significant others involved in these interactions. It follows that altered emotional experience and social interactions in the ABI survivor will be encoded, recognised and internally simulated in significant others' subjective emotional experience. This process has been already described in psychoanalytic accounts of intersubjective *identification*, where an individual's felt sense of closeness and knowing of a person in an intimate and familiar way is actually dependent on the recognition and interactions of the other (Freud, 1957/1917, 1961/1923; Lacan, 1949, 1953). It follows that altered emotional experience and social behaviour arising from the aforementioned differing lesions results in significant others not getting the same "feel" of the survivor with ABI, hence the very real sense of personality change. This may be especially pronounced with even more elemental changes in social engagement following ABI, such as a tendency reported in the famous case of EVR not to initiate shifts of attention to the eyes of others (Vecera & Rizzo, 2006).

Psychosocial interventions. In conceptualising both the interaction of distinct neuropsychological, psychological and social processes, or the exclusive influence of the social dimension, a number of psychosocial interventions can then be applied in clinicians' responses to personality change judgements.

Given the association of personality change judgements and mental distress in either the survivor of ABI and/or relatives (McGrath, 1997; Weddell & Leggett, 2006), there is an ethical impetus to identify such mental health difficulties during assessment. A psychological intervention such as cognitive-behavioural therapy (Dewar & Gracey, 2007; McGrath, 1997) or family therapy (Johnson & McCown, 1997; Yeates, 2007) addressing these issues may serve to re-establish the social manifestation of personhood in the survivor of ABI through renewed social functioning (e.g., a reduction in social disengagement or withdrawal) and/or changed interpersonal relationships between those system members who had defined the change initially.

When an influential social neuropsychological deficit has been identified, an important family and/or social intervention would be a psycho-educational conversation with significant others, identifying specific social neuropsychological impairments and corresponding strategies. This specificity could be a more empowering sense-making resource than a broad language of personality change. This conversation would require careful negotiation with the family, as differing families may take up different meanings of standard neuropsychological information as a function of their own idiosyncratic sense-making (Johnson & McCown, 1997; Yeates et al., 2007). Some existing approaches that focus on the neuro-cognitive and intrapsychic dimensions to identity reconstruction following ABI also prioritise social contextual resources and meanings in rehabilitation (Dewar & Gracey, 2007; Ylvisaker & Feeney, 2000).

Family interventions following ABI can be used to attend to conversational processes, in particular those that mark out discontinuity in the personhood of the ABI survivor (Yeates, 2007; Yeates et al., 2007). Allowing families to reflect on the inter-relationship of their languages of pre-injury selves versus a medicalised emphasis on the brain-injury (Cloute, Mitchell, & Yates, 2008 this issue; Yeates et al., 2007) may highlight the exact conditions and meanings in which a loss of personhood is identified, and from whose perspective. Explorations can be made to identify what needs to be seen or undertaken for a re-establishment of continuity to be achieved within a family or social system. To re-establish continuity in personhood does not necessarily equate to a recovery of pre-injury self, which given the aforementioned neuropsychological factors is often impossible, although often romanticised by self or others (McGrath, 2004). Rather continuity may be achieved if a link can be found between pre-injury self and current personhood as part of a life-growth process (McGrath, 2004). Central to this endeavour may be the aim of achieving role re-negotiation within the family system (Maitz & Sachs, 1995) and establishing meaningful employment and/or other productivity roles (Petrella et al., 2005).

Similarly, conversational processes may be crucial for neuropsychological-social interactions that may undermine personhood. It may be necessary to attend to conversational repair by others that further exclude someone with memory or language impairments from inserting their preferred self into the exchanges. When recall difficulties are primarily the result of executive or attentional difficulties, conversations can be guided to include necessary cues to prompt the insertion of survivors' autobiographical memories into conversations.

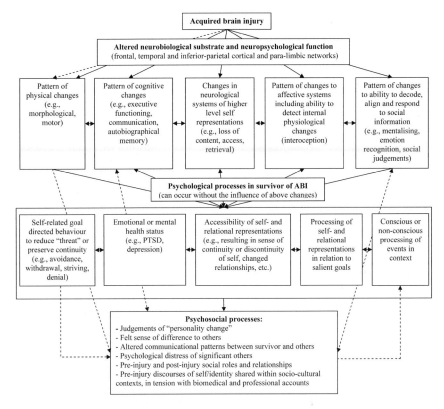

Figure 1. Summary and integration of literature reviewed to describe some possible biopsychosocial influences on, and by, judgements of personality change following brain injury. (Note: the processes pertaining to the individual with brain injury are prioritised for the purposes of clarity).

CONCLUSIONS

In contrast to a unitary, unspecified notion of personality change following ABI, a range of interacting and interdependent causal mechanisms have been identified across neuropsychological, psychological and psychosocial levels. The potential impact of disruption to these mechanisms on subjective experience of change in "self", judgement of personality change by others, and altered experience of personhood in social interactions has been described. The argument presented above is summarised and integrated in Figure 1.

In short, through subjecting the term "personality change" to a critical review in relation to a sample of relevant literature, we have highlighted how interacting processes set in motion following brain injury can lead to maintenance of subjective and/or observed changes described as "personality change". We also suggest that at times judgement of personality change itself, or other form of social meaning or action may serve to challenge post-injury adjustment at individual and systemic levels. However, the connections and interactions between these mechanisms require empirical validation through further research.

The contemporary concepts introduced and integrated in this paper do contain some theoretical and epistemological tensions in relation to each other. However, the relative value of this collection is defined in terms of clinical utility: the invitation of multiple interventions that can be used separately or in combination. Innovative rehabilitation interventions are described that suggest promise addressing cognitive and social-cognitive deficit, subjective experience (including "felt sense") and meaning, auto-biographical memory, goal processes and social relational context. These theoretical sources and applications are not claimed to be definitive or exclusive. We accept that alternative collections of literature from other areas of affective and cognitive neuroscience, social psychology or critical social theory can be drawn for a similar purpose and would embrace such projects to generate further clinical applications in this area.

Finally, this review places greater emphasis on psychological and psycho-social processes over altered biology as (1) influences on the experience and judgement of personality change following ABI and as (2) mediums for inter-vention. This is consistent with wider critiques of biopsychosocial approaches that implicitly promote a biological dominance (e.g., Armstrong, 1987), and the study by Weddell and Legget (2006) offers some empirical support for this emphasis. Further research employing both cross-sectional and longitudi-nal methodologies is required carefully to compare the relative predictive utility of direct injury-related and psychosocial variables for personality change judgements across time, in both survivors and significant others. Simi-larly, the value of psychological therapies in combination with neuro-rehabilitative interventions, for restoring continuity in identity for survivors and others requires future systematic evaluation beyond isolated case reports.

REFERENCES

Adolphs, R., Damasio, H., Tranel, D., Cooper, G., & Damasio, A. R. (2000). A role for soma-tosensory cortices in the visual recognition of emotion as revealed by three- dimensional lesion mapping. *Journal of Neuroscience*, *20(7)*, 2683–2690.

Adolphs, R., Tranel, D., Damasio, H., & Damasio, A. R. (1994). Impaired recognition of emotion in facial expressions following bilateral damage to the human amygdala. *Nature*, *372*, 669–672.

Anderson, A. K., & Phelps, E. A. (2000). Expression without recognition: Contributions of the human amygdala to emotional communication. *Psychological Science*, *11*, 106–111.

Antaki, C., & Widdicombe, S. M. (1998) *Identities in Talk*. London: Sage.

Armstrong, D. (1987). Theoretical tensions in biopsychosocial medicine. *Social Science & Medicine, 25(11)*, 1213–1218.

Baddeley, A. (1986). *Working Memory*. New York: Oxford University Press.

Baird, A., Dewar, B. K., Critchley, H., Dolan, R., Shallice, T., & Cipolotti, L. (2006). Social and emotional functions in three patients with medial frontal lobe damage including the anterior cingulated cortex. *Cognitive Neuropsychiatry, 11(4)*, 369–388.

Bechara, A., Damasio, A. R., Damasio, H., & Anderson, S. W. (1994). Insensitivity to future consequences following damage to human prefrontal cortex. *Cognition, 50*, 7–15.

Bennett, M., & Hacker, P. (2003). *Philosophical Foundations of Neuroscience*. Oxford: Blackwell.

Bennett-Levy, J., Westbrook, D., Fennell, M., Cooper, M., Rouf, K., & Hackmann, A. (2004) Behavioural experiments: historical and conceptual underpinnings. In J. Bennett-Levy, G. Butler, M. Fennell, & A. Hackmann (Eds.), *The Oxford Guide to Behavioural Experiments in CBT*. Oxford: Oxford University Press.

Ben-Yishay, Y. (1996). Reflections on the evolution of the therapeutic milieu concept. Historical aspects of neuropsychological rehabilitation. *Neuropsychological Rehabilitation, 6(4)*, 327–343.

Ben-Yishay, Y. (2000). Postacute neuropsychological rehabilitation. A holistic perspective. In A. L. Christensen & B. P. Uzzell (Eds.), *Critical Issues in Neuropsychology, International Handbook of Neuropsychological Rehabilitation*. Netherlands: Kluwer Academic.

Blair, R., & Cipolotti, L. (2000). Impaired social response reversal: A case of acquired sociopathy. *Brain, 123*, 1122–1141.

Boake, C. (1996). Social skills training following head injury. In J. S. Kreutzer & P. H. Wehman (Eds.), *Cognitive Rehabilitation for Persons with Traumatic Brain Injury: A Functional Approach*. Baltimore: P.H. Brookes.

Brewin, C. (2001). A cognitive neuroscience account of posttraumatic stress disorder and its treatment. *Behaviour Research and Therapy, 39(4)*, 373–393.

Brooks, N., Campsie, L., Symington, C., Beattie, A., & McKinlay, W. (1987). The effects of severe head injury on patient and relative within several years of injury. *Journal of Head Trauma Rehabilitation, 2*, 1–13.

Burgess, P. W., & Wood, R. Ll. (1990). Neuropsychology of behaviour disorders following brain injury. In R. Ll. Wood (Ed.), *Neurobehavioural Sequelae of Traumatic Brain Injury* (pp. 110–133). Hove, UK: Lawrence Erlbaum Associates Ltd.

Calder, A. J., Keane, J., Manes, F., Antoun, N., & Young, A. W. E. (2000). Impaired recognition and experience of disgust following brain injury. *Nature Neuroscience, 3*, 1077–1078.

Cantor, J., Ashman, T., Schwartz, M. E., Gordon, W. A., Hibbard, M. R., Brown, M., Spielman, L., Charatz, H. J., & Cheng, Z. (2005) The role of self-discrepancy theory in understanding post-traumatic brain injury affective disorders: A pilot study. *Journal of Head Trauma Rehabilitation, 20(6)*, 527–543.

Carver, C., & Scheier, M. (1990). Origins and function of positive and negative affect: A control process view. *Psychological Review, 97*, 19–36.

Channon, S. (2004). Frontal lobe dysfunction and everyday performance: Social and non-social contributions. *Acta Psychologia, 115*, 235–254.

Channon, S., & Crawford, S. (1999). Problem-solving in real-life-type situations: The effects of anterior and posterior lesions on performance. *Neuropsychologia, 37*, 757–770.

Channon, S., & Crawford, S, (2000). The effects of anterior lesions on performance on a story comprehension test: Left anterior impairment on a theory of mind task. *Neuropsychologia, 38*, 1006–1017.

Cicerone, K., & Tanenbaum, L. (1997). Disturbances of social cognition after traumatic orbitofrontal brain injury. *Achives of Clinical Neuropsychology, 12*, 173–188.

Cloute, K., Mitchell, A., & Yates, P. (2008). Traumatic brain injury and the construction of identity: A discursive approach. *Neuropsychological Rehabilitation, 18*, 651–670.

Collicutt McGrath, J. (2007). *Ethical Practice in Brain Injury Rehabilitation*. Oxford: Oxford University Press.

Collicutt McGrath, J. (2008). Recovery from brain injury and positive rehabilitation practice. In S. Joseph & P. A. Linley (Eds.), *Trauma, recovery and growth: positive psychological perspectives on posttraumatic stress* (pp. 259–274). New York: John Wiley.

Conway, M. A. (2005). Memory and the Self. *Journal of Memory and Language, 53(4)*, 594–628.

Conway, M., & Pleydell-Pearce, C. W. (2000). The construction of autobiographical memories in the self-memory system. *Psychological Review, 107(2)*, 261–288.

Curran, C. A., Ponsford, J. L., & Crowe, S. (2000). Coping strategies and emotional outcome following traumatic brain injury: A comparison with orthopedic patients. *Journal of Head Trauma Rehabilitation, 15*, 1256–1274.

Damasio, A. R. (1994). *Descartes' Error: Emotion, Reason and the Human Brain*. New York: Grosset/Putnam.

Damasio, A. (1999). *The Feeling of What Happens*. San Diego, CA: Harcourt.

Damasio, A. R. (2003). *Looking for Spinoza: Joy, Sorrow and the Feeling Brain*. London: Heinemann.

Damasio, A. R., Grabowoski, T. J., Bechara, A., Damasio, H., Ponto, L. L. B., Parvizi, J., & Hichwa, R. D. (2000). Subcortical and cortical brain activity during the feeling of self-generated emotions. *Nature Neuroscience, 3(10)*, 1049–1056.

Dennett, D. (2004). *Consciousness Explained*. Harmondsworth, UK: Penguin.

Derrida, J. (1977). *Of Grammatology*. Baltimore: Johns Hopkins University Press.

Dewar, B. K., & Gracey, F. (2007). "Am not was": Cognitive behavioural therapy for adjustment and identity change following herpes simplex encephalitis. *Neuropsychological Rehabilitation, 17(4/5)*, 602–620.

Dewey, J. (1922/2002). *Human Nature and Conduct*. Mineola, NY: Dover.

Dimitrov, M., Grafman, J., & Hollnagel, C. (1996). The effects of frontal lobe damage on everyday problem solving. *Cortex, 32*, 357–366.

Dunn, B. D., Dalgleish, T., & Lawrence, A. D. (2006). Somatic marker hypthesis: A critical evaluation. *Neuroscience & Behavioural Reviews, 30*, 239–271.

Ehlers, A., & Clark. D. M. (2000). A cognitive model of PTSD. *Behaviour Research and Therapy, 38(4)*, 319–345.

Emmons, R. (1999). *The Psychology of Ultimate Concerns*. New York: Guilford Press.

Eslinger, P. J., Parkinson, K., & Shamay, S. G. (2002). Empathy and social–emotional factors in recovery from stroke. *Current Opinion in Neurology, 15*, 91–97.

Eysenck, H. J. (1967). *The Biological Basis of Personality*. Springfield, IL: Charles C Thomas.

Fotopoulou, A., Solms, M., & Turnbull, O. (2003). Wishful reality distortions in confabulation: A case report. *Neuropsychologia, 42(6)*, 727–744.

Frith, C. D. (2003). Neural hermeneutics: How brains interpret minds. [Keynote Lecture], *9th Annual Meeting of the Organization of Human Brain Mapping*, New York.

Frith, C. D., & Wolpert, D. M. (Eds.) (2003). *The Neuroscience of Social Interaction: Decoding, Imitating and Influencing the Actions of Others*. Oxford, UK: Oxford University Press.

Freud, S. (1957). *Mourning and Melancholia*. In J. Strachey (Ed. & Trans.), *The standard edition of the complete psychological works of Sigmund Freud* (Vol. 14, pp. 237–259). London: Hogarth Press. (Original work published 1917)

Freud, S. (1961). *The Ego and the Id*. In J. Strachey (Ed. & Trans.), *The standard edition of the complete psychological works of Sigmund Freud* (Vol. 19, pp. 3–66). London: Hogarth Press. (Original work published 1923)

Gallese, V. (1999). From grasping to language: Mirror neurons and the origin of social communication. In S. Hameroff, A. Kazniak, & D. Chalmers (Eds.) *Towards a Science of Consciousness* (pp. 165–178). Cambridge, MA: MIT Press.

Godfrey, H. P. D., Knight, R. G., & Partridge, F. M. (1996). Emotional adjustment following traumatic brain injury: A stress-appraisal coping formulation. *Journal of Head Trauma Rehabilitation, 11*, 29–40.

Gracey, F. (2005). No room for error? Identity, cognitive therapy and rehabilitation of executive impairment. An illustrative single case. *Journal of the International Neuropsychological Society, 11(S2)*, 77–78.

Gracey, F., Oldham, P., & Kritzinger, R. (2006). Finding out if the 'me' will shut down: Successful cognitive-behavioural therapy of seizure related panic symptoms following subarachnoid haemorrhage, a single case report. *Neuropsychological Rehabilitation, 17(1)*, 106–119.

Grafman, J. (1994). Alternative frameworks for the conceptualization of prefrontal lobe functions. In F. Boller, F., & J. Grafman (Eds.), *Handbook of Neuropsychology, Vol 9.* (pp. 187–202). Amsterdam: Elsevier.

Grafman, J., Schwab, K., Warden, D., Pridgen, B. S., Brown, H. R., & Salazar, A. M. (1996). Frontal lobe injuries, violence and aggression: A report of the Vietnam Head Injury Study. *Neurology, 46*, 1231–1238.

Haslam, C., Holme, A., Haslam S. A., Iyer, A., Jetten, J., & Williams, W. H. (2008). Maintaining group memberships: Social identity continuity predicts well-being after stroke. *Neuropsychological Rehabilitation, 18*, 671–691.

Hatfield, E., Cacioppo, J., & Rapson, R. L. (1994). *Emotional Contagion.* New York: Cambridge University Press.

Hornak J., Rolls, E. T., & Wade, D. (1996). Face and voice expression identification in patients with emotional and behavioural changes following ventral frontal lobe damage. *Neuropsychologia, 34*, 247–261.

Horowitz, M. J. (1986) Stress-response syndromes: A review of posttraumatic and adjustment disorders, *Hospital and Community Psychiatry 37*, 241–249.

Jackson, H., & Manchester, D. (2001). Towards the development of brain injury specialists. *Neurorehabilitation, 16*, 27–40.

Janoff-Bulman, R. (1989). Assumptive worlds and the stress of traumatic events: Applications of the schema construct. *Social Cognition, 7(2)*, 113–136.

Johnson, J., & McCown, W. (1997). *Family Therapy of Neurobehavioral Disorders: Integrating Neuropsychology and Family Therapy.* New York: Haworth Press.

Krefting, L. (1990). Double bind and disability: The case of traumatic head injury. *Social Sciences & Medicine, 30(8)*, 859–865.

Lacan, J. (1949). The mirror stage as formative of the I as revealed in psychoanalytic experience. In J. Lacan (Ed.), *Écrits: A Selection.* London: Tavistock Publications.

Lacan, J. (1953). The function and field of speech and language in psychoanalysis. In J. Lacan (Ed.), *Écrits: A Selection.* London: Tavistock Publications.

Lazarus, R. S., & Folkman, S. (1989). Transactional theory and research on emotions and coping. *European Journal of Personality, 1(3)*, 141–169.

Lishman, W. A. (1998). *Organic Psychiatry: The Psychological Consequences of Cerebral Disorder.* Oxford: Blackwell.

Maitz, E. A., & Sachs, P. R. (1995). Treating families of individuals with traumatic brain injury from a family systems perspective. *Journal of Head Trauma Rehabilitation, 10(2)*, 1–11.

Markus, H. (1977). Self-schemata and processing information about the self. *Journal of personality and Social Psychology, 35*, 63–78.

Martin, R., & Macdonald, S. (2003). Weak coherence, no theory of mind, or executive dysfunction? Solving the puzzle of pragmatic language disorders. *Brain & Language, 85*, 451–466.

Mazaux, J. M., Masson, F., Levin, H.S., Alaoui, P., Maurette, P., & Barat, M. (1997). Long-term neuropsychological outcome and loss of social autonomy after traumatic brain injury. *Archives of Physical Medicine & Rehabilitation 78(12)*, 1316–1320.

McAdams, D. (1990). Unity and purpose in human lives: The emergence of identity as the life story. In A. Rabin, R. Zucker, R. Emmons, & S. Franck (Eds.), *Studying Persons and Their Lives* (pp. 148–200). New York: Springer.

McAdams, D. (1993). *The Stories We Live By: Personal Myths and the Making of the Self.* New York: Morrow.

McCrae, R. R., & Costa, P. T. (1996). Towards a new generation of personality theories: Theoretical contexts for the five-factor model. In J. S. Wiggins (Ed.), *The Five Factor Model of Personality: Theoretical Perspectives* (pp. 51–87). New York: Guilford Press.

McGrath, J. (1997) Cognitive impairment associated with post-traumatic stress disorder and minor head injury: A case report. *Neuropsychological Rehabilitation, 7(3)*, 231–239.

McGrath, J. (2004). Beyond restoration to transformation: Positive outcomes in the rehabilitation of acquired brain injury. *Clinical Rehabilitation, 18(2)*, 761– 775.

McGrath, J., & Adams, L. (1999). Patient-centred goal planning: A systemic psychological therapy? *Topics in Stroke Rehabilitation, 6*, 43–50.

McGrath, J., & King, N. (2004). Acquired brain injury. In J. Bennett-Levy, G. Butler, M. Fennell, A. Hackmann, M. Mueller, & D. Westbrook (Eds.), *The Oxford Guide to Behavioural Experiments in CBT*. Oxford: Oxford University Press.

McMillan, T. M., Williams, W. H., & Bryant, R. (2003). Post-traumatic stress disorder and traumatic brain injury: A review of causal mechanisms, assessment and treatment. *Neuropsychological Rehabilitation, 13(1/2)*, 149–164.

Melamed, S., Stern, M., Rahmani, L., Groswasser, Z., & Najenson, T. (1985). Attention capacity limitation, psychiatric parameters and their impact on work involvement following brain injury. *Scandinavian Journal of Rehabilitation Medicine, 12*, 21–26.

Milders, M., Fuchs, S., & Crawford, J. R. (2003). Neuropsychological impairments and changes in emotional and social behaviour following severe traumatic brain injury. *Journal of Clinical & Experimental Neuropsychology, 25(2)*, 157–172.

Moore, A. D., & Stambrook, M. (1992) Coping strategies and locus of control following traumatic brain injury: Relationship to long-term outcome, *Brain Injury, 6(1)*, 89–94.

Moorey, S. (1996). When bad things happen to rational people: Cognitive therapy in adverse circumstances. In P. Salkovskis (Ed.), *Frontiers of Cognitive Therapy* (pp. 450–469). New York: Guilford Press.

Morin, C., Thibierge, S., Bruguière, P., Pradat-Diehl, P., & Mazevet, D. (2005). "Daughter-somatoparaphrenia" in women with right hemisphere syndrome: A psychoanalytic perspective on neurological body knowledge disorders. *Neuro-psychoanalysis, 7(2)*, 171–184,

Nochi, M. (1997). Dealing with the "Void": Traumatic brain injury as a story. *Disability & Society, 12(4)*, 533–555.

Nochi, M. (1998). Struggling with the labeled self: People with traumatic brain injuries in social settings. *Qualitative Health Research, 8(5)*, 665–681.

Nochi, M. (2000). Reconstructing self-narratives in coping with traumatic brain injury. *Social Science & Medicine, 51(12)*, 1795–1804.

Obonsawin, M. C., Jefferis, S., Lowe, R., Crawford, J. R., Fernandes, J., Holland, L., et al. (2007). A model of personality change after traumatic brain injury and the development of the Brain Injury Personality Scales. *Journal of Neurology, Neurosurgery, and Psychiatry, 78*, 239–1247.

Oddy, M. (1995). He's no longer the same person: How families adjust to personality change after head injury. In N. V. T. Chamberlain (Ed.), *Traumatic Brain Injury Rehabilitation* (pp. 197–180). London: Chapman and Hall.

Oddy, M., Humphrey, M., & Uttley, D. (1978). Stresses upon the relatives of head-injured patients. *British Journal of Psychiatry, 133*, 507–513.

Panksepp, J. (1999). The periconscious substrates of consciousness: Affective states and the evolutionary origins of the self. In S. Gallagher & J. Shear (Eds.), *Models of the Self* (pp. 113–130). Exeter, UK: Imprint Academic.

Park, N. W., Conrod, B., Rewilak, D., Kwon, C., Gao, F., & Black, S. (2001). Automatic activation of positive but not negative attitudes after traumatic brain injury. *Neuropsychologia, 39*, 7–24.

Petrella, L., McColl, M. A., Krupa, T., & Johnston, J. (2005). Returning to productive activities: Perspectives of individuals with long-standing brain injuries. *Brain Injury, 19(9)*, 643–655.

Ponsford, J., Sloane, S., & Snow, P. (1995) *Traumatic Brain Injury: Rehabilitation for Everyday Adaptive Living.* Hove, UK: Lawrence Erlbaum Associates.

Potter, J., & Wetherell, M. (1987). *Discourse and Social Psychology: Beyond Attitudes and Behaviour.* London: Sage.

Power, M. J., & Dalgeish, T. (1999). Two routes to emotion: Some implications of multi-level theories of emotion for therapeutic practice. *Behavioural and Cognitive Psychotherapy, 27*, 129–141.

Prigatano, G. P., & Weinstein, E. A. (1996). Edwin A. Weinstein's contribution to neuropsychological rehabilitation. *Neuropsychological Rehabilitation, 6(4)*, 305–326.

Rath, J. F., Simon, D., Langenbahn, D. M., Sherr, R. L., & Diller, L. (2003). Group treatment of problem-solving deficits in outpatients with traumatic brain injury: A randomised outcome study *Neuropsychological Rehabilitation, 13*, 461–488.

Robertson, I. H. (1996). *Goal Management Training: A Clinical Manual.* Cambridge, UK: PsyConsult.

Sabat, S. R., & Harré, R. (1992). The construction and deconstruction of self in Alzheimer's disease. *Ageing and Society, 12*, 443–461.

Saver, J. L., & Damasio, A. R. (1991). Preserved access and processing of social knowledge in a patient with acquired sociopathy due to ventromedial frontal damage. *Neuropsychologia, 39*, 1241–1249.

Schulte-Ruther, M., Markowitsch, H. J., Fink, G. R., & Piefke, M. (2007). Mirror neuron and theory of mind mechanisms involving face to face interactions: A functional magnetic resonance imaging approach to empathy. *Journal of Cognitive Neuroscience, 8*, 1354–1372.

Segal, Z. V., Williams, J. M. G., & Teasdale, J. D. (2003). *Mindfulness-Based Cognitive Therapy for Depression: A New Approach to Preventing Relapse.* New York: Guilford Press.

Shallice, T., & Burgess, P. (1996). The domain of the supervisory process and temporal organisation of behaviour. *Philosophical Transactions of the Royal Society of London, Series B: Biological Sciences, 351*, 1404–1412.

Shamay-Tsoory, S., Tomer, R., Berger, B. D., & Aharon-Peretz, J. (2003). Characterisation of empathy deficits following prefrontal brain damage: The role of the right ventromedial prefrontal cortex. *Journal of Cognitive Neuroscience, 15*, 324–337.

Sheldon, K., & Kasser, T. (1995). Coherence and congruence: Two aspects of personality integration. *Journal of Personality and Social Psychology, 68*, 531–543.

Siegert, R., McPherson, K., & Taylor, W. (2004). Toward a cognitive-affective model of goal setting in rehabilitation: Is self-regulation theory a key step? *Disability & Rehabilitation, 26*, 1175–1183.

Singer J. A., & Salovey, P. (1993). *The Remembered Self: Emotion and Memory in Personality.* New York: The Free Press.

Solomon, M., Goodlin-Jones, B. L., & Anders, T. F. (2004). A social adjustment enhancement intervention for high functioning autism, Asperger's syndrome, and pervasive developmental disorder NOS. *Journal of Autism & Developmental Disorders, 34,* 649–668.

Stuss, D. T., Gow, C. A., & Hetherington, C. R. (1992). "No Longer Gage": frontal lobe dysfunction and emotional changes. *Journal of Consulting & Clinical Psychology, 60(3),* 349–359.

Tajfel, H., & Turner, J. C. (1979). An interactive theory of intergroup conflict. In W. G. Austin & S. Worchel (Eds.), *The Social Psychology of Intergroup Relations* (pp. 33–47). Monterey, CA: Brooks/Cole.

Tate, R. L. (1999). Executive dysfunction and characterological changes after traumatic brain injury: Two sides of the same coin? *Cortex, 35,* 39–55.

Tate, R.L. (2003). Impact of pre-injury factors on outcome after severe traumatic brain injury: Does post-traumatic personality change represent an exacerbation of premorbid traits? *Neuropsychological Rehabilitation 13*(1/2), 43–64.

Teasdale, J. D. (1999). Emotional processing, three modes of mind and the prevention of relapse in depression, *Behaviour Research and Therapy, 18,* 51–60.

Teasdale, J. D., & Barnard, P. J. (1993). *Affect, Cognition and Change: Re-Modelling Depressive Thought.* Hove, UK: Lawrence Erlbaum Associates.

Turnbull, O. (2002). Implicit awareness of deficit in anosognosia? An emotion-based account of denial of deficit. *Neuro-Psychoanalysis, 4(1),* 69–87.

Turnbull, O., Evans, C. E. Y., & Owen, V. (2005). Negative emotions and anosognosia. *Cortex, 41(1),* 67–75.

Turk, D., Heatherton, T., Macrae, C. N., Kelley, W., & Gazzaniga, M. (2003). Out of contact out of mind. The distributed nature of the self. *Annals of the New York Academy of Science, 1001,* 65–78.

Vecera, S. P., & Rizzo, M. (2006). Eye gaze does not produce reflexive shifts of visual attention: Evidence from frontal lobe damage. *Neuropsychologia, 44,* 150–159.

Villki, J., Ahola, K., Holst, P., Ohman, J., Servo, A., & Heiskanen, O. (1994). Prediction of psychosocial recovery after head injury with cognitive test and neurobehavioural ratings. *Journal of Clinical & Experimental Neuropsychology, 16,* 325–338.

Von Cramon, D. Y., & Mattes-von Cramon, G. (1994). Back to work with a chronic dysexecutive syndrome? *Neuropsychological Rehabilitation, 4,* 399–417.

Watt, D. (2007). Towards a neuroscience of empathy: Integrating affective and cognitive perspectives. *Neuropsychoanalysis, 9(2),* 119–140.

Weddell, R., & Leggett, J. (2006). Factors triggering relatives' judgements of personality change after traumatic brain injury. *Brain Injury, 20(12),* 1221–1234.

Weddell, R., Oddy, M., & Jenkins, D. (1980). Social adjustment after rehabilitation: A two year follow-up of patients with severe head injury. *Psychological Medicine, 10,* 257–263.

Williams, W. H. (2003). Neuropsychological rehabilitation and CBT for emotional disorders after acquired brain injury. In B. A. Wilson *Neuropsychological Rehabilitation: Theory and Practice.* Abingdon, UK: Swets and Zeitlinger.

Williams W. H., Williams J. M. G., & Ghadiali, E. J. (1998) Autobiographical memory in traumatic brain injury: Neuropsychological and mood predictors of recall. *Neuropsychological Rehabilitation, 8(1),* 43–60.

Wilson, B. A., Emslie, H., Quirk, K., & Evans, J. J. (2001). Reducing everyday memory and planning problems by means of a paging system: A randomised control crossover study. *Journal of Neurosurgery, Neurology & Psychiatry, 70,* 477–482.

Yeates, G. N. (2007). Avoiding the skull seduction in post-acute acquired brain injury (ABI) services: Individualist invitations and systemic responses. *Clinical Psychology Forum, 175*, 33–36.

Yeates, G. N., Hamill, M., Sutton, L., Psaila, K., Gracey, F., Mohamed, S., & O'Dell, J. (2008). Dysexecutive problems and interpersonal relating following frontal brain injury: Reformulation and compensation in Cognitive-Analytic Therapy (CAT). *Neuropsychoanalysis, 10*(1), 43–58.

Yeates, G. N., Henwood, K., Gracey, F., & Evans, J. J. (2006). Awareness of disability after acquired brain injury: Subjectivity within the psychosocial context. *Neuro-Psychoanalysis, 8(2)*, 175–189.

Yeates, G. N., Henwood, K., Gracey, F., & Evans, J. J. (2007). Awareness of disability and the family context. *Neuropsychological Rehabilitation, 17(2)*, 151–173.

Ylvisaker, M., & Feeney, T. (2000). Reconstruction of identity after brain injury. *Brain Impairment, 1*, 12–28.

Ylvisaker, M., McPherson, K., Kayes, N., & Pellett, E. (2008). Metaphoric identity mapping: Facilitating goal setting and engagement in rehabilitation after traumatic brain injury. *Neuropsychological Rehabilitation, 18*, 713–741.

NEUROPSYCHOLOGICAL REHABILITATION
2008, 18 (5/6), 590–606

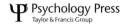

Awareness of memory functioning, autobiographical memory and identity in early-stage dementia

Emma Naylor and Linda Clare

University of Wales Bangor, Gwynedd, Wales, UK

Sense of identity is thought to be closely related to autobiographical memory. Theoretical models of awareness suggest that both may also be related to level of awareness of memory functioning among people with early-stage dementia. This study explores the relationships between autobiographical memory, identity and awareness in early-stage dementia. Thirty participants with Alzheimer's disease, or vascular or mixed dementia were assessed using the Autobiographical Memory Interview, with an additional section eliciting recall for the mid-life period, the Tennessee Self-Concept Scale, and the Memory Awareness Rating Scale. Lower levels of awareness of memory functioning were associated with poorer autobiographical recall for the mid-life period and with a more positive and definite sense of identity. Reduced awareness may serve a protective function against the threats to self posed by the onset and progression of dementia.

INTRODUCTION

There is considerable variability in the extent to which people with early-stage dementia show awareness of aspects of their functioning, of their current

Correspondence should be addressed to Linda Clare, Reader in Psychology, School of Psychology, University of Wales Bangor, Bangor, Gwynedd LL57 2AS, Wales, UK. E-mail: l.clare@bangor.ac.uk

We are grateful to Kate Jones and Nia Williams for assistance with participant recruitment; to Caroline Parkinson, Sue Evans and Jorien van Paasschen for contributions to assessment; to Kate Jones and Bob Woods for permission to use their assessment of autobiographical recall for the mid-life period; to staff of the North Wales Clinical Psychology Programme; and most of all to our participants for taking the time to contribute to the study. We would like to thank Professor Michael Kopelman for helpful comments on an earlier draft of this paper.

situation, and of the disorder itself. This has significant practical implications. For example, higher levels of awareness seem to be related to higher levels of depression, but better outcomes following cognitive rehabilitation, in the person with dementia (Clare, Wilson, Carter, Roth, & Hodges, 2004), and lower levels of stress, burden, and depression in caregivers (De Bettignies, Mahurin, & Pirozzolo, 1990). Consequently, it is important to consider why this variability might arise and to explore what factors might influence level of awareness.

Clare (2004) proposed a biopsychosocial framework for understanding awareness, which emphasises the interplay between neurological damage relating directly to the dementia process and the psychological resources that the individual brings to the situation, and views this interplay within a wider social context. This framework highlights the importance of the sense of self as the context within which awareness of functioning and situation is experienced and expressed.

Within a social cognitive approach, self is viewed as a complex, multi-dimensional construct, comprising beliefs, attitudes and information and providing a schematic framework for information processing (Greenwald & Pratkanis, 1984; Gergen, 1984; Markus & Wurf, 1987). Identity forms one sub-component of self, and is likewise viewed as multi-dimensional, incorporating a range of self-relevant domains (Fitts, 1965). Identity is a dynamic construct, and may be presented differently across different social contexts or at different life-periods (Damasio, 1999; Deaux, 1992). Despite this multi-dimensional and dynamic nature, identity is characterised by a sense of coherence and continuity over time, providing a unifying context for personal experience (Baars, 1997) as life changes are integrated into one's identity and a coherent self-narrative is constructed and reconstructed (McAdams, 1988).

It has been noted that sense of self may alter in early-stage dementia (Orona, 1990). The degree to which previous information about the self can be drawn upon to provide a sense of continuity, and the extent to which new information about the self can be incorporated into a revised sense of identity, are likely to be influenced by changes in autobiographical memory, the store of personally relevant semantic and episodic memories (Baddeley, 1992). Conway and Pleydell-Pearce (2000) propose a bi-directional relationship between sense of self and autobiographical memory. In this model, autobiographical knowledge is encoded through the goal structure of the working self, which then plays a role in constructing specific memories during autobiographical remembering. However, autobiographical memory is typically impaired from the early stages of Alzheimer's disease (AD) and vascular dementia, with a disproportionate impairment of recent, relative to remotely acquired, autobiographical memories (e.g., Graham & Hodges, 1997; Greene, Hodges & Baddeley, 1995; Kopelman, 1989). Addis and Tippett

(2004) investigated the impact of changes in autobiographical memory on identity in people with mild to moderate AD, using multiple measures of both constructs. Personal semantic and personal incident aspects of autobiographical memory were impaired in those with AD, relative to a healthy control group. Identity was weaker, less definite, and more negative in the group with AD. People with AD also evidenced less complexity of identity relative to the control group, although this trend failed to reach significance. Analysis of the relationships between various measures of identity and autobiographical memory led to the conclusion that degree of impairment on some measures of autobiographical memory directly influenced some components of identity.

One recent cognitive model of awareness in dementia, the Cognitive Awareness Model (CAM; Morris & Hannesdottir, 2004) proposes a mechanism linking awareness of memory functioning with autobiographical memory and potentially indirectly also with sense of self. A key element in this model is the personal database (PDB), the necessary store of events containing instances of success or failure on tasks. The model suggests that accurate appraisal of abilities is based on the perception of success or failure on cognitive or behavioural tasks. Information regarding the outcome of tasks can be stored in episodic memory, but is also consolidated in the PDB within semantic memory. The PDB is updated when comparator mechanisms within a central executive system detect a mismatch between the information held in the PDB and current experiences of success or failure. Conscious awareness of failure is generated when a signal regarding this mismatch is sent to a metacognitive awareness system (MAS). Awareness problems can result from an error in updating the PDB, as an impairment of memory prevents the creation of a permanent record relating to evaluation of self-ability. Alternatively, a breakdown in the executive system or comparator mechanisms can prevent the detection of a mismatch between incoming information and the PDB. Finally, a global impairment in the MAS can result in information being detected and stored in the PDB, but not reaching conscious awareness (Agnew & Morris, 1998). In the CAM model, autobiographical memories are stored both in episodic memory and in the semantic store of the PDB. Although the PDB is primarily viewed in the specific context of the model as a store of information relating to ability or impairment, it is described as having the potential to be influenced by social and cultural inputs, and it could also contain memory for more general personal information. In this sense the PDB could be seen as similar to the personal semantic component of autobiographical memory, containing self-relevant knowledge related to sense of identity. A somewhat broader construct is suggested by Kopelman (1999, 2000). Presenting a model that draws together social factors and brain systems influencing autobiographical memory and identity, Kopelman proposes the operation of a "personal semantic belief system". This is conceptualised as equivalent to the "self", and is viewed as interacting with both executive control systems and the autobiographical memory store.

Thus, there are theoretical arguments to suggest that the constructs of self and autobiographical memory are closely related, both to each other and to the level of awareness of memory functioning. These relationships are likely to be bi-directional, with self being involved in the encoding and recon-struction of autobiographical memories, but also being dependent on autobio-graphical memory as a store of self-relevant information. Self provides the context within which awareness is demonstrated, but accurate appraisal of one's abilities is necessary for the formation of realistic goals, which the self utilises to guide behaviour. Based on these arguments we can hypothesise that there should be an association between better autobiographical memory performance, stronger sense of identity (as a component of self), and higher level of awareness of memory functioning. The present study aimed to explore the relationships between autobiographical memory, identity, and awareness of memory functioning in a sample of people with early-stage dementia, in order to test these hypothesised associations.

METHOD

Design

Relationships between autobiographical memory, identity and awareness of memory functioning in early-stage dementia were explored using a correla-tional design. Power analysis (Cohen, 1992) indicated that a minimum sample size requirement of 28, based on a large effect size would provide 80% power to detect significant effects at $\alpha = .05$. A favourable ethical opinion for the present study was granted by the local research ethics commit-tee of the North West Wales NHS Trust.

Participants

Participants were recruited from a local memory clinic. Inclusion criteria were that participants should be in the early stages of dementia, as defined by a score of 18 and over on the Mini-Mental State Examination (MMSE, Folstein, Folstein, & McHugh, 1975) and/or a Clinical Dementia Rating Scale (CDR; Hughes, Berg, Danziger, Cobe,n & Martin, 1982) score of 0.5 or 1, fluent in English, and without concurrent severe mental health problems. Thirty-six indi-viduals were approached, 30 were recruited and provided written consent, and 29 completed all the assessments. The 30 participants included 6 men and 24 women aged between 64 and 91 years ($M = 78.20$ years, $SD = 6.18$). Twenty participants had a diagnosis of AD, 8 had a diagnosis of mixed AD and vascular dementia, and 2 had a diagnosis of vascular dementia, based on the Diagnostic and Statistical Manual of Mental Disorders – Fourth Edition (DSM-IV, American Psychiatric Association, 1994). Diagnoses were assigned following multidisciplinary assessment by the memory clinic team, based on medical history and examination, neuropsychological assessment, functional assessment, electroencephalogram and computed tomography scan. MMSE scores ranged from 16 to 29 (M = 22.40, SD = 3.61). Twelve participants lived alone in their own home, 16 lived with a spouse, and 2 lived with another family member. Where possible, and with the consent of the person with dementia, an informant was also recruited. In total, 26 informants became involved with the study: 13 spouses, 1 sister, 8 daughters, 2 sons, and 2 other family members.

Measures

Participants were assessed on standardised measures of autobiographical memory, identity, and awareness of memory functioning.

Autobiographical memory was assessed using the Autobiographical Memory Interview (AMI; Kopelman, Wilson, & Baddeley, 1990). This is a structured interview that assesses personal semantic and personal incident (episodic) memory over three lifetime periods: childhood, early adulthood and recent life. The measure yields a total semantic memory score and a total incident memory score, along with semantic and incident scores for each of the three lifetime periods. As none of the participants was seen in a hospital setting, questions from the recent life section, which relates to "present hospital or institution", were re-worded to ask about the home environment and recent visits to hospital, as advised by Kopelman et al. (1990). The AMI has good inter-rater reliability, construct validity, and discriminant validity (Kopelman et al., 1990). However, it has been noted that the AMI does not assess the period between early adulthood and recent life (e.g., Graham & Hodges, 1997), and that this may represent a possible limitation when participants are in the older age range. Therefore, a "middle to late adulthood" section, developed specifically for use with people who have a dementia diagnosis at the Dementia Services Development Centre, University of Wales Bangor (Jones & Woods, 2006), was also included. While it is acknowledged that this additional section is not standardised and may differ from the main measure in level of difficulty, it was considered to be of interest to explore the accessibility of autobiographical information about the mid-life period in the present sample.

Self-concept was assessed using the Tennessee Self-Concept Scale – Second Edition (TSCS-II; Fitts & Warren, 1996). The TSCS-II consists of 82 statements, which are rated for self-descriptiveness on a 5-point scale. One item was reworded from "I treat my parents as well as I should" to "I treat my family as well as I should", since the parents of most participants were deceased. Scores can be calculated for overall self-concept, for three components (identity, satisfaction and behaviour), and for five domains (personal, family, social, moral and physical). A response distribution score can also be calculated; this is a measure of the number of "always true" and "always false" responses made, and indicates the degree of certainty about the way one sees oneself, thus reflecting the extent to which a definite sense of identity is expressed. The TSCS-II scales have good internal consistency, test-retest reliability, construct validity, and discriminant validity (Coopersmith, 1981; Fitts & Warren, 1996). For the purposes of the present study the TSCS-II identity score and TSCS-II response distribution score were used as measures of identity. The identity component score correlated highly with the total self-concept score ($r = .886$, $p < .001$).

Awareness of memory functioning was assessed using the Memory Awareness Rating Scale (MARS; Clare, Wilson, Carter, Roth, & Hodges, 2002). This scale is administered together with the subtests of the Rivermead Behavioural Memory Test – Second Edition (RBMT-II; Wilson, Cockburn, & Baddeley, 2003), which represent analogues of everyday memory tasks. The Memory Functioning Scale (MFS) of the MARS compares self-ratings and informant ratings of everyday memory functioning in relation to the kinds of everyday activities tested in the RBMT-II, while the Memory Performance Scale (MPS) compares actual performance on the RBMT-II sub-tests with self-ratings of performance made after completing each subtest. Discrepancy scores are calculated in each case, indicating whether the participant rates his or her memory more or less favourably than the informant in the case of the MFS (MFS-D score), and whether the participant's self-rating is an over- or underestimate compared to the objective test results in the case of the MPS (MPS-D score). A positive discrepancy score indicates the participant's self-rating is higher, and vice versa. The component scales of the MARS have good internal consistency, test-retest reliability, and construct validity (Clare et al., 2002).

Procedure

Participants were offered the choice of being seen at home or at the University of Wales Bangor; all 30 chose to be seen at home. Sixteen completed the assessments in one session and the remaining 14 were seen for two sessions. The MARS was always administered first and the other two measures were administered in counterbalanced order.

Data analysis

Preliminary descriptive analyses used independent t-tests to explore possible differences among diagnostic sub-groups, Pearson's product-moment correlations to assess the impact of cognitive ability on performance, and repeated-measures analysis of variance (ANOVA) to assess the temporal gradient of autobiographical memory recall. In addressing the main research questions, partial correlations were used to investigate the relationships between autobiographical memory, identity and awareness, controlling for general cognitive ability as assessed by MMSE scores. Bonferroni corrections were applied to adjust for multiple comparisons.

RESULTS

The analysis examined the relationships between autobiographical memory (scores on the AMI), identity (identity and definite responses scores on the TSCS-II), and awareness (discrepancy scores on the MARS). All participants completed the AMI and the MARS MPS, 26 participants had informants available, permitting calculation of the MARS MFS-D score, and 29 completed the TSCS-II. Missing data constituted less than 5% of the total; where data were missing, cases were excluded on a pair-wise basis. Analysis using the one-sample Kolmogorov-Smirnov test indicated that data for all variables were suitable for parametric analysis ($z = .420$-1.275, $p \geq .05$).

Mean scores on measures of autobiographical memory, identity and awareness are presented in Table 1. Preliminary analyses explored the temporal gradient of autobiographical memory, the extent to which differences were

TABLE 1
Mean scores on measures of autobiographical memory, awareness, and identity

		N	Maximum possible score	Mean	SD
AMI Personal Semantic	Total +	30	63	45.9	9.0
	New Total +	30	78	55.5	11.4
	Childhood	30	21	16.5	4.1
	Early Adulthood	30	21	15.5	3.4
	Mid-Life	30	15	9.6	3.0
	Recent Life	30	21	13.9	4.2
AMI Personal Incident	Total +	30	27	11.1	4.8
	New Total +	30	33	12.5	5.2
	Childhood	30	9	5.2	2.1
	Early Adulthood	30	9	3.6	2.2
	Mid-Life	30	6	1.4	1.3
	Recent Life	30	9	2.3	1.9
MARS	MFS-D	26	52	14.5	14.8
	MPS-D	30	52	13.1	7.1
TSCS-II	Definite Responses	29	100*	55.9	6.9
	Identity	29	100*	50.2	9.5

*T-scores, +Total gives the total score for the original test; New total includes the added mid-life section as well.

observed among diagnostic sub-groups, and the impact of cognitive ability level on participants' scores.

Figure 1 illustrates the mean percentage recall scores on both the personal semantic and personal incident aspects of the AMI for each time period plus the additional mid-life section (percentages were used here because the score range for the new section differed from that for the pre-existing sections). Repeated-measures ANOVAs revealed significant main effects of time period both for personal semantic memory ($F = 7.185$, $p < .05$, partial $\eta^2 = .199$) and for personal incident memory ($F = 20.513$, $p < .001$, partial $\eta^2 = .414$), indicating a significant difference in recall of autobiographical memories across the lifetime periods. The gradients obtained follow the same pattern as those in other published studies (e.g., Kopelman, 1989), in that the greatest number of memories recalled related to the earliest time periods, with scores declining in a linear fashion over time. The number of memories recalled for the mid-life period was slightly lower than for the recent life period; however, as the mid-life section is not part of the standardised test, and may differ in difficulty level, no firm conclusions can be drawn from this.

The scores of participants with AD ($n = 20$) were compared to those of participants with vascular or mixed AD and vascular dementia ($n = 10$), as shown in Table 2. Following Bonferroni correction for multiple comparisons, there were no significant differences between the two groups. However, although not statistically significant, it should be noted that the Alzheimer's group did have a higher mean MMSE score (23.3 as opposed to 20.6).

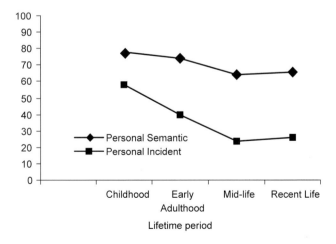

Figure 1. Mean percentage recall of personal semantic and personal incident memories.

TABLE 2
Comparison of mean scores for the Alzheimer's disease and "other dementia" groups

		Alzheimer's groupMean (SD)		Other dementia groupMean (SD)		t	p
MMSE		23.3	(3.8)	20.6	(2.5)	2.04	.051
AMI Personal	Childhood	15.9	(4.6)	17.7	(2.6)	−1.34	.190
Semantic	Early Adulthood	15.9	(3.2)	14.7	(3.8)	0.95	.351
	Mid-Life	10.3	(2.7)	8.3	(3.1)	1.77	.088
	Recent Life	15.2	(3.7)	11.4	(4.1)	2.59	.015
AMI Personal	Childhood	5.4	(2.0)	5.0	(2.4)	0.43	.672
Incident	Early Adulthood	3.7	(2.3)	3.3	(2.0)	0.47	.646
	Mid-Life	1.6	(1.5)	1.2	(0.8)	0.85	.403
	Recent Life	2.9	(1.9)	1.2	(1.5)	2.43	.022
MARS	MFS-D	14.3	(14.4)	15.0	(16.5)	−0.11	.911
	MPS-D	12.3	(7.0)	14.8	(7.2)	−0.93	.362
TSCS − II	Definite Responses	56.0	(6.4)	55.7	(8.3)	0.10	.920
	Identity	50.6	(8.9)	49.6	(11.3)	0.26	.800

Bonferroni correction applied (p threshold set at .004).

The impact of level of cognitive functioning on participants' scores was explored by investigating the correlations between the MMSE score and the scores on the AMI, TSCS-II definite responses and identity scores, and the two MARS discrepancy scores. Following Bonferroni correction, MMSE score was significantly correlated with the AMI semantic memory score for the early adulthood ($r = .482$, $p = .004$, $r^2 = .232$) and recent life ($r = .549$, $p = .001$, $r^2 = .3$) periods, indicating that, as might be expected, a higher level of cognitive functioning was associated with significantly greater recall of recent autobiographical semantic information (Table 3). Level of cognitive functioning did not significantly affect scores on the identity or awareness measures.

Relationships between autobiographical memory, identity and awareness were then explored using partial correlations with Bonferroni correction for multiple comparisons, controlling for level of cognitive functioning (MMSE score) in each case given the significant association between MMSE score and recent semantic memory score on the AMI.

Following Bonferroni correction there were no significant correlations between AMI and TSCS-II scores when controlling for level of cognitive functioning (Table 4). There was a significant negative correlation between the MARS MFS-D score and the score for mid-life personal incident memory ($r = −.56$, $p = .002$, $r^2 = .314$) on the additional section of the AMI (Table 5). Thus a lower discrepancy between an individual's perception of his/her memory functioning and the perception of an informant, taken to

TABLE 3
Correlations between MMSE scores and scores on the autobiographical memory, awareness, and identity measures.

		MMSE score	
		r	p
AMI Personal Semantic	Childhood	−.015	.468
	Early Adulthood	.482	.004*
	Mid-Life	.380	.019
	Recent Life	.549	.001*
AMI Personal Incident	Childhood	.111	.279
	Early Adulthood	.071	.355
	Mid-Life	.230	.110
	Recent Life	.153	.209
MARS	MFS-D	−.218	.142
	MPS-D	−.353	.028
TSCS-II	Definite Responses	−.258	.088
	Identity	−.037	.423

*Significant following Bonferroni correction (p threshold set at .004).

indicate greater awareness, was associated with greater recall of personal incidents from the mid-life period.

Significant positive correlations were found between the MARS-MFS-D score and both the TSCS-II identity score ($r = .498$, $p = .006$, $r^2 = .248$) and the TSCS-II definite responses score ($r = .55$, $p = .002$, $r^2 = .303$). This suggests that a greater discrepancy score, indicative of a less accurate appraisal

TABLE 4
Correlations between autobiographical memory and identity scores, controlling for level of cognitive functioning

		TSCS Identity		TSCS Definite Responses	
		r	p	r	p
AMI Personal Semantic	Childhood	.1309	.253	.1759	.185
	Early Adulthood	.1992	.155	.4252	.012
	Mid-Life	.0599	.381	−.0020	.496
	Recent Life	.0617	.378	.0275	.445
AMI Personal Incident	Childhood	.0644	.372	.2037	.149
	Early Adulthood	.0970	.312	.3524	.033
	Mid-Life	−.3877	.021	−.4102	.015
	Recent Life	−.0458	.408	.0392	.421

Bonferroni correction applied (p threshold set at .006).

TABLE 5
Correlations between autobiographical memory and awareness scores, controlling for level of cognitive functioning

		MARS-MFS-D		MARS-MPS-D	
		r	p	r	p
AMI Personal Semantic	Childhood	.0646	.380	.0719	.355
	Early Adulthood	.1868	.186	−.0461	.406
	Mid-Life	−.0321	.439	.0608	.377
	Recent Life	−.1710	.207	−.1935	.157
AMI Personal Incident	Childhood	−.1485	.239	−.1056	.293
	Early Adulthood	.0158	.470	−.1011	.301
	Mid-Life	−.5603	.002*	−.2049	.143
	Recent Life	−.2414	.123	−.1328	.246

*Significant following Bonferroni correction (p threshold set at .006).

TABLE 6
Correlations between identity and awareness scores, controlling for level of cognitive functioning

	TSCS Identity		TSCS Definite Responses	
	r	p	r	p
MARS-MFS-D	.4980	.006*	.5503	.002*
MARS-MPS-D	.2196	.131	.1901	.166

*Significant following Bonferroni correction (p threshold set at .006).

of functioning on the part of the individual with dementia, is associated with more positive and more definite sense of identity (Table 6). There were no significant correlations between MARS-MPS-D scores and TSCS scores.

DISCUSSION

This study explored the relationships between autobiographical memory, identity, and awareness of memory functioning in people with early-stage dementia. Characterising the autobiographical memory performance of the sample indicated that temporal gradients were similar to those reported in other studies (Addis & Tippett, 2004; Graham & Hodges, 1997; Greene, Hodges, & Baddeley, 1995; Kopelman, 1989), with greater recall from earlier life periods. Participants with higher levels of cognitive functioning, as indicated by higher MMSE scores, were more successful in recalling early adult and recent semantic information. Level of cognitive functioning was therefore partialled out in the subsequent analyses. Autobiographical memory perform-ance was not related to identity scores, suggesting that there was no straight-forward connection between impairment in autobiographical memory and self-report of identity. Autobiographical memory performance was, however, related to awareness of memory functioning, in that people with better recall of mid-life incidents showed greater awareness of memory functioning as indicated by lower discrepancies between self-ratings and informant reports. Awareness of memory functioning was also related to identity, in that people with lower awareness, as indicated by greater discrepancies between self-ratings and informant reports, also demonstrated a more positive and more definite sense of identity.

We hypothesised that better autobiographical memory performance would be associated with a stronger sense of identity. In fact we found no significant associations between performance on the original AMI and scores for sense of identity. There was a trend towards a positive association between better recall of early adulthood semantic and incident memories and a more definite sense of identity, but following Bonferroni correction this was not significant. Such a finding is contrary to that of Addis and Tippett (2004) who, using the TSCS and the AMI, found a negative relationship between recall for personal semantic memories from childhood and definite sense of identity in people with AD. This finding was at odds with their initial expectations and with their other findings of positive relationships between strength of identity and autobiographical fluency for early adulthood names and childhood events, and between fewer abstract identity responses and recall of childhood personal incident memories. The literature suggests that autobiographical memories relating to the early period of adulthood are encoded during a time of intense self-orientated activity, and underpin the construction of a stable identity and life narrative (Fitzgerald, 1988, 1996, 1999). Thus, it would be expected that impairment of memories from this period would have the greatest negative impact on sense of self and identity.

Our hypothesis that better autobiographical recall would be associated with a higher level of awareness of memory functioning was supported only in terms of a significant association between recall of mid-life incident memories and lower discrepancies between self- and informant ratings of memory functioning, suggesting higher awareness on the part of the partici-pant. The ability to recall personal experiences when evaluating memory functioning in response to questionnaire items may help to produce more accurate ratings. There were no associations with awareness when assessed in terms of discrepancy between objectively-scored and self-rated task per-formance, but this method of evaluating awareness involves different kinds of judgements, effectively requiring on-line monitoring of performance. The lack of any other significant relationships was surprising given the importance placed on the role of the PDB, reflecting the operation of autobio-graphical memory, in the Morris and Hannesdottir (2004) model of aware-ness. The CAM focuses on specific information relating to success or failure on memory-related tasks, which is quite different to the types of auto-biographical information sampled by the AMI, although one might expect that the self-rating of objective test performance would provide the kind of information about experiences of success or failure assumed to be used by the PDB. Again, the effect was only observed for the mid-life period, and was thus based on performance on the additional section rather than the orig-inal test. If the mid-life period does have special characteristics in this regard, it may be because this is a time of subtle changes in memory functioning. It has been suggested (Barsalou, 1988; Conway, 1992) that autobiographical memories could be viewed primarily as records of success or failure in goal attainment. Thus, the mid-life period may contain a larger proportion of memory failure experiences relative to earlier periods of life, supporting its particular relevance for awareness.

The final hypothesis, which proposed an association between higher levels of awareness of memory functioning and a stronger sense of identity, was not supported. In fact the opposite pattern was found; a greater discrepancy between self- and informant rating of memory functioning, indicative of a lower level of awareness, was associated with more positive and more definite sense of identity. A number of possible explanations may help to account for this finding. Addis and Tippett (2004) suggest that any degradation of seman-tic memory erodes access to general information about identity and therefore forces a search of episodic memory for self-relevant information. Identity decisions are then based on the recall of a single relevant incident, resulting in more "all or none" responses. The CAM model (Morris & Hannesdottir, 2004) proposes that, in the absence of recent perceptual input, decisions regarding ability would be based on the information contained within the PDB. If the PDB is not updated then it will support the belief that functioning remains at previous levels; therefore, individuals will not be prompted to inte-grate changes into their sense of identity and will feel more definite as regards identity, but ongoing awareness will be compromised. Alternatively, the relationship between lower awareness and more definite identity responses could indicate the operation of psychological defences, designed to protect the self from the psychological distress associated with failure. This would be consistent with previous studies demonstrating that psychological factors may play a role in determining level of awareness (Clare, 2003; Seiffer, Clare, & Harvey, 2005; Weinstein, Friedland, & Wagner, 1994).

In interpreting the present findings, a number of issues must be borne in mind. Although the study was adequately powered and the sample size was generally consistent with other studies in this area (e.g., Addis & Tippett, 2004), the need to control for multiple comparisons using Bonferroni corrections meant that several associations that would have been significant at the $p = .05$ level were missed. Future studies could limit the number of comparisons (for example, by using only the MFS scale of the MARS) and include larger numbers of participants in order to counteract this limitation. In so doing, it might be advantageous to identify a sample with a smaller range of MMSE scores, less heterogeneity with respect to age and diagnosis, and a better gender balance. Over and above these sampling issues, autobiographical memory, sense of identity and awareness of memory functioning are all complex constructs, and both conceptualisation and measurement are far from straightforward.

In the present study, using the AMI to assess autobiographical memory, the only significant correlations were found with the mid-life section, which was not part of the original task, but was appended to the measure for the purposes of this study. It is possible that this additional section, which has not been standardised with the overall measure, performed differently to the sections of the original test, and therefore the results are difficult to interpret. Nevertheless, it is conceivable that the mid-life period may be of particular relevance when assessing autobiographical memory in people with dementia. A fully-standardised task incorporating questions about the middle years of adulthood could be valuable. In the absence of such a task, future studies could consider incorporating multiple measures of autobiographical memory. Nevertheless, it should be noted that in terms of assessing the temporal gradient of autobiographical memory the original AMI serves its original purpose well with this group.

Few studies have attempted to measure aspects of self or identity in people with mild to moderate dementia, and consequently there is little evidence regarding the suitability of particular approaches. The TSCS was used by Addis and Tippett (2004) together with the Twenty Statements Test (Kuhn & McPartland, 1954). We could find no previous instances of either measure being used with people who have dementia. Pilot work in our group indicated that participants found it very difficult to generate statements about themselves as required by the Twenty Statements Test; while many found the TSCS demanding, most were able to complete it, suggesting that this was a more suitable, albeit not ideal, measurement approach. Future research may help to identify optimal methods of assessing identity in this group.

Awareness was assessed for the present study specifically in relation to memory functioning. Significant effects were found only in respect of the discrepancies between self- and informant ratings on the MARS, with lower discrepancies (higher awareness) associated with better recall from the mid-life period and higher discrepancies (lower awareness) associated with stronger and more definite sense of identity. No such effects were found for the discrepancy between self-rated and objective task performance, which is sometimes considered to provide a more accurate measure of awareness (Dalla Barba, Parlato, Iavarone, & Boller, 1995), and which arguably reflects the kinds of cognitive judgements embodied in the CAM model in terms of the operation of the PDB. Consequently we cannot generalise from the findings to make statements about awareness in general. The findings tell us only about awareness of memory functioning when measured in terms of discrepancies between self- and informant rating. Future research might aim to identify which aspects of awareness are most relevant when evaluating associations with other variables (Clare, 2004; Clare, Markova, Verhey, & Kenny, 2005).

CONCLUSIONS

The present study is the first to explore the relationships between identity, autobiographical memory, and awareness of memory functioning. The results provide preliminary evidence that awareness of memory functioning is associated with both autobiographical memory and sense of identity. People with lower levels of awareness had poorer autobiographical recall for events from the mid-life period and expressed a stronger and more definite sense of identity. This may reflect a failure to update the store of personally-relevant information (Morris & Hannesdottir, 2004), thus reducing the degree to which sense of identity is challenged by perceived changes in ability and functioning. Consistent with the biopsychosocial framework for understanding awareness in dementia (Clare, 2004), this could be interpreted as reflecting an interaction between cognitive impairments, evident in compromised autobiographical memory performance, and the operation of psychological defensive strategies aimed at maintaining the prior sense of self. Reduced awareness may serve a protective function against the threats to sense of self posed by the onset and progression of dementia.

REFERENCES

Addis, D. R., & Tippett, L. J. (2004). Memory of myself: Autobiographical memory and identity in Alzheimer's disease. *Memory, 12*, 56–74.

Agnew, S. K., & Morris, R. G. (1998). The heterogeneity of anosognosia for memory impairment in Alzheimer's disease: A review of the literature and a proposed model. *Aging and Mental Health, 2*, 7–19.

American Psychiatric Association (1994). *Diagnostic and statistical manual of mental disorders. Fourth Edition.* Washington, DC: American Psychiatric Association.

Baars, B. J. (1997). *In the theater of consciousness: The workspace of the mind.* New York: Oxford University Press.

Baddeley, A. D. (1992). What is autobiographical memory? In M. A. Conway, D. C. Rubin, H. Spinnler, & W. A. Wagenaar (Eds.), *Theoretical perspectives on autobiographical memory* (Vol. 65, pp. 13–29). Dordrecht, Netherlands: Kluwer.

Barsalou, L. W. (1988). The content and organisation of autobiographical memories. In U. Neisser & E. Winograd (Eds.), *Remembering reconsidered: Ecological and traditional approaches to the study of memory* (pp. 193–243). New York: Cambridge University Press.

Clare, L. (2003). Managing threats to self: Awareness in early-stage Alzheimer's disease. *Social Science and Medicine, 57,* 1017–1029.

Clare, L. (2004). Awareness in early-stage Alzheimer's disease: A review of methods and evidence. *British Journal of Clinical Psychology, 43,* 177–196.

Clare, L., Markova, I. S., Verhey, F., & Kenny Y. G. (2005). Awareness in dementia: A review of assessment methods and measures. *Aging and Mental Health, 9,* 394–413.

Clare, L., Wilson, B. A., Carter, G., Roth, I., & Hodges, J. R. (2002). Assessing awareness in early-stage Alzheimer's disease: Development and piloting of the Memory Awareness Rating Scale. *Neuropsychological Rehabilitation, 12,* 341–362.

Clare, L., Wilson, B. A., Carter, G., Roth, I., & Hodges, J. R. (2004). Awareness in early-stage Alzheimer's disease: Relationship to outcome of cognitive rehabilitation. *Journal of Clinical and Experimental Neuropsychology, 26,* 215–226.

Cohen, J. (1992). A power primer. *Psychological Bulletin, 112,* 155–159.

Conway, M. A. (1992). A structural model of autobiographical memory. Cited in Conway, M. A., & Pleydell-Pearce, C. W. (2000). The construction of autobiographical memories in the Self-Memory System. *Psychological Review, 107,* 261–288.

Coopersmith, S. (1981). *The antecedents of self-esteem.* Palo Alto, CA: Consulting Psychologists Press.

Dalla Barba, G., Parlato, V., Iavarone, E., A., & Boller, F. (1995). Anosognosia, intrusions and 'frontal' functions in Alzheimer's disease and depression. *Neuropsychologia, 33,* 247–259.

Damasio, A. R. (1999). *The feeling of what happens. Body and emotion in the making of consciousness.* New York: Harcourt Brace and Company.

Deaux, K. (1992). Personalizing identity and socializing self. In G. M. Breakwell (Ed.), *Social psychology of identity and the self concept* (pp. 9–33). London: Surrey University Press.

De Bettingnies, B. H., Mahurin, R. K., & Pirozzolo, F. J. (1990). Insight for impairment in independent living skills in Alzheimer's disease and multi-infarct dementia. *Journal of Clinical and Experimental Neuropsychology, 12,* 355–363.

Fitts, W. H. (1965). *Tennessee Self-Concept Scale.* Nashville, TN: Counselor Recordings and Tests.

Fitts, W. H., & Warren, W. L. (1996). *Tennessee Self-Concept Scale.* (2nd ed.) Los Angeles, CA: Western Psychological Services.

Fitzgerald, J. M. (1988). Vivid memories and the reminiscence phenomenon: The role of a self-narrative. *Human Development, 31,* 261–273.

Fitzgerald, J. M. (1996). The distribution of self-narrative memories in younger and older adults: Elaborating the self-narrative hypothesis. *Aging, Neuropsychology and Cognition, 3,* 229–236.

Fitzgerald, J. M. (1999). Autobiographical memory and social cognition. In T. M. Hess & F. Blanchart-Fields (Eds.), *Social cognition and aging* (pp. 143–171). San Diego, CA: Academic Press.

Folstein, M. F., Folstein, S. L., & McHugh, P. R. (1975). 'Mini-Mental State', practical methods for grading the cognitive state of patients for clinicians. *Journal of Psychiatry Research, 12,* 189–198.

Gergen, K. J. (1984). Theory of the self: Impasse and evolution. In L. Berkowitz (Ed.), *Advances in experimental social psychology* (Vol. 17, pp. 49–115). New York: Harcourt Brace Jovanovich.

Graham, K. S., & Hodges, J. R. (1997). Differentiating the roles of the hippocampal complex and the neocortex in long-term memory storage: Evidence from the study of semantic dementia and Alzheimer's disease. *Neuropsychology, 11,* 77–89.

Greene, J. D. W., Hodges, J. R., & Baddeley, A. D. (1995). Autobiographical memory and executive function in early dementia of Alzheimer type. *Neuropsychologia, 33,* 1647–1670.

Greenwald, A. G., & Pratkanis, A. R. (1984). The self. In J. Robert, S. Wyer & T. K. Skrull (Eds.), *Handbook of social cognition* (Vol. 3). Hillsdale, NJ: Lawrence Erlbaum Associates.

Hughes, C. P., Berg, L., Danziger, W. L., Coben, L. A., & Martin, R. L. (1982). A new clinical scale for the staging of dementia. *British Journal of Psychiatry, 140,* 566–572.

Jones, C., & Woods, R. T. (2006). *The Autobiographical Memory Interview: Development of a mid-life section.* Unpublished document. University of Wales Bangor: Dementia Services Development Centre.

Kopelman, M. D. (1989). Remote and autobiographical memory, temporal context memory and frontal atrophy in Korsakoff and Alzheimer's patients. *Neuropsychologia, 27,* 431–460.

Kopelman, M. D. (1999). Varieties of false memory. *Cognitive Neuropsychology, 16,* 197–214.

Kopelman, M. D. (2000). Focal retrograde amnesia and the attribution of causality: An exceptionally critical view. *Cognitive Neuropsychology, 17,* 585–621.

Kopelman, M., Wilson, B., & Baddeley, A. (1990). *The Autobiographical Memory Interview.* Bury St Edmunds, UK: Thames Valley Test Company.

Kuhn, M. H., & McPartland, T. S. (1954). An empirical investigation of self-attitudes. *American Sociological Review, 19,* 68–76.

Markus, H., & Wurf, E. (1987). The dynamic self-concept: A social-psychological perspective. *Annual Review of Psychology, 38,* 299–337.

McAdams, D. P. (1988). *Power, intimacy, and the life story: Personalogical inquiries into identity.* New York: Guilford Press.

Morris, R. G., & Hannesdottir, K. (2004). Loss of awareness in Alzheimer's disease. In R. Morris & J. Becker (Eds.), *Cognitive neuropsychology of Alzheimer's disease.* (2nd ed.). Oxford: Oxford University Press.

Orona, C. J. (1990). Temporality and identity loss due to Alzheimer's disease. *Social Science and Medicine, 30,* 1247–1256.

Seiffer, A., Clare, L., & Harvey, R. (2005). The role of personality and coping style in relation to awareness of current functioning in early-stage dementia. *Aging and Mental Health, 9,* 535–541.

Weinstein, E., Friedland, R., & Wagner, E. (1994). Denial/unawareness of impairment and symbolic behaviour in Alzheimer's disease. *Neuropsychiatry, Neuropsychology and Behavioural Neurology, 7,* 176–184.

Wilson, B. A., Cockburn, J., & Baddeley, A. D. (2003). *The Rivermead Behavioural Memory Test* (2nd ed.). Bury St Edmunds, UK: Thames Valley Test Company.

NEUROPSYCHOLOGICAL REHABILITATION
2008, 18 (5/6), 607–626

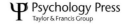

Self-esteem as a predictor of psychological distress after severe acquired brain injury: An exploratory study

Samantha Cooper-Evans[1], Nick Alderman[2], Caroline Knight[1], and Michael Oddy[3]

[1]*St Andrew's Healthcare, Townsend Division, Northampton, UK;* [2]*St Andrew's Healthcare, Kemsley Division, Northampton, UK and University of Swansea, UK;* [3]*Brain Injury Rehabilitation Trust, Horsham, West Sussex, UK and University of Swansea, UK*

This study explored the effects of severe acquired brain injury (ABI) on self-esteem. A within-subjects design investigated 22 severe ABI survivors' self-reported responses on measures of self-esteem, mood and awareness of deficit. Data on cognitive ability and awareness of degree of executive impairment were included in the analysis. Self-esteem was measured using Rosenberg's Self-Esteem Scale (Rosenberg) and psychological distress by the Hospital Anxiety and Depression Scale (HADS). Self-esteem was found to be consistent over a two-week interval. Participants reported that their self-esteem had suffered following ABI when contrasting their current self-esteem with their retrospective perceptions. Self-esteem was highly correlated with psychological distress. More intact cognitive functioning and awareness of deficit were associated with lower self-esteem. The paradoxical finding that survivors who were more impaired cognitively and/or less aware of their deficits reported higher self-esteem poses an ethical dilemma for clinicians. It is hoped that this finding, along with the consistency of self-esteem ratings sparks further debate about how best to address issues of self-esteem among severe ABI survivors, particularly in the context of psychological distress, during rehabilitation.

Correspondence should be sent to Samantha Cooper-Evans, Principal Clinical Psychologist, St Andrew's Healthcare, Townsend Division, St Andrew's Hospital, Billing Road, Northampton, NN1 5DG, UK. E-mail: scooper-evans@standrew.co.uk and Professor Nick Alderman, St Andrew's Healthcare, Kemsley Division, Billing Road, Northampton, NN1 5DG, UK. E-mail: nalderman@standrew.co.uk

INTRODUCTION

The complex and pervasive impairments following a severe acquired brain injury (ABI) are well documented, yet just how such an injury impacts on the "self" and what this means to the survivor remains relatively unexplored (Howes, Edwards, & Benton, 2005; Judd & Wilson, 2005; Keppel & Crowe, 2000; Man, Tam, & Li, 2003; Nadell, 1994; Ownsworth, McFarland, & Young, 2000; Pollens, McBratnie, & Burton, 1998; Tyerman, 1987; Tyerman & Humphrey, 1984; Wood, Liossi, & Wood, 2005; Wright & Telford, 1996; Ylvisaker, Jacobs, & Feeney, 2003). This study aimed to further research into this area, investigating the impact of severe ABI on self-esteem.

Self-esteem is viewed as an emotional and subjective evaluation of the self, providing an indication of how individuals fundamentally experience themselves and has hence been used as a measure of the subjective experience of the "self" (Coopersmith, 1967; Fennell, 1999; Guindon, 2002; Mrurk, 1999; Robson, 1989; Rosenberg, 1965). It is relatively stable during adulthood with the exception of times of acute crisis and is usually referred to as a global construct, although it has also been researched according to specific domains of functioning (Guindon, 2002; Hamacheck, 1978; Torrey, Mueser, McHugo, & Drake, 2000; Trezesniewski, Donnellan, & Robins, 2003). However, for the purposes of this study, self-esteem will be defined as an overall, personal estimation of the self and hence a potentially useful platform from which to explore how the changes associated with a severe ABI are experienced by survivors (Garske & Thomas, 1992; Guindon, 2002; Keppel & Crowe, 2000). One limitation when researching self-esteem is the variability among definitions and that it has been used interchangeably with other concepts such as self-concept (Guindon, 2002; Strein, 1993). Self-concept and self-esteem have been associated with similar clinical outcomes and are considered to be closely associated in general and ABI populations (Kravetz et al., 1995; Man et al., 2003; Tyerman & Humphrey, 1984; Vickery, Gontkovsky, & Caroselli, 2005). However, this literature review focused solely on self-esteem with the exception of the landmark study by Tyerman and Humphrey (1984) which investigated changes in self-concept following severe ABI. As this was the only directly related study found researching subjective meaning among severe ABI survivors, it was used to inform the research hypotheses for this study (Tyerman & Humphrey, 1984).

Self-esteem and ABI

Self-esteem seems to have powerful motivational significance with respect to behaviour, particularly in selecting and attaining goals (Coopersmith, 1967;

Guindon, 2002; Rosenberg, 1965). How consistent goals are with an individual's self-esteem impacts on motivation and could therefore be an important factor to consider in severe ABI rehabilitation programmes (Brown & Marshall, 2001; Guindon, 2002; Robson, 1988; Rosenberg, 1965; Vickery et al., 2005).

Self-esteem has been associated with functional behaviour and life satisfaction as well as with physical and mental well-being (Bednar & Peterson, 1995; Witmer & Sweeney, 1992). For example, a high self-esteem has been linked with positive outcomes such as occupational success, healthy social relationships, and subjective well-being (Brown & Dutton, 1995; Robson, 1988; Trzesniewski et al., 2003). In contrast, low self-esteem has been linked to many problematic outcomes such as depression, health problems and anti-social behaviour (Kernis, Grannemann, & Barclay, 1989; Robson, 1988, 1989; Silverston, Lemay, Elliot, Hsu, & Starko, 1996; Trzesniewski et al., 2003). It would appear that very little research has been conducted exploring how self-esteem relates to outcome, particularly with regard to healthy emotional adjustment in severe ABI survivors (Curran, Ponsford, & Crowe, 2000; Keppel & Crowe, 2000; Kernis et al., 1989; Kravetz et al., 1995; Lubuskso, Moore, Stambrook, & Gill, 1994; Moore & Stambrook, 1992, 1995; Robson, 1988, 1989; Trzesniewski, et al., 2003; Tyerman, 1987; Tyerman & Humphrey, 1984; Vickery et al., 2005).

Despite the paucity of research, there is evidence to suggest that ABI survivors report that their injury has a negative impact on their self-esteem (Curran et al., 2000; Kravetz et al., 1995; Wright & Telford, 1996). Keppel and Crowe (2000) found that when male and female stroke survivors were asked to rate their retrospective perceptions of body image and self-esteem, body image was significantly negatively affected and this was associated with lowered self-esteem. Based on these findings, Howes et al. (2005) explored the effect of ABI on female body image and included self-esteem as a variable. They (Howes et al., 2005) found that both body image and self-esteem were significantly lower among ABI survivors when compared with a control group. Interestingly, they (Howes et al., 2005) also measured the impact of cognitive ability on self-esteem ratings and found that more cognitively able ABI female survivors reported lower self-esteem.

Low self-esteem has also been associated with increased rates of psychological distress (measured by depression and anxiety) following ABI (Curran et al., 2000; Howes et al., 2005; Judd & Wilson, 2005; Keppel & Crowe, 2000; Kravetz et al., 1995; Man et al., 2003; Tyerman & Humphrey, 1984). This suggests that, despite the difficulties ABI survivors may have in reporting their level of impairment accurately, they have definite internal assumptions about themselves that impact on mood (Curran et al., 2000; Guindon, 2002; Howes et al., 2005; Vickery et al., 2005). High rates of psychological distress among ABI survivors and how seriously this can impact upon long-term rehabilitation outcomes has been well documented (Hibbard, Uysal, Keple, Bogdany & Silver, 1998; Lubusko et al., 1994; Morton & Wehman, 1995; Tyerman & Humphrey, 1984; Wallace & Bogner, 2000; Wells, 1997). The most widely reported mood disturbance following ABI is depression, although anxiety is also common (Harris & Barraclough, 1997; Williams, 2003). Thus, it seems important to explore the link between psychological distress and self-esteem following ABI. Furthermore, it would appear that the greater the discrepancy between ABI survivors' current perceptions of self-esteem and their perceptions of their pre-injury self-esteem, the greater the reported levels of psychological distress (Tyerman & Humphrey, 1984; Wright & Telford, 1996).

Why then, has research into ABI survivors' self-esteem lagged behind? A number of reasons have been cited in the literature. Firstly, the cognitive deficits, particularly with regards to memory, associated with severe ABI have brought the reliability of self-report measures into question given that these could vary significantly upon each administration (for example, Man et al., 2003; Tyerman & Humphrey, 1984). Secondly, impaired self-awareness (also sometimes referred to as "insight") resulting in unrealistic self-appraisals and the tendency for ABI survivors to under-report their difficulties has also cast doubt on the validity of self-report measures to inform treatment (Ezrachi, Ben-Yishay, Kay, Diller, & Rattok, 1991; Hillier & Metzer, 1997; Port, Willmott, & Charlton, 2002; Prigatano & Fordyce, 1986; Sbordone, Seyranian, & Ruff, 1998). While individuals who are more aware of their deficits recognise their need for treatment and tend to have better rehabilitation outcomes, those with severely impaired awareness tend to resist treatment (Deaton, 1986; Ezrachi et al., 1991; Hillier & Metzer, 1997).

Thus, the question remains, can survivors of severe ABI meaningfully report their self-esteem in the light of the cognitive deficits and impaired awareness arising from their injuries (Curran et al., 2000; Gordon, Haddad, Brown, Hibbard, & Silwinski, 2000; Judd & Wilson, 2005; Malia, Powell, & Torode, 1995; Ownsworth et al., 2000; Vickery et al., 2005)? More recently, in contrast with previous research, there have been a limited number of studies demonstrating that people with severe ABI are able to use self-report measures effectively to report a wide range of their problems (Ezrachi et al., 1991; Giacino & Cicerone, 1998; Gordon et al., 2000; Green, Felmingham, Baguley, Slewa-Younan, & Simpson, 2001; Ponsford, Olver, & Curran, 1995a; Ponsford, Olver, Nelms, & Curran, 1996; Ponsford, Sloan, & Snow, 1995b).

However, despite issues raised about the reliability of self-report measures among severe ABI survivors, focusing on such issues can obscure the real task of understanding their personal perspective and meaning during rehabilitation. The pioneering work by Tyerman and Humphrey (1984) coupled with the more recent research suggests that severe ABI survivors are more able to report perceived changes to their "self" than has previously been accounted for. More recently, there has been an emphasis that personal meaning, irrespective of reliability, seems a central issue in understanding and helping ABI survivors adjust to their injury and to motivate them to engage in their rehabilitation (Judd & Wilson, 2005; Man et al., 2003; Moore & Stambrook, 1995; Ponsford et al., 1995b; Vickery et al., 2005).

Perhaps one way of determining the validity of self-reported self-esteem would be to investigate its stability among severe ABI survivors. While the change in "self" has been reported in the literature, it would appear that neither the stability of these changes nor the potential role of awareness underlying such ratings has been investigated (Keppel & Crowe, 2000; Tyerman & Humphrey, 1984). Furthermore, it would appear that the impact of ABI on self-esteem has not been comprehensively or directly explored. Instead, it has been investigated as a variable in relation to other outcomes such as quality of life or body image (Howes et al., 2005; Keppel & Crowe, 2000). The impact of severe ABI on survivors' self-esteem has attracted even less attention and it would appear, in a narrative literature review, that there are no direct studies to date. This seems extraordinary, given that survivors of a severe ABI have even greater changes to adjust to. If the relationship between self-esteem and severe ABI could be more fully understood in relation to awareness, cognitive functioning and degree of psychological distress experienced, then this may lead to future implications for treatment and rehabilitation (Curran et al. 2000; Howes et al., 2005; Judd & Wilson, 2005; Kravetz et al., 1995; Man et al., 2003; Tyerman & Humphrey, 1984).

Hence, the specific hypotheses to be explored in this study are:

- Given the cognitive and awareness deficits associated with severe ABI, it is predicted that ratings of self-esteem will be inconsistent over time in contrast with findings in the general and psychiatric populations (Ezrachi et al., 1991; Hillier & Metzer, 1997; Prigatano & Fordyce, 1986; Sbordone et al., 1998; Torrey et al., 2000; Trezesniewski et al., 2003).

- It is expected, in keeping with previous research, that when asked to contrast current self-esteem with that prior to injury, severe ABI survivors will report that self-esteem had reduced (Howes et al., 2005; Keppel & Crowe, 2000; Tyerman & Humphrey, 1984; Vickery et al., 2005).

- Existing research among mild and severe ABI survivors suggests that low self-esteem is associated with higher levels of psychological distress and thus it was anticipated that this finding will be repeated in this study (Howes et al., 2005; Tyerman & Humphrey, 1984; Vickery et al., 2005).

- A relationship between low self-esteem was found with more intact cognitive functioning among survivors of mild to moderate ABI (Howes et al., 2005). Hence it is expected that more intact cognitive functioning will be associated with lowered self-esteem.

- Survivors with more intact awareness will be more likely to detect differences in their functioning following injury (Deaton, 1986; Ezrachi et al., 1991; Hillier & Metzer, 1997). Hence it is predicted that greater awareness of deficit and more intact executive functioning will be associated with low self-esteem.

METHOD

Design

A within-subjects design methodology was used similar to that employed by Keppel and Crowe's (2000) investigation of changes in self-esteem among stoke survivors. In order to facilitate comparisons with other studies, only measures that have been reported in the ABI literature were used.

Participants

The neurobehavioural service within which participants resided (Kemsley Division, St Andrew's Healthcare, Northampton, UK) provides rehabilitation to people with acquired, non-progressive neurological damage. It has been comprehensively described in the literature (for example, Alderman, Davies, Jones, & McDonnell, 1999; Fluharty & Glassman, 2001). The majority of admissions to the service have received very severe brain injuries. Referrals to the service are characteristically (but not exclusively) survivors whose challenging behaviour prevents attainment of their full rehabilitation potential. Stage of rehabilitation ranged from active rehabilitation enabling community reintegration to slow stream residential rehabilitation. Participants were aged between 18 and 70, spoke English as a first language and had no gross language impairments.

The study was subjected to mandatory ethical review prior to recruiting participants. Twenty-nine participants were identified. Twenty-three consented to participate in the study and 22 participated throughout. The majority of injuries were traumatic brain injuries (TBI) of which 13 (59%) had resulted from a road traffic accident (RTA) or falls. The other categories of injury constituted assault ($n = 3$, 14%) and anoxia ($n = 3$, 14%) while stroke (CVA)

($n = 1, 5\%$), viral infections and combinations of these categories constituted the remaining two injuries (8%). Extent of neurological damage for
all patients was classified as at least "severe" using either duration of post-
traumatic amnesia (24 hours or more) or the Glasgow Coma Scale (8 or
less when first seen in hospital: see King, 1997, pp.169–170). The average
time since injury was 122.05 months ($SD = 102.74$) with the range
varying from 16 months to 348 months. 17 (77%) participants were male
and five (23%) were female. They were aged between 20 and 61 years
($M = 43.00, SD = 11.82$).

Measures

Self-esteem

The Rosenberg Self-Esteem Scale (Rosenberg, 1965) is a 10-item questionnaire that requires the respondent to report feelings about the self in
response to 10 questions using a 4-point Likert-type scale ranging from
strongly agree (4) to strongly disagree (1). The Rosenberg was selected
because it has a strong research base and has been used with ABI populations
(Dobson, Goudy, Keith, & Powers, 1979; Fleming & Courtney, 1984a, b;
Howes et al., 2005; Keppel & Crowe, 2000; Robson, 1989; Silber &
Tippet, 1965; Vickery et al., 2005). The Rosenberg is a widely used
measure with high reliability and construct validity (Keppel & Crowe,
2000). Previous research in the general population has indicated that the
Rosenberg has a high test-retest correlation at both one and two week intervals (Fleming & Courtney, 1984a, b; Silber & Tippet, 1965).

Psychological distress

The Hospital Anxiety and Depression Scale (HADS; Snaith & Zigmond,
1994; Zigmond & Snaith, 1983) is a brief, 14-item, self-report questionnaire
used to measure psychological distress. It yields an overall score and also separate scores for anxiety and depression which may be compared to cut off
scores. Zigmond and Snaith (1994) recommend that the scores yielded for
the two subscales should be interpreted separately with raw scores of
between 8 and 10 identifying mild cases, 11 and 15 moderate cases and 16
and above indicating severe cases. It was developed originally for use in
general medical outpatient clinics but is now widely used in clinical practice
and research (Hermann, 1997). The HADS has sound psychometric properties (Zigmond & Snaith, 1983). It is particularly useful for measuring psychological distress in individuals with ABI because of the emphasis placed on
affective and behavioural symptoms and the exclusion of items relating to
physical difficulties.

Executive functioning

The Behavioural Assessment of Dysexecutive Syndrome (BADS; Wilson, Alderman, Burgess, Emslie, & Evans, 1996) was selected to assess executive functioning. This was used as it is reported to be ecologically valid and reflect everyday abilities (Burgess, Alderman, Evans, Emslie, & Wilson, 1998). The BADS consists of six subtests from which an age corrected standard score is devised. Adequate inter-rater and test-retest reliability is reported and performance on the BADS gave an indication of current level of executive functioning (Burgess et al., 1998; Norris & Tate, 2000; Wilson et al., 1996).

Awareness

The Dysexecutive Questionaires (DEX), which forms part of the BADS battery (Wilson et al., 1996) was administered to determine levels of awareness. There are two forms, one for self-rating (DEX-S) which was completed by the participants and another for independent rating by someone who knows the patient well (DEX-O), in this case, rehabilitation staff. Both forms ask the same questions hence an ABI survivors' degree of insight/awareness regarding their executive difficulties can be determined by the degree of difference between the two sets of answers (Norris & Tate, 2000).

Items are rated on a 6-point Likert scale ranging from 0 (never) to 5 (very often) with a higher score indicating higher frequency of dysexecutive problems in everyday life. A single score is produced for each questionnaire as well as five factor scores (inhibition, intentionality, executive memory, positive affect and negative affect). Lower scores on the DEX represent fewer perceived disabilities. The DEX aims to cover 20 of the most commonly reported symptoms of the dysexecutive syndrome based on the broad areas of dysfunction defined by Stuss and Benson (1984, 1986).

Cognitive ability

The Wechsler Test of Adult Reading (WTAR; Weschler, 2001) produces an error score that can be converted to a WTAR predicted WAIS-III Full Scale IQ. Normative data from the WAIS-III then apply. This score estimates the level of cognitive functioning an individual had prior to brain injury (Wechsler, 2001).

The Wechsler Adult Intelligence Scale – Third Edition (WAIS-III) Full Scale IQ (FSIQ) measures general cognitive functioning and yields a full scale IQ which is calculated from the scores of the individual subtests. Normative data exist for randomised samples in age bands of the general population (Wechsler, 1999).

Procedure

All participants were interviewed individually. Each participant was interviewed twice with each interview lasting no more than an hour in order to minimise fatigue levels. The second interview was held two weeks after the first with the objective of administering the self-esteem questionnaire again to test whether reported self-esteem remained stable over time. The Rosenberg was administered three times, twice during the initial interview and once during the second. All other questionnaires were administered once. Information regarding cognitive and executive functioning was gathered from participants' case notes. A carer who knew the participant well was asked to complete the DEX-O.

Interview 1

At the first administration, participants were asked to rate their self-esteem retrospectively (i.e., how they thought it was prior to their ABI) and currently. The use of retrospective perceptions of change following a severe ABI has proved a useful way of exploring subjective change in this population (Tyerman & Humphrey, 1984). The HADS and DEX-S were also administered.

Interview 2

The third administration of the Rosenberg took place during the second interview when participants were asked to rate their current level of self-esteem only. The HADS and DEX-S were completed in this interview if not completed during the first interview.

Data analysis

Data were found to be reasonably normally distributed when examined by visual inspection. Analysis was conducted using SPSS (version 12). Relationships between variables were explored using Pearson's product moment correlation coefficient. Differences between means were explored using paired samples t-tests. Where a definite direction could be predicted in the results based on existing research, one-tailed tests were applied (Dyer, 1995).

RESULTS

Stability of self-esteem ratings

The total scores on the Rosenberg range from 10 (highest self-esteem) to 40 (lowest self-esteem) (Torrey et al., 2000). These scores were reversed to help the reader more readily interpret the findings (that is, low scores were associated with low self-esteem rather than high scores being associated with low self-esteem). There are no discrete cut-off points to delineate high and low self-esteem on the Rosbenberg (Rosenberg, 1965). However, in keeping with previous studies (Kneckt, 2000), self-esteem scores were divided at the median (21.5). Thus scores of 10–21 equated to high self-esteem and scores of 22–40 equated to low self-esteem. The stability of self-esteem over a two-week period was analysed by calculating Pearson product moment correlations between administrations.

In order to investigate whether ratings of self-esteem by severe ABI survivors remain consistent over time, the total Rosenberg scores were compared across a two-week interval. They were found to be highly correlated ($r =$ .86; $p < .01$) and marginally higher than those found by Torrey et al. (2000) who found correlations of .70, .71 and .72 respectively at six month intervals over an 18 month period with mentally ill adults.

To determine whether the mean scores differed between administrations (see Table 1), paired sampled t-tests were carried out. No significant difference was found when the means for each item were compared, $t(21) = 1.03$; $p = ns$. This finding suggests that not only do self-esteem scores on first administration predict scores at the second administration but also that the level of self-esteem does not vary over time.

TABLE 1
Mean, standard deviation (SD) and range of variables

Variable	Mean	SD	Range
Age	**43**	**11.32**	**20–61**
Time since injury	**122.05**	**102.74**	**16–348**
Self-esteem			
Retrospective Rosenberg	18.59	7.00	10–30
Rosenberg interview 1	21.86	8.14	10–35
Rosenberg interview 2	21.23	7.87	10–37
Psychological distress			
HADS anxiety scores	7.86	5.01	0–16
HADS depression scores	7.23	4.99	0–18
Cognitive functioning			
FSIQ			
WTAR FSIQ	103.11	10.01	85–120
WAIS-III-R FSIQ	89.45	14.25	62–110
Executive functioning			
DEX–others	38.91	13.06	19–61
DEX–self	20.59	11.44	0–39
BADS	67.17	17.91	22–112
Awareness co-efficient	−18.32	17.91	−60–11

Due to the strong correlation and lack of discrepancy between the two administrations of the Rosenberg, the scores obtained from the initial administration of the Rosenberg were used in the remaining analyses.

Comparison of retrospective ratings of self-esteem prior to injury and current self-esteem

In order to investigate whether survivors reported lowered self-esteem following ABI, the differences in the mean scores between the pre and post ratings on the Rosenberg were analysed using a one-tailed, paired samples t-test (see Table 1). A significant difference was found, $t = -3.43$; $df(21)$; $p < .01$, indicating that current self-esteem scores were lower than retrospective ratings of self-esteem prior to injury.

Association between self-esteem and psychological distress

It was hypothesised that lower self-esteem would be associated with higher levels of psychological distress. Both depression ($r = .65$; $p < .01$) and anxiety ($r = .71$; $p < .01$) were positively correlated with current self-esteem indicating that those participants who reported low self-esteem also reported higher rates of psychological distress.

Low self-esteem will be associated with more intact cognitive functioning

It was further hypothesised that low self-esteem would be associated with more intact cognitive functioning (WTAR mean FSIQ and the mean WAIS-III-R FSIQ are included in Table 1). Magnitude of cognitive deterioration was determined by subtracting the current FSIQ from the WTAR predicted FSIQ.

To explore whether present self-esteem ratings were associated with magnitude of cognitive deterioration following brain injury, this difference between predicted pre-morbid IQ and current full scale IQ was correlated with the Rosenberg. No clear relationship was evident ($r = .26$; $p > .05$) suggesting that levels of current self-esteem was not associated with magnitude of acquired cognitive impairment.

When general cognitive ability was correlated with the Rosenberg, the relationship was significantly positive ($r = .43$; $p < .05$) suggesting that lower current cognitive ability was associated with high self-esteem.

Low self-esteem will be associated with greater awareness and more intact executive functioning

In order to investigate whether low self-esteem was associated with greater awareness, an "awareness coefficient" was calculated by subtracting the total sum of ratings made by participants on the DEX-S from those reported by their carers on the DEX-O (see Table 1). A paired t-test was calculated to determine whether there was a significant difference between ratings made by "others" and the participant's ratings on the DEX. There was a highly significant difference between "others" and "self" ratings, $t = 4.8$, $df(21)$; $p < .01$. Thus participants reported significantly less difficulties than their carers. In order to investigate the association between awareness and self-esteem, the awareness coefficient and the Rosenberg scores were correlated. The relationship was significant and negative ($r = -.49$; $p < .05$). Thus those with higher self-esteem had less awareness of their executive difficulties.

Association between self-esteem and executive functioning

To explore the relationship between executive functioning and current levels of self-esteem, performance on the BADS was correlated with the Rosenberg (see Table 1 for age-related BADS profile score). A significant, negative relationship ($r = -.48$; $p < .05$) was found suggesting that greater impairment in executive functioning was associated with higher self-esteem. This finding was consistent with the finding outlined above that lower current cognitive ability is associated with higher self-esteem.

DISCUSSION

Summary of findings

Despite the presence of variable levels of cognitive impairment, self-esteem ratings of participants remained consistent over a two-week period. Thus, participants' perceptions of themselves were stable. As far as we are aware, this is the first study to demonstrate that self-reported self-esteem can be rated in a reliable manner by survivors of severe ABI. This finding was contrary to expectation and adds weight to the emerging argument to take the subjective experience of the survivor into account during rehabilitation (Howes et al., 2005; Judd & Wilson, 2005; Keppel & Crowe, 2000; Man et al., 2003; Nadell, 1994; Ownsworth et al., 2000; Pollens et al., 1998; Ylvisaker, et al., 2003).

Furthermore, participants reported, in keeping with previous research, that their current self-esteem was lower than their retrospective perceptions of self-esteem prior to injury (Fleming & Courtney, 1984; Howes et al., 2005; Kravetz et al., 1995; Silber & Tippett, 1965; Tyerman & Humphrey, 1984, Wright & Telford, 1996). Low self-esteem was also strongly correlated with higher levels of psychological distress (Curran et al., 2000; Robson, 1988; Silverstone et al., 1996; Trzesniewski et al., 2003).

More intact cognitive functioning was associated with lower self-esteem although no clear association was found between current self-esteem and magnitude of deterioration following injury (Howes et al., 2005). Similarly, more intact executive functioning was associated with lower self-esteem as was greater awareness of executive difficulties. As a group, and consistent with the existing literature, the participants reported significantly less problems than those observed by carers (Gordon et al., 2000; Port et al., 2002; Moore & Stambrook, 1995). The relationship between cognitive functioning and awareness was not investigated. Thus, it cannot be assumed that participants who were more cognitively intact were also more aware of their deficits. However, what has been established in this study is that lower self-esteem tends to be associated with a higher degree of awareness of impairment, more intact cognitive and/or executive functioning as well as with higher rates of psychological distress.

Application of present finding and implications for future research

The finding that self-esteem remains stable among severe ABI survivors highlights the relevance of taking this into account during rehabilitation. Despite the diversity of their injuries, the participants' perceptions of self-esteem remained consistent. This supports the validity and value of self-reported self-esteem in understanding the experience of severe ABI (Judd & Wilson 2005; Man et al., 2003 Tyerman & Humphrey, 1984). Furthermore, this consistency is identical to that found in general and psychiatric populations (Guindon, 2002; Torrey et al., 2000; Trzesniewski et al., 2003). Given that mean length of time post-injury in this sample was 10 years this result is perhaps not surprising but it highlights the significance of internal evaluative processes like self-esteem for survivors. Given the association between self-esteem and motivation in the general population, this finding would suggest that further investigation is needed in order to understand more about how internal belief systems, such as self-esteem, could be impacting on motivation during rehabilitation of severe ABI survivors (Guindon, 2002; Howes et al., 2005; Keppel & Crowe, 2000; Tyerman & Humphrey, 1984).

The stability of current self-esteem ratings and the finding that severe ABI survivors report lowered self-esteem following injury further strengthens the argument that subjective meaning needs to be taken into account during rehabilitation (Howes et al., 2005; Judd & Wilson, 2005; Keppel & Crowe, 2000; Man et al., 2003; Nadell, 1994; Ownsworth et al., 2000; Pollens et al., 1998; Ylvisaker et al., 2003). Surviving an ABI is a traumatic experience and often involves immense loss, not least of self (Petrella, McColl, Krupa, & Johnston, 2005). It would appear that the complexity of an ABI has hindered progress in the development of psychological approaches aimed at helping ABI survivors reconcile these losses (Judd & Wilson, 2005). However, this study highlights the importance of such approaches being developed. Qualitatively, all participants emphasised that they felt that very little had been done to take their personal meaning of the injury into account during rehabilitation.

While this study did not investigate the concept of awareness of deficit, it highlighted a potential relationship between self-esteem and awareness that could add to current theories (Gasquione & Gibbons, 1994; Giacino & Cicerone, 1998; Ownsworth et al., 2002; Petrella et al., 2005). While research suggests that those who have greater awareness of deficit fare better in rehabilitation, this study found that those with greater awareness of deficit suffer worse self-esteem. How subjective reality among ABI survivors will influence outcome in rehabilitation is of particular interest to the clinician (Anderson & Tranel, 1989; Ponsford, 1995; Prigatano, 1991). While it may be that ABI survivors who recognise and appreciate their limitations will be motivated to work towards realistic goals, it would appear that their sense of self is also more vulnerable than ABI survivors who are less aware of their deficits (Prigatano et al., 1986). In addition, survivors who are more intact cognitively are also more likely to have lower self-esteem and hence, according to the findings, are more likely to experience higher rates of psychological distress. Thus, these findings suggest that while self-esteem may not be related to functional outcome in rehabilitation, it may be related to subjective outcome for the ABI survivor. This seems a relatively unexplored area within the ABI literature but it could have important implications for rehabilitation particularly in terms of adjustment and quality of life outcomes within this population (Howes et al., 2005; Judd & Wilson, 2005).

The paradoxical relationship found in this study was that those with more impaired awareness and cognitive functioning had higher self-esteem and the lowest incidence of psychological distress. While no causal relationship was established, this finding raises further questions about the role of awareness in more impaired survivors. Psychological theories argue that awareness deficits reflect the use of psychological defence mechanisms to buffer emotional distress resulting from the injury (Petrella et al., 2005). Thus this finding is suggestive of the potentially buffering role impaired awareness could play among more severely impaired survivors in protecting them from higher rates of psychological distress through the maintenance of higher self-esteem. Indeed, lack of insight and good self-esteem may be important coping mechanisms following severe brain injury. Research within adult psychiatry has proposed that delusions result from individuals' attempts to maintain their underlying self-esteem and self-concepts (Garety, Kuipers, Fowler, Freeman, & Bebbington, 2001). Perhaps this need to preserve self-esteem is also evident and more pronounced among more impaired survivors. This may explain why threats presented to their self-esteem during rehabilitation, such as trying to increase their awareness, could be met with resistance

(Garety et al., 2001; Kinderman & Bentall, 1996). Thus, an interesting area of research in this regard would be to explore the content of confabulations and how these relate to self-esteem. Furthermore, this finding suggests that self-esteem could be an implicit process that is not impacted on by magnitude of cognitive deterioration. However, this warrants further, more robust investigation.

In terms of practical application, the findings of this study suggest that prior to therapeutic intervention, an assessment of self-esteem, degree of awareness and cognitive ability could enable the therapist to predict which clients may be at risk of developing increased psychological distress if their awareness of deficit was increased. For those clients who report awareness of deficit and low self-esteem it may be advisable for the therapeutic process to focus on redefining personal strengths and coping skills prior to, or as an alternative to increasing awareness (aimed at improving rehabilitation outcome) in order to reduce the risk of increasing the psychological distress (Petrella et al., 2005; Klonoff, 1997). Additionally, it offers a tenuous suggestion that perhaps therapeutic outcome would be improved if the process of redefining the self was addressed at the initial rather than the end stages of therapy and that this was used to promote the development of coping and compensation strategies (Bennett & Raymond, 1997; Howes et al., 2005).

Methodological considerations

As exploratory research, it is acknowledged that the sample size is small and heterogeneous. Consequently, replication of this study would be useful to increase generalisation of the findings to the ABI population (Keppel & Crowe, 2000; Lubusko et al., 1994). However, it nevertheless parallels sample sizes in similar studies (Howes et al., 2005; Keppel & Crowe, 2000). Secondly, it may also have been the case that findings were influenced by excluding those participants with severe language deficits (Alderman, Knight, & Henman, 2002; Alderman, Knight, & Morgan, 1997, Keppel & Crowe, 2000). The contribution of other variables that potentially could be related to self-esteem such as physical impairments, functional ability, age, education, time since injury or length of time in rehabilitation were also not investigated. A future study might also investigate how pre-morbid, as well as current personality factors and coping styles influence self-esteem following a severe ABI (Brown & Dutton, 1995; Malia et al., 1995; Moore & Stambrook, 1995). Additionally, this research did not explore the relationship between coping styles and self-esteem (Moore & Stambrook, 1995). Another option for future research could be to conduct a longitudinal study which could shed light on how self-esteem changes during the process of recovery and adjustment to an ABI (Curran et al., 2000; Howes et al., 2005). A series of assessments conducted over a period of at least 2 years following ABI would enhance understanding of the effects of ABI on self-esteem and the impact on the recovery process (Keppel & Crowe, 2000).

CONCLUSION

This exploratory study provides evidence that severe ABI survivors report that their self-esteem has suffered as a result of their injury. It has further demonstrated that self-reported self-esteem shows consistency in this population even a number of years after brain injury. Clear links were found between cognitive functioning, awareness, self-esteem and mood. While this study attempted to begin unravelling these links, further investigation is clearly required to understand them more clearly. Notwithstanding, this study suggests that ABI survivors have an established and consistent self-esteem. Given that subjective, rather than accurate self-appraisal is a powerful influence in predicting psychological outcome, this finding suggests that understanding the role of self-esteem during rehabilitation warrants further attention (Keppel & Crowe, 2000; Howes et al., 2005; Prigatano, 1997; Tyerman & Humphrey, 1984). The paradoxical finding that survivors who were more impaired cognitively and/or less aware of their deficits report higher self-esteem poses an ethical dilemma for clinicians. While attempting to engage them in rehabilitation would require raising their awareness of deficit, this may result in lowering their self-esteem and increasing their psychological distress. Should clinicians focus instead on maintaining the higher self-esteem in order to promote subjective well-being? It is hoped that the consistency of self-esteem ratings among this population of severe ABI survivors sparks further ethical debate about which direction clinicians should take when faced with this paradox.

REFERENCES

Alderman, N., Davies, J. A., Jones, C., & McDonnell, P. (1999). Reduction of severe aggressive behaviour in acquired brain injury: Case studies illustrating clinical use of the OAS-MNR in the management of challenging behaviours. *Brain Injury, 13*, 669–704.

Alderman, N., Knight, C., & Henman, C. (2002). Aggressive behaviour within a neurobehavioral rehabilitation service: Utility of the OAS-MNR in clinical audit and applied research. *Brain Injury, 16*, 469–489.

Alderman, N., Knight, C., & Morgan, C. (1997). Use of a modified version of the Overt Aggression Scale in the measurement and assessment of aggressive behaviours following brain injury. *Brain Injury, 11*(7), 503–523.

Anderson, S. W., & Tranel, D. (1989). Awareness of disease states following cerebral infarction, dementia and head trauma: Standardised assessment. *Clinical Neuropsychologist, 3*, 327–339.

Bednar, R. L. & Peterson, S. R. (1995). *Self-esteem: Paradoxes and innovations in clinical theory and practice* (2nd ed.). Washington, DC: American Psychological Association.

Bennett, T. L., & Raymond, M. J. (1997). Individual psychotherapy and minor head-injury. *Applied Neuropsychology*, *4*, 55–61.

Brown, J. D., & Dutton, K. A. (1995). The thrill of victory, the complexity of defeat: Self-esteem and people's emotional reactions to success and failure. *Journal of Personality and Social Psychology*, *68*(4), 712–722.

Brown, J. D., & Marshall, M. A. (2001). Self-esteem and emotions: Some thoughts about feelings. *Personality and Social Psychology Bulletin*, *27*(5), 575–584.

Burgess, P. W., Alderman, N., Evans, J., Emslie, H., & Wilson, B. A. (1998). The ecological validity of tests of executive function. *Journal of the International Neuropsychological Society*, *4*, 547–558.

Coopersmith, S. (1967). *The Antecedents of Self-Esteem.* San Fransisco, CA: W.H. Freeman.

Curran, C. A., Ponsford, J. L., & Crowe, S. (2000). Coping strategies and emotional outcome following traumatic brain injury: A comparison with orthopaedic patients. *Journal of Head Trauma Rehabilitation*, *1*(6), 1256–1274.

Deaton, A.V. (1986). Denial in the aftermath of traumatic head injury: Its manifestations, measurement and treatment. *Rehabilitation Psychology*, *31*, 231–240.

Dobson, C., Goudy, W. J., Keith, P. M., & Powers, E. (1979). Further analysis of Rosenberg's self-esteem scale. *Psychological Reports*, *44*, 639–641.

Dyer, C. (1995). *Beginning research in psychology: A practical guide to research methods and statistics.* Oxford: Blackwell Publishers.

Ezrachi, O., Ben-Yishay, Y., Kay, T., Diller, L., & Rattock, J. (1991). Predicting employment in traumatic brain injury following neuropsychological rehabilitation. *Journal of Head Trauma Rehabilitation*, *6*(3), 71–84.

Fennell, M. (1999). *Overcoming low self-esteem.* London: Robinson.

Fleming, J. S., & Courtney, B. E. (1984a). The dimensionality of self-esteem. II. Heirarchical facet model for revised measurement scales. *Journal of Personality and Social Psychology*, *46*, 404–421.

Fleming, J. S., & Courtney, B. E. (1984b). The dimensionality of self-esteem: Some results for a college sample. *Journal of Personality and Social Psychology*, *39*, 921–929.

Fluharty, G., & Glassman, N. (2001). Use of antecedent control to improve the outcome of rehabilitation for a client with frontal lobe injury and intolerance for auditory and tactile stimuli. *Brain Injury*, *15*, 995–1002.

Garety, P., Kuipers, E., Fowler, D., Freeman, D., & Bebbington, P. (2001). A cognitive model of the positive symptoms of psychosis. *Psychological Medicine*, *31*, 198–195.

Garske, G., & Thomas, K. R. (1992). Self-reported self-esteem and depression: Indexes of psychosocial adjustment following severe traumatic brain injury. *Rehabilitation Counselling Bulletin*, *36*, 44–52.

Gasquione, P. G., & Gibbons, T. A. (1994). Lack of awareness of impairment in institutionalized, severely and chronically disabled survivors of traumatic brain injury: A preliminary investigation. *Journal of Head Trauma Rehabilitation*, *9*(4), 16–24.

Giacino, J. T., & Cicerone, K. D. (1998). Varieties of deficit unawareness after brain injury. *Journal of Head Trauma Rehabilitation*, *12*(5), 1–15.

Gordon, W. A., Haddad, L., Brown, M., Hibbard, M. R., & Sliwinski, M (2000). The sensitivity and specificity of self-reported symptoms in individuals with traumatic brain injury. *Brain Injury*, *14*(1), 21–33.

Green, A., Felmingham, K., Baguley, I. J., Slewa-Younan, S., & Simpson, S. (2001). The clinical utility of the Beck Depression Inventory after traumatic brain injury. *Brain Injury*, *15*(12), 1021–1028.

Guindon, M. H. (2002). Toward accountability in the use of the self-esteem construct. *Journal of Counselling and Development, 80*(2), 204–214.

Hamacheck, D. E. (1978). *Encounters with the Self* (2nd ed.). New York: Holt Rinehart and Winston.

Harris, E. C., & Barraclough, B. (1997). Suicide as an outcome for mental disorders: A meta-analysis. *British Journal of Psychiatry, 170*, 205–228.

Hermann, C. (1997). International experiences with the Hospital Anxiety and Depression Scale: A review of validation data and clinical results. *Journal of Psychosomatic Research, 42*, 17–41.

Hibbard, M. R., Uysal, S., Keple, K., Bogdany, J., & Silver, J. (1998). Axis I psychopathology in individuals with traumatic brain injury. *Journal of Head Trauma Rehabilitation, 13*, 24–39.

Hillier, S. L., & Metzer, J. (1997). Awareness and perceptions of outcomes after traumatic brain injury. *Brain Injury, 11*, 525–536.

Howes, H. F. R., Edwards, S., & Benton, D. (2005). Female body image following acquired brain injury. *Brain Injury, 19*(6), 403–415.

Judd, D., & Wilson, S. L. (2005). Psychotherapy with brain injury survivors: An investigation of the challenges encountered by clinicians and their modifications to therapeutic practice. *Brain Injury, 19*(6), 437–449.

Keppel, C. C., & Crowe, S. F. (2000). Changes to body image and self-esteem following stroke in young adults. *Neuropsychological Rehabilitation, 10*(1), 15–31.

Kernis, M. H., Grannemann, B. D., & Barclay, L. C. (1989). Stability and level of self-esteem as predictors of anger arousal and hostility. *Journal of Personality and Social Psychology, 56*(6), 1013–1022.

Kinderman, P., & Bentall, R. P. (1996). Self-discrepancies and persecutory delusions: Evidence for a defensive model of paranoid ideation. *Journal of Abnormal Psychology, 105*, 106–114.

King, N. S. (1997). Mild head injury: Neuropathology, sequelae, measurement and recovery. A literature review. *British Journal of Clinical Psychology, 36*, 161–184.

Klonoff, P. S. (1997). Individual and group psychotherapy in milieu-orientated neurorehabilitation. *Applied Neuropsychology, 4*, 107–118.

Kneckt, M. (2000). *Psychological features characterizing oral health behaviour, diabetes self-care health status among IDDM patients.* Oulu, Finland: Oulu University Library.

Kravetz, S., Gross, Y., Weiler, B., Ben-Yaker, M., Tadir, M., & Stern, M. J. (1995). Self-concept, marital vulnerability and brain damage. *Brain Injury, 9*(2), 131–139.

Lubusko, A. A., Moore, A. D., Stambrook, M., & Gill, D. D. (1994). Cognitive beliefs following severe traumatic brain injury: Association with post-injury employment status. *Brain Injury, 8*(1), 65–70.

Malia, K., Powell, G., & Torode, S. (1995). Personality and psychosocial function after brain injury. *Brain Injury, 9*(7), 697–712.

Man, D. W. K., Tam, A. S. F., & Li, E. P. Y. (2003). Exploring self-concepts of persons with brain injury. *Brain Injury, 17*(9), 775–788.

Moore, A. D., & Stambrook, M. (1992). Coping strategies and locus of control following traumatic brain injury: Relationship to long term outcome. *Brain Injury, 6*, 89–94.

Moore, A. D., & Stambrook, M. (1995). Cognitive moderators of outcome following traumatic brain injury: A conceptual model and implications for rehabilitation. *Brain Injury, 9*, 109–130.

Morton, M. V., & Wehman, P. (1995). Psychosocial and emotional sequelae of individuals with traumatic brain injury: A literature review and recommendations. *Brain Injury, 9*, 81–92.

Mrurk, C. (1999). *Self-esteem: Research, theory and practice* (2nd ed.). New York: Springer.

Nadell, J. (1994). Towards an existential psychotherapy with the traumatically brain injured patient. *Cognitive Rehabilitation, 9*, 8–13.

Norris, G., & Tate, R. L. (2000). The Behavioural Assessment of the Dysexecutive Syndrome (BADS): Ecological, concurrent and construct validity. *Neuropsychological Rehabilitation*, *10*(1), 33–45.

Ownsworth, T. L., McFarland, K., & Young, R. M. (2000). Self-awareness and psychosocial functioning following acquired brain injury: An evaluation of a group support programme. *Neuropsychological Rehabilitation*, *10*(5), 465–484.

Petrella, L., McColl, M. A., Krupa, T., & Johnston, J. (2005). Returning to productive activities: Perspectives of individuals with long-standing acquired brain injuries. *Brain Injury*, *19*(9), 643–655.

Pollens, R. D., McBratnie, B. P., & Burton, P. L. (1998). Beyond cognition: Executive functions in closed head injury. *Cognitive Rehabilitation*, *6*, 26–32.

Ponsford, J., Olver, J., & Curran, C. (1995a). A profile of outcome: 2 years after traumatic brain injury. *Brain Injury*, *9*, 1–10.

Ponsford, J., Olver, J., Nelms, R., & Curran, C. (1996). Self-report of problems and emotional adjustment 2–5 years following traumatic brain injury. In J. Ponsford, P. Snow, & V. Anderson (Eds.), *International perspectives in traumatic brain injury.* Proceedings of the 5th conference of the International Association for the Study of Brain Injury and the Study of Brain Impairment (pp. 434–437). Bowen Hills, Australia: Australian Academic Press.

Ponsford, J., Sloan, S., & Snow, P. (1995b). *Traumatic brain injury: Rehabilitation for everyday adaptive living.* Hove UK: Lawrence Erlbaum Associates.

Port, A., Willmott, C.. & Charlton, J. (2002). Self-awareness following traumatic brain injury and implications for rehabilitation. *Brain Injury*, *16*(4), 277–289.

Prigatano, G. P. (1991). Disturbance of self-awareness of deficit after traumatic brain injury. In G. P. Prigatano, & D. L. Schacter (Eds). *Awareness of deficit after brain injury: Clinical and theoretical issues.* New York, Oxford: Oxford University Press.

Prigatano, G. P. (1997). Learning from our successes and failures: Reflections and comments on "cognitive rehabilitation": How it is and how it might be. *Journal of the International Neuropsychological Society*, *3*, 497–499.

Prigatano, G. P., & Fordyce, D. J. (1988). Cognitive dysfunction and psychosocial adjustment after brain injury. In G. P. Prigatano, D. J. Fordyce, H. K. Zeiner, J. R. Roueche, M. Pepping, & B. C. Wood (Eds.), *Neuropsychological rehabilitation after brain injury.* (pp. 1–17). Baltimore, MD: Johns Hopkins University Press.

Robson, P. (1988). Self-esteem – A psychiatric review. *British Journal of Psychiatry*, *153*, 6–15.

Robson, P. (1989). Development of a new self-report questionnaire to measure self-esteem. *Psychological Medicine*, *19*, 513–518.

Rosenberg, M. (1965). *Society and the adolescent self image.* Princeton, NJ: Princeton University Press.

Sbordone, R. J., Seyranian, R., & Ruff, R. M. (1998). Are the subjective complaints of traumatically brain injured patients reliable? *Brain Injury*, *11*, 505–515.

Silber, E., & Tippett, J. (1965). Self-esteem: Clinical assessment and measurement validation. *Psychological Reports*, *16*, 1017–1071.

Silverstone, P. H., Lemay, T., Elliott, J., Hsu, V., & Starko, R. (1996). The prevalence of major depressive disorder and low self-esteem in medical inpatients. *Canadian Journal of Psychiatry*, *41*, 67–74.

Snaith, R. P., & Zigmund, A. S. (1994). *HADS: Hospital Anxiety and Depression Scale.* Windsor, UK: NFER Nelson.

Strein, W. (1993). Advances in research on academic self-concept: Implications for school psychology. *School Psychology Review*, *22*, 273–284.

Stuss, D. T., & Benson, D. F. (1984). Neuropsychological studies of the frontal lobes. *Psychological Bulletin*, *95*(1), 3–28.

Stuss, D. T., & Benson, D. F. (1986). *The frontal lobes*. New York: Raven Press.

Torrey, W. C., Mueser, K. T., McHugo, G. H., & Drake, R. E. (2000). Self-esteem as an outcome measure in studies of vocational rehabilitation for adults with severe mental illness. *Psychiatric Services*, *51*, 229–233.

Trezesniewski, K. H., Donnellan, M. B., & Robins, R. W. (2003). Stability of self-esteem across the life span. *Journal of Personality and Social Psychology*, *84*(1), 205–220.

Tyerman, A. (1987). *Self-concept and psychological change in the rehabilitation of the severely head injured person*. Unpublished Doctoral Thesis: University of London.

Tyerman, A., & Humphrey, M. (1984). Changes in self-concept following severe head injury. *International Journal of Rehabilitation Research*, *7*(1), 11–23.

Vickery, C. D., Gontkovsky, S. T., & Caroselli, J. S. (2005). Self-concept and quality of life following acquired brain injury: A pilot investigation. *Brain Injury*, *19*(9), 657–665.

Wallace, C. A., & Bogner, J. (2000). Awareness of deficits: Emotional implications for persons with brain injury and their significant others. *Brain Injury*, *14*(6), 549–562.

Wells, A. (1997). *Cognitive therapy of anxiety disorders: A practice manual and conceptual guide*. Chichester, UK: John Wiley & Sons.

Weschler, D. (1999). *The Weschler Adult Intelligence Scale Third Edition (UK)*. Oxford: Harcourt Assessment.

Weschler, D. (2001). *The Weschler Test of Adult Reading: Adapted for UK Use*. Oxford: Harcourt Assessment.

Williams, W. H. (2003). Neurorehabilitation and cognitive behaviour therapy for emotional disorders in acquired brain injury (pp. 115–135). In B. A. Wilson (Ed.), *Neuropsychological rehabilitation: Theory and practices*. Lisse: Swets & Zeitlinger.

Wilson, B. A., Alderman, N., Burgess, P. W., Emslie, H., & Evans, J.J. (1996). *Behavioural Assessment of the Dysexecutive Syndrome*. London: Harcourt Assessment.

Witmer, J. M., & Sweeney, T. J. (1992). A holistic model for wellness and prevention over the life span. *Journal of Counselling and Development*, *71*, 140–147.

Wood, R. Ll., Liossi, C., & Wood, L. (2005). The impact of head injury neurobehavioural sequelae on personal relationships: Preliminary findings. *Brain Injury*, *19*(10), 845–851.

Wright, J. C., & Telford, R. (1996). Psychological problems following minor head injury: A prospective study. *British Journal of Clinical Psychology*, *35*, 399–412.

Ylvisaker, M., Jacobs, H. E., & Feeney, T. (2003). Positive supports for people who experience behavioural and cognitive disability after brain injury. *Journal of Head Trauma Rehabilitation*, *18*(1), 7–32.

Zigmond, A., & P. Snaith (1983). The Hospital Anxiety and Depression Scale. *Acta Psychiatrica Scandinavica*, *67*, 361–370.

NEUROPSYCHOLOGICAL REHABILITATION
2008, 18 (5/6), 627–650

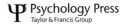

"Feeling part of things": Personal construction of self after brain injury

Fergus Gracey[1], Siobhan Palmer[1], Becky Rous[1], Kate Psaila[2], Kendra Shaw[3], Juliette O'Dell[1], Jo Cope[1], and Shemin Mohamed[4]

[1]*Oliver Zangwill Centre for Neuropsychological Rehabilitation, Princess of Wales Hospital, Ely, UK;* [2]*Cambridgeshire Learning Disability Partnership, Ida Darwin Hospital, Fulbourn, Cambridge, UK;* [3]*Neuropsychology Department, Charing Cross Hospital, London, UK;* [4]*Cambridgeshire and Peterborough Mental Health Trust, Fulbourn, Cambridge, UK*

There is a growing body of literature on the nature of subjective changes experienced following brain injury. This study employs personal construct and qualitative research methods to address the question of how people make sense of, or construe, themselves after brain injury. Thirty-two individuals who had experienced acquired brain injury engaged in small group exercises based on a personal construct approach. Bipolar constructs were elicited through systematic comparison of pre-injury, current and ideal selves. The constructs elicited in this way were subjected to a thematic analysis. Nine themes were derived and an acceptable level of reliability of the definitions of these themes achieved. The highest proportion of constructs fell into the theme "experience of self in the world", followed by "basic skills" (cognitive, sensory, physical, social) and "experience of self in relation to self ". It is concluded that following brain injury, people make sense of themselves in terms of the meanings and felt experiences of social and practical activity. This is consistent with social identity theory and stands in contrast to traditional neuropsychological sense making in terms of impairments and abilities alone, or activity or social participation alone. The implications of these findings for future research and rehabilitation are briefly considered.

Keywords: Brain injury; Rehabilitation; Identity; Personal construct psychology.

Correspondence should be sent to: Dr Fergus Gracey, Oliver Zangwill Centre for Neuropsychological Rehabilitation, Princess of Wales Hospital, Lynn Road, Ely, Cambridgeshire, CB6 1DN, UK. E-mail: Fergus.gracey@ozc.nhs.uk

INTRODUCTION

Self and identity changes after brain injury

Kurt Goldstein (1959) was among the first to highlight the devastating emotional impact of brain injury, and how this can further impact on functioning in the world, describing the "catastrophic reaction". Ben-Yishay (2000) has described this as "the behavioural manifestation of a threat to the person's very existence, due to the failure to cope" (p. 128). Examples in the literature where understanding of the meaning and experience of the person with brain injury informs or is informed by psychological theory remains under-developed (Nadell, 1991), although a small number of studies are helpful in this regard.

Tyerman and Humphrey (1984) attempted to quantify and characterise the nature of changes in self-concept after brain injury. Asking traumatically brain injured participants to rate their current, pre-injury and future selves according to a list of pairs of adjectives (the Head Injury Semantic Differential Scale, HISD), they found current self-ratings to differ greatly from pre and future self, as well as a "striking similarity" between pre and future self-ratings. They interpret this in terms of the sense of current discrepancy and hope for future return of the past self, commenting on the capacity for people with brain injury to be able to reflect on subjective aspects of themselves despite a common perception of lack of awareness. Ellis-Hill and Horn (2000) applied the same approach to stroke survivors, finding a similar negative view of current self, compared with pre-stroke self. While the HISD has established an acceptable list of psychometric properties with brain injured participants, the adjectives that make up the rating scale were selected by clinicians rather than derived from participants. As such, they may not capture the most salient or subtle dimensions of sense making for all people following brain injury.

Qualitative research methods are especially designed to generate rich data that can communicate the perspective of the research participants and can be most informative where the views and experiences of those being studied may have been marginalised or neglected in research (e.g., Pidgeon & Henwood, 1996). Nochi (Nochi, 1998, 2000; Nochi, Jansson, & Norberg, 1997) carried out a series of qualitative interviews with survivors of traumatic brain injury with the aim of identifying key themes in the narratives of survivors. Nochi (1998) identified a key narrative of "loss of self" further analysed into three domains: loss of clear knowledge of self (e.g., through memory loss), loss of self by comparison (e.g., of pre- and post-injury selves) and loss of self in the eyes of others. Nilsson, Jansson, and Norberg (1997) employed qualitative methods to discover the experiences of stroke victims in the acute phase of recovery. They describe five interpretative themes, one of which captures sense of identity (in past activity and achievements) and potential current identity confusion. Yeates, Henwood, Gracey, and Evans (2007) looked at the discourses of individuals with brain injury seen as lacking awareness, and of a significant other. This study identified how, at times, the person with brain injury may draw upon discourses from pre-injury (e.g., viewing a characteristic in terms of a work skill, one participant described how, "We don't do detail in marketing") to make sense of her changed abilities after injury. In response this person's relative presented an alternative account (e.g., as a result of the injury the individual is seen as lacking an ability to plan and make sound decisions). Such "contesting accounts" may be played out in interactions such that individuals with brain injury feel they are defending their identity, while their significant others perceive a worrying lack of awareness. Also in the realm of social relating, Gutman and Napier-Klemic (1995) explored the impact of head injury on gender role and identity through detailed interviewing of four participants. The personal importance of ability to participate in activities that support strong meanings associated with gender roles was highlighted. These methodologies, while informative, are very time consuming and would be difficult to implement for assessing or measuring aspects of identity change in clinical practice. Furthermore, while revealing meanings and experiences that might otherwise not be uncovered by quantitative methods, potential for generalisability may be limited by sample size in such studies.

Cantor et al. (2005) tested predictions from self-discrepancy theory (Higgins, 1987) regarding types of self-discrepancy after brain injury and prediction of anxiety and depression. Self-discrepancy, as defined in self-discrepancy theory, is the degree of difference between a person's self-concept or "actual self" and other self-representations that relate to some desired or aspired-to state (ideal self and ought self). Such discrepancies are thought to give rise to anxiety or depression. In order to adapt the theory to be relevant to individuals after brain injury, Cantor et al. added a further aspect of self that may be discrepant from actual self, the person's "pre-injury self". They employed both an adjective checklist measure derived from established methods in self-discrepancy theory research (the Selves Adjective Checklist, SAC: similar to that employed by Tyerman & Humphrey, 1984), and an interview in which adjectives were elicited from the participants. Pre- to post-injury actual self-discrepancy scores derived from the interview measure were not related to emotional outcome, although interview-based discrepancy scores were arrived at through use of a thesaurus to quantify "distance" between adjectives relating to different selves. SAC pre- to post-injury actual self-discrepancy scores did predict anxiety and depression. Thus, although the elicited adjectives may have been pertinent to the participants, the method for measuring discrepancy was not based on subjective experience, and this may account for the inconsistency in results here.

In summary, loss of self and self-discrepancy (between actual and pre-injury selves) have emerged as key problems following brain injury. Quantitative measures used in research may be sensitive to assessing and measuring identity change. However, they lack the specificity of qualitative approaches that have identified ways in which self and identity change is experienced as both a subjective and social phenomenon. Qualitative methods would be too time-consuming to be clinically practical.

Personal construct psychology

Personal construct psychology was developed by Kelly (1955) to attempt to bring together a humanist orientation with rigorous and quantifiable methods to personality theory and psychotherapy. A complete account of Kelly's personal construct psychology and the specific terminology used is beyond the scope of the present paper (see Winter, 1992, for a helpful summary). Personal construct psychology could be seen as an early type of cognitive approach, in that the psychological representation of external reality is central (Blowers & O'Connor, 1995; Nevid, 2007). Kelly proposed that each of us actively makes sense of or interprets all the things we encounter. A cognitive model such as that proposed by Beck (1972) proposes that repeated experiences lead to the development of beliefs, assumptions and rules, which may then be used to anticipate or interpret situations. However, for Kelly, repeated interpretations of experiences are made on the basis of, and form *dichotomous* constructs (e.g., good – evil, warm hearted – cold, serious – fun) that become hierarchically organised. It is proposed that the logic of ascribing meaning via the application of a uni-dimensional concept (e.g., pain, love, bravery – as in traditional cognitive approaches) is flawed as these concepts only make sense in relation to their absence or opposite (pain-free, hate, cowardice, for example). Sets of constructs will develop for specific sets of situations, people or other aspects of reality. This means that for a given encounter (e.g., with a new acquaintance) our sense making is restricted (or "channelised" in Kelly's terms) by constructs formed from past encounters with people and relationships, so we tend to make sense of the person according to, for example, their goodness, warmth and seriousness as mapped on dichotomous constructs such as "good – evil", "warm hearted – cold", "serious – fun"). Kelly (1955) presented a number of theoretical statements about personal construal that allow consideration of issues such as the range of situations a particular personal construct covers, the number of constructs one may have related to something, and the variability, flexibility and complexity of our construing of particular things.

The theory of personal construct psychology is realised in the methods used for finding out or "eliciting" and rating constructs about certain target items of interest ("elements" in the language of personal construct psychology) such as people or situations. This approach to assessment aims to be both quantitative and rigorous, and at the same time sensitive to the subjectivity of the individual (or group) and his or her particular patterns of construing in relation to a set of elements. While there are a range of approaches to identifying or eliciting personal constructs, and interpreting the outcomes (see Fransella, Bell, & Bannister, 2004), the procedure typically involves the comparison of "elements" making up a set (e.g., people) that are of particular interest (e.g., in understanding the person's relationships with others). The individual is asked to compare two or three elements from such a set at a time (e.g., self, father, best friend at university), and then asked to identify similarities and differences and if necessary, their opposites (e.g., "father is serious, compared to myself and best friend who are fun loving"; or "my father and I are both politically motivated, the opposite of this would be politically naïve"). Arrangement of all the constructs together with all the elements forms a kind of personal questionnaire called a repertory grid. Using this, it becomes possible to rate the people making up the set of elements according to all the bi-polar constructs elicited from the exercise, usually done on a 7-point Likert scale. Analysis of these ratings provides a map of how the individual makes sense of or construes other people, and repeated ratings over time can be used to measure change, for example, in psychotherapy. The approach can be applied to eliciting constructs from individuals, or from groups to develop standardised or consensus grids which represent the commonalities in construing of a group or of a wide range of people in relation to a specific topic or set of elements (Fransella et al, 2004; Winter, 1992).

In addition to the qualitative aspects of the content of constructs, and repertory grid ratings, other useful aspects of the data elicited from the technique include variability of construing over time, or hierarchical organisation of constructs. The number of constructs relating to an element or set of elements is thought to indicate the degree of elaboration of construal. For example, an experienced wine taster is likely to have a larger number of wine-related constructs and therefore more elaborated construal of wine than a pure beer drinker (whose constructs may not extend beyond "drinkable – unpleasant", "red – white", and "sweet – dry").

Current study

The study described here forms part of a longer-term research project aiming to develop a sensitive and meaningful, yet convenient way of assessing and measuring self-construal and self-discrepancy changes following brain injury and through rehabilitation. Our assumption for this study is that social identity arises from community membership and culture, that personal identity provides a sense of definition of self in the context of social identity, and that identities can be internalised into the self-concept as relatively stable and enduring patterns, consistent with social identity theory (Turner, 1982). Kelly's notion of self-construal in this study is seen as a means of operationalising self-concept, as a set of internalised dichotomous representations of personal and social identity.

The aim of this study is to find out the salient patterns of self-construing engaged in by individuals when making sense of changes after brain injury.

METHOD

Participants

Participants were recruited as consecutive admissions to a holistic neuropsychological rehabilitation programme. Selection for the study was thus consistent with selection for this programme. All individuals who attended the programme over the study period were recruited and completed the study. The inclusion criteria were:

- Adult of working age.

- Acquired, non-progressive brain injury at least one year ago.

- Clear functional difficulties or social participation restrictions associated with interacting cognitive, emotional, social, family and communicative difficulties.

- No significant unmanaged severe mental health problem.

- No significant unmanaged substance misuse disorder.

- No significant behavioural disturbance such that the individual would not be able to participate in group sessions.

- Sufficient communication abilities, with use of aids if required, to allow participation in group-based rehabilitation.

Selection of programme clients and thus study participants followed initial screening of referral by a clinical neuropsychologist, screening assessment including cognitive assessment, and interdisciplinary detailed assessment over eight consecutive days followed by team formulation to check programme inclusion criteria. The sample was thus a range of individuals with acquired brain injury who attended a milieu oriented or holistic rehabilitation programme. Table 1 presents a summary description of the sample. This shows that most participants were in full-time paid employment prior to

TABLE 1
Description of two sub-samples and total sample

	First sub-sample (Group 1)	Second sub-sample (Group 2)	Total sample
Sample size	18	14	32
Age: mean (range)	36.6 years (21–59 years)	39.5 years (21–57 years)	38 years (21–59 years)
Male	13	10	23
Type of injury	TBI = 12 (closed 11, open 1) Haemorrhage = 2 Encephalitis = 2 Other = 2	TBI = 10 (closed 10) Haemorrhage = 3 Other = 1 (post-surgical clipping of aneurysm)	TBI = 22 (closed 21; open 1), Haemorrhage = 5 Encephalitis = 2 Other = 3
Severity of injury*	> = severe = 7 < severe = 4 Not recorded = 1 Not applicable = 6	> = severe = 9 < severe = 1 Not recorded = 0 Not applicable = 4	> = severe = 16 < severe = 5 Not recorded = 1 Not applicable = 10
Years post-injury: mean (range)	2 years (1.5–10 years)	4 years (1–10 years)	3 years (1–10 years)
Pre-injury employment status	Education = 2 Unemployed = 0 Full-time paid = 16 Part-time paid = 0	Education = 0 Unemployed = 0 Full-time paid = 12 Part-time = 2	Education = 2 Unemployed = 0 Full-time paid = 28 Part-time = 2
Employment status at time of study	Education = 0 Unemployed = 16 Full-time paid = 2 Part-time = 0	Education = 0 Unemployed = 11 Full-time paid = 0 Part-time = 3	Education = 0 Unemployed = 27 Full-time paid = 2 Part-time = 3
Pre-injury education level attained	Minimum = 5 Further/voc = 4 Diploma = 4 Degree = 3 Masters = 1 Doctorate = 1	Minimum = 3 Further/voc = 6 Diploma = 1 Degree = 3 Masters = 1 Doctorate = 0	Minimum = 8 Further/voc = 10 Diploma = 5 Degree = 6 Masters = 2 Doctorate = 1
Estimated pre-injury intellectual functioning (SCOLP Spot the Word scaled score)	Mean = 10.125 SD = 2.12 (missing data for 2)	Mean = 10.29 SD = 3.17	Mean = 10.2 SD = 2.62

*severity as recorded in medical notes; TBI = traumatic brain injury; "minimum" education level = leaving school at age 16 years; "further" = leaving school at age 18 years; "voc" = leaving school at 16 for 1–2 years vocational training; SCOLP = Speed and Capacity of Language Processing

their injury, and most were unemployed at the time of the study. There was a range of educational backgrounds represented ranging from minimal (25% of the sample leaving school at age 16 to 3.1%, one individual, achieving doctoral level). On average the sample fell into the average range of estimated pre-injury intellectual functioning on the Speed and Capacity of Language Processing "Spot the Word" subtest (SCOLP; Baddeley, Emslie, & Nimmo-Smith, 1992; mean scaled score = 10.2; $SD = 2.6$), with scaled scores ranging from 6 to 15.

The data collection occurred in a clinical group session run in the first week of a 24-week rehabilitation programme, prior to the delivery of any intervention. Within the programme, the group exercise aimed to facilitate individuals' discussion of their identity and adjustment post-injury. The constructs elicited and subsequent ratings made through rehabilitation were used as an idiographic assessment and outcome measure, but these data were not included in the current study. All participants gave informed consent to take part.

Data were collected continuously over a 29 month period. The data collected over the first 14 months were analysed first (described as the first sub-sample). The data collected following this (second sub-sample) were used for development of initial themes derived from the first sub-sample, and for verification and reliability of coding. Description of the two sub-sample groups is presented in Table 1.

Design

In this study, a constructivist epistemology (Neimeyer and Neimeyer, 1993) emphasising an assumption that individuals actively construct meaning from experience, was used to provide a foundation to understanding self and identity changes post-brain injury. Definitions of self and identity were taken from social identity theory (Turner, 1982). This describes identities as negotiated in social contexts, consistent with social constructionism, in which there is attention to the importance of context and social interaction on the construction of meaning (e.g., Gergen & Davis, 1985). Social identity theory also notes how such identities may become internalised as representations within the self-concept. Representations making up the self-concept are operationalised in this study as personal constructs, as defined in Kelly's personal construct psychology. The dichotomous constructs elicited are taken to indicate an aspect of internal representation of self and identity. These constructs were the unit of analysis, and were in turn subjected to qualitative data reduction methods to identify themes. The elaboration or salience of themes was established through quantification of the number of constructs making up a theme, thus a theme with a greater proportion of constructs was taken to represent a theme of more general importance to self-construal or self-concept after brain injury. This was considered the most appropriate background to the qualitative design because the epistemology behind it assumes a physical reality (which in this sample might be considered to be the reality of the brain injury), while acknowledging that representations of this reality are mediated through individual interpretation (such as perceived change to self and the meaning of this, consistent with the personal construct literature previously described), and social interaction.

As discussed previously, a personal construct elicitation method (Fransella et al., 2004) was used to identify constructs relating to self that involved three elements: pre-injury, current (post-injury) and ideal (post-injury) selves. The specific procedure used for qualitative data reduction was the inductive phenomenological thematic analysis procedure of Boyatzis (1998). Boyatzis describes thematic analysis as a process of "translating" (Boyatzis, 1998, p.145) qualitative data into quantitative data, thereby having the potential to combine the "richness and uniqueness of qualitative information with precision and discipline of quantitative methods" (Boyatzis, 1998, p.145). This is a systematic process of transformation that organises data and allows for interpretation of aspects of a phenomenon.

Paterson and Scott-Findlay (2002) provide guidance on qualitative interviewing with people with brain injury, noting the difficulty some individuals have responding to open questioning. The personal construct elicitation method employed here, in our view addressed potential problems of interviewing people following brain injury by being both structured and allowing expression of personal perspectives. The group context was also important as individuals developed their ideas in relation to the comments of others with a brain injury. In this way the method aimed to account for the cognitive effects of brain injury on qualitative data collection.

In social constructionist qualitative research it is recognised that researchers' own theoretical and socio-cultural perspectives will influence the analysis, and so making explicit possible influences through researcher reflexivity is recognised as good practice (Yardley, 2000). All researchers were experienced in working with people with brain injury through either research (BR) or clinical practice. The qualified clinical psychologists involved had, between them, specific knowledge, interest and expertise in neuropsychology, cognitive therapy, positive psychology, systemic practice, and neurosciences. One member of the research group was male. White, European, middle class, as well Asian and North American backgrounds were represented.

Procedure

Data collection and analysis was conducted in accordance with the guidelines for reliability and validity of qualitative research, as outlined by Elliot, Fischer, and Rennie (1999) and Yardley (2000), aspects of which will be highlighted in the description below.

Structured group discussion of one-hour duration was facilitated with small groups of participants (varying in size between two and five individuals). A clinical psychologist and assistant psychologist facilitated group discussion according to a procedure covering the following steps:

- The notion of changes in how people see themselves after injury was introduced.

- The ideas of "how I saw myself before my injury, how I see myself now and how I'd like to be" were introduced and a small amount of time allowed for group discussion to establish clarity regarding the nature of the topic.

- Throughout, the group facilitators prompted the group to enable equity of contribution to the discussions by participants.

- The group was asked to think about current and pre-injury selves, specifically responding to the questions: "In what ways do you see your self pre-injury (or current self) as similar to your current self (or self pre-injury)" and "In what ways do you see your self pre-injury (or current self) as different from your current self (or self pre-injury)", consistent with the dyadic comparison method described by Fransella et al. (2004). The group was prompted with more closed or specific questions if required. The group was asked to identify the opposite to each idea or construct and this was also written up on the white-board. Clarification and agreement of the elicited personal constructs was sought from the participant group for each construct.

- After 15 minutes the group was asked to do the same, this time considering current and ideal selves, again for about 15 minutes.

- Finally, pre-injury and ideal selves were compared and contrasted to elicit constructs.

- The assistant psychologist transcribed the constructs identified from the exercise for later analysis.

To carry out the thematic analysis, the five stages of data analysis described by Boyatzis (1998) were conducted. The process of analysis is summarised in Figure 1.

Reducing the raw information.   Initial data reduction occurred during the group exercise. As described above, the facilitated discussions of participants were not fully transcribed and analysed, rather the elicitation of personal constructs from the discussion was seen as an exercise in "in vivo" data reduction. In this way involvement of participants in checking the initial data analysis was ensured, and enhanced the sensitivity of data to its context (Yardley, 2000). Following this, all constructs were entered into a

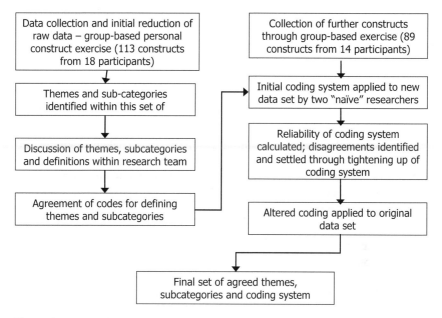

Figure 1. Process of data collection, analysis and development of themes, sub-categories and definitions.

spreadsheet, allowing tracking of decisions and progress in the analysis and contributing to trustworthiness (Elliot et al., 1999) and transparency (Yardley, 2000) of the analysis. An example list of constructs is provided in the appendix.

Identifying themes within the sub-sample groups. A clinical psychologist working on the rehabilitation programme and familiar with the methodology (KP) identified an initial set of manifest themes based on the data collected from sub-sample group 1 ($n = 18$). The themes were reviewed and adapted by two other psychologists (SP and FG). A focus on the overall sense of the bipolar construct was maintained in order to aid categorisation of constructs containing words that could be logically coded under different themes. At times this meant reference back to the context of the initial discussion with participant groups. The themes were then discussed within the team and the theme descriptions and definitions further developed. In accordance with Boyatzis (1998) an attempt was made to provide a rigorous and clear description of each theme, written as a heading with description of what the theme captured, a definition, inclusions and exclusions, examples, and sub-categories of the theme. This was written in such a way as to provide a clear template for further categorisation of data. A final agreed set of themes was established, the headings for which were traceable to the original data and not an abstract interpretation of the data, as recommended by Boyatzis (1998).

Comparing themes across subsamples.   A clinical psychologist (KS) and research assistant (BR), both naïve to the initial data analysis or collection re-categorised a selection of constructs from the first sub-sample of data to check the coding system and identify any potential difficulties in applying it. They then categorised the second sub-sample group ($n = 14$) data by applying the previously devised definitions and descriptions for themes and sub-categories. The aim of this was to develop and adapt the themes if necessary (by seeking further cases through which themes can be tested and developed), establish clarity and rigour of the system for categorising constructs, and tighten up the theme definitions, consistent with Elliot et al.'s (1999) rec-ommendation for using additional researchers to conduct a "credibility check" of the data and analysis.

Creating themes.   Further discussion with the research team enabled clarification of aspects of the coding system, honing and clarifying definitions and the means by which these were arrived at.

Determining the reliability of a theme.   Two of the research team (KS and BR) established reliability of the coding system through comparison of their coding of constructs. This was found to be 89.9% agreement for the main themes, and 76.9% for the subcategories. This is arguably a second "credi-bility check" (Elliot et al., 1999) of the coding system and confirmation of data saturation. During this process, major subcategory disagreements were identified as relating to two issues. There were different interpretations of the term "role" in the subcategory "active self" of the theme "self in the world" such that one researcher themed the constructs as "active self", the other "relationships with others". Also, variation in coding constructs under the theme "self in the world" arose due to different views about the need for subjective experience to be mentioned in the construct.

These discrepancies were discussed further within the research team and definitions developed in order to agree a final set of themes. The final coding key was then applied to the initial sub-sample group 1 ($n = 18$) set of constructs, and amendments made to the categorisation and count of constructs per theme as necessary. The final set of themes is reported as the outcome of the analysis (a shortened form of the coding key including the list of themes, definitions and subcategories is provided in the appendix). Counts of constructs in each theme and sub-category were calculated.

In applying the themes to the second group, then recoding the first group, no new themes were required. In this respect, for this analysis, rigour of the coding system was confirmed and the coding could be seen as having reached "saturation" as described by Glaser and Strauss (1967).

RESULTS

The counts of constructs identified under each theme and subcategory are displayed in Table 2.

Approximately 25% of the constructs elicited fell into the theme relating to "self in the world". This theme was defined in terms of constructs that include reference to both an aspect of activity or social participation (including practical tasks, social interactions, etc.) as well as reference to subjective experience or perception of self in this context. One of these features needed to be present in both poles of the construct, whereas the second feature need only be present in one of the poles. A construct might, for example, include reference to feelings of self-worth, but if reference is also made to the context in which that is felt, the construct was coded accordingly and assigned to the subcategory best representing the nature of the context referred to. This is evident in the constructs described below where there is overlap in some of the words included in constructs across sub-categories. However, given that the overall sense of the whole construct was the focus for categorisation, apparent discrepancies in interpretation based on single words/phrases could be resolved. For example, under each sub-category:

TABLE 2

Count and percentage of constructs elicited per theme for the two sub-sample groups and total sample

Theme	Sub-categories	Gp 1	Gp 2	Total (%)
Experience of self in the world	Belonging, independence, active self, assertiveness, relating	30	21	51 (25.2)
Basic skills	Physical, sensory, cognitive, social	19	18	37 (18.3)
Experience of self in relation to self	Acceptance, sense of self, (awareness)	13	18	31 (15.3)
Coping/outlook	Emotional outlook, strategies	6	14	20 (10)
Emotions	Quality, type	12	5	17 (8.4)
Social relating	Quality of relationships (competence moved to "basic skills: social")	9	5	14 (6.9)
Activity	Physical, practical, social, lifestyle	8	4	12 (6)
Motivation	Interest, effort, caring (bothered)	8	3	11 (5.4)
Uncertainty	Future, finances, past	8	1	9 (4.5)
Total constructs		113	89	202 (100)

Self in the world – Activity

- "engaged, doing things that reinforce who I am – loss of key activities, not doing personally important things"

This clearly describes activity and relates this to 'reinforcement' of identity.

- "can't rely on myself to do things properly – Very organised, skilled and confident"

Doing is mentioned in the first pole of the construct, along with skills in the second, and reference to sense of confidence, so coded under "activity" rather than "confidence".

Self in the world - Assertion, confidence

- "Positive in myself/believe in myself – Not confident"
- "Standing up for myself – Helpless"

Both these constructs imply a social context, and highlight feelings of assertiveness to others.

Self in the world - Belonging

- "Don't feel I fit in, belong – Feeling part of things"
- "Feeling equal with my friends – Feeling betrayed"
- "Struggle to be part of a group, a burden – Feel useful and able to contribute"

Here, connection with social context is the overarching meaning, articulated slightly differently in each of these constructs.

Self in the world - Independence

- "Capable, able, making a contribution – Feel like a waste of space"

While activity and social contexts are both implied in this construct, the overall sense of being an independent person with a contribution to make, fitted more strongly with the "independence" subcategory.

The second most commonly identified constructs were themed as "basic skills", with subcategories relating to cognitive, sensory, physical and social domains. Under this theme, participants' self-construal was clearly related to specific changes in such skills or abilities. For example:

- "Hard to make decisions – Decisive"
- "Energetic – Always tired"
- "Self-centered – Noticing others"

- "Appearing to be rude – Polite"
- "No visual deficits – Visual deficit"

Representing 15.3% of the constructs, the theme "experience of self in relation to self" was defined to describe those constructs in which there was some aspect of self-reflection or dialogue with self stated or implied. Subcategories identified in both sub-groups of data were "sense of self" and "self-acceptance". The subcategory "self-awareness" only arose in the coding of constructs elicited from the first subgroup. Example constructs from this theme include:

Self-acceptance:

- "Happy with how I am – Discontent with myself"
- "Accepting of losses or difficulties – Why me?"
- "Acceptance, moving on – Denial, hatred of what's happened"

Sense of self:

- "I know me, predictable – I've lost me"
- "Can't articulate who I am – Not preoccupied with who I am"

Although "articulation" may imply a context that would lead this to be coded under "self-in the world" theme, the mention of preoccupation in the second pole brings a different overall sense highlighting a more internal process or experience.

- "Feeling out of control – Being in control"
- "Knowledge is power – Ignorance is bliss"

Self-awareness:

- "Not aware of my behaviour – Aware of my behaviour"

Constructs themed as relating to "emotions" included subcategories for "type of emotion" including constructs such as:

- "Get embarrassed easily/quickly – Takes a lot to get embarrassed"
- "Happy – Depressed, sad"
- "Stressed – Relaxed"

The "nature of emotion" subcategory was developed for constructs where participants described altered quality of emotion such as speed, intensity, range of emotion, such as:

- "Enthusiasm, range of emotion, 'wow factor' – emotionally flat, grey, don't get the best out of experiences"

- "More emotional – Less emotional"

- "Familiar, expected controllable feelings – Odd, unexpected, unusual feelings"

Other less frequent themes related to changes in practical aspects of life:

- "Staying in a lot – Going out",

- "Structure to life – No structure"

and motivation:

- "Happy to give up – Determined to see things through"

- "Feeling motivated, getting things done – Lack of motivation"

DISCUSSION

The analysis presented in this study suggests that following brain injury individuals predominantly make sense of themselves in terms of both subjective experience and activity together, highlighting how "meaning and doing" are linked for the participants. Within personal construct theory, a high frequency of a particular type of construct can be considered indicative of a higher level of complexity or elaboration in relation to this aspect of construing. The high proportion of constructs elicited that fall under the "experience of self in the world" theme could thus be considered an indication that following brain injury individuals may be especially concerned with the personal meanings and feelings associated with activity, both practical and social. Perhaps more predictably, the second most frequent constructs fell under the "basic skills" category, suggesting that, in self-construal post-injury cognitive, physical, sensory and social ability changes are significant. Thus construal of self involves perception or experience of changes arising as a result of the injury. The third most common construct fell into the "experience of self in relation to self" theme. Within these constructs participants described the highly personal reflections or dialogues they have with themselves, indicating that existential concerns feature strongly in the process of self-construal after injury. The remaining themes touch on the other ways in which individuals actively construe themselves in terms of their outlook on life, emotional experiences, motivation, lifestyle and uncertainty, reflecting the range of ways in which people make sense of themselves. Reliability and validity of the analysis was pursued through application of principles identified by Elliot et al. (1999) and Yardley (2000).

This, the first study of its kind to elicit and analyse personal constructs of individuals following brain injury endorses the need in rehabilitation to focus on skills in the domains of cognitive, physical, sensory and social functioning. However, from the client's point of view, the need to focus on meaning and activity together might be more important in rehabilitation. For example, in functional goal setting in relation to independent living, one might want to add questions regarding the meaning of the goal. Constructs from this study indicate questions relating to belonging, capability, the extent to which the activity "reinforces who I am", or how the activity helps to "feel part of things" may be pertinent. Alternatively, if emotional adjustment post-injury is the topic of discussion, questions relating personal meanings to examples in specific contexts (including social and interpersonal), goals or activities might be helpful. This notion is already present in some descriptions of clinical practice. For example, William's "twin track approach" notes how psychological therapy (e.g., cognitive-behavioural therapy, CBT) and functionally oriented rehabilitation can reinforce one another, as illustrated by Williams, Evans, and Fleminger (2003). Furthermore, McGrath and King (2004) describe application of "behavioural experiments" in CBT following brain injury, where meanings associated with certain aspects of doing (e.g., "If I try to cook for my family it'll go wrong and they'll laugh at me") are made explicit with the client in advance and then explored, challenged or reinforced through planned activities or tasks (e.g., planning to carry out an achievable cooking task with appropriate strategies to see if this assumption is the case). It is thought that carrying out, then reflecting on the outcome of these experiments with the therapist addresses change at a deeper level of cognitive representation of self (Bennett-Levy et al., 2004). Ylvisaker and Feeney (2000) also describe an approach to brain injury rehabilitation in which reconstruction of identity is central, and the focus of this therapeutic work is always in specific communication or activity contexts. Drawing elements from these approaches, together with Wilson's (2002) emphasis on the systematic application of models in rehabilitation, and Ben-Yishay's holistic approach, Dewar and Gracey (2007) describe a case illustrating how systematically linking activity with personal meanings in interdisciplinary rehabilitation facilitated reduced subjective self-discrepancy.

The study is not without its weaknesses. The sample used here is both small and relatively narrow given the selection of participants via a specific rehabilitation programme, limiting generalisability of findings in terms of both the themes developed, and the frequencies of constructs occurring within each theme. For example, in a sample from a population with higher levels of unawareness or denial of deficit, one might predict fewer constructs relating to cognitive and social "basic skills", as many regarding subjective changes, and a greater number under the "activities" theme (noting for example not being in work, going out less, etc.). This would be consistent with the notion that unawareness especially affects cognitive and social or emotional changes while such individuals may be able to recognise and describe changes in their lifestyle or physical abilities (e.g., Fordyce & Roueche, 1986). Further data collection following the principle of purposive sampling and analysis of this type with a variety of subgroups of individuals would allow further development of the themes arrived at here. Furthermore, the data reduction occurred in vivo, which was helpful in that participants contributed to the derivation of the initial constructs. However, during the coding process and in the research group discussions, disagreements about the application or definition of some themes to specific constructs were resolved by discussing the context of the discussion from which the construct was identified. As such, some contextual data that may have been helpful in supporting theme development was lost. Retention of contextual data through note taking or audio taping during the construct elicitation exercise would have been helpful here at improving relation of constructs elicited and themes derived to the data collection context. It should be recognised that, to an extent, the constructs and themes arrived at from this study are a specific product of the interaction between a set of individuals in one context. Therefore, it is possible that in other contexts alternative results could be arrived at. In order to address this issue, we have endeavoured to demonstrate transparency and trustworthiness of our data and analysis, in keeping with Elliot et al.'s (1999) and Yardley's (2000) guidelines on reliability and validity in qualitative research. The usual approach in deriving a repertory grid is to use a larger number of "elements" (about 10 would be typical), in this case only thre were used: pre-injury, current and ideal self. It is thus possible that the range of constructs elicited is narrower than the range employed by individuals in their self-construal. However, it is nevertheless possible to conclude that the range of constructs elicited, while perhaps not exhaustive, are relevant to self-construal based on these three aspects of self. Finally, the results presented here are restricted to themes derived from group-based data collection and analysis. Analysis of individual ratings of constructs would be required to determine variation in constructs most salient to different aspects of self at different times.

With these caveats in mind, the findings of this study are nevertheless broadly consistent with previous research in that the exercise of self-comparison is evidently meaningful to individuals post-injury, as argued by Tyerman and Humphrey (1984) who suggest that people with brain injury may have more insight than is typically appreciated. By taking as the starting point a presumption that the brain injured individual has subjective experiences, including capacity to comment on their sense of self (even if "lost", altered, discrepant or at odds with others' views), it is possible to develop a finer understanding of the "phenomenological field" (Prigatano, 2000) of our brain injured clients. While Prigatano (2000) expresses the importance of understanding the brain injured person's experience, little guidance is offered for how to do this, given the unique ways in which people are affected by brain injury. Nochi's (Nochi, 1998; Nochi et al., 1997) series of qualitative studies also indicated significant subjective changes that brain injured participants were able to comment on. Consistent with this study, loss of self in one's own eyes (perhaps akin to the "experience of self in relation to self" theme), and in the eyes of others ("experience of self in the world" theme, "belonging" and "relating" sub-categories) emerged as important themes. It could be argued that these studies have included smaller proportions of individuals with impaired self-awareness, thus findings may not be relevant to such individuals. However, findings of a small sample qualitative study by Yeates et al. (2007) suggest that individuals with brain injury identified as having poor awareness were able to reflect on their experiences of themselves in relation to past self and others. It could tentatively be suggested that the findings of the current study, in which subjective experience of self in activities and social contexts is central to sense making, converge with others regarding the possible relationships between interpersonal relating, sense of identity or belonging, and awareness (Shoenberger, Humle, Zeeman, & Teasdale, 2006; Yeates et al., 2007). Further research on this topic, and development of clinical and research tools to help support systematic understanding and intervention of subjective experiences of self following brain injury is required.

A further question we are interested in relates to the capacity for an individual to be able to construe in a certain way given specific areas of organic damage (Rous & Gracey, 2007). For example, Lieberman's (2000) recent review of social neuroscience literature suggests medial frontal areas are associated with understanding internal states. One might predict fewer constructs where reflection on internal, experienced states is required for those with medial frontal damage. There are clearly further applications of a development of this method in research and clinical practice as a tool for assessment of phenomenological experience and evaluation of changes in self-construal after injury and through rehabilitation.

REFERENCES

Baddeley, A., Emslie, H., & Nimmo-Smith, I. (1992). *The speed and capacity of language processing*. Bury St Edmunds, UK: Thames Valley Test Company.
Beck, A. T. (1972). *Depression: Causes and treatment*. Philadelphia: University of Pennsylvania Press.

Bennett-Levy, J., Butler, G., Fennell, M., Hackman, A., Mueller, M., & Westbrook, D. (Eds.) (2004). *Oxford guide to behavioural experiments in cognitive therapy.* Oxford: Oxford University Press.

Ben-Yishay, Y. (2000). Post-acute neuropsychological rehabilitation: A holistic perspective. In A. L. Christensen & B. P. Uzzell (Eds.), *Critical issues in neuropsychology: International handbook of neuropsychological rehabilitation.* Amsterdam: Kluwer Academic.

Blowers, G. H., & O'Connor, K. P. (1995). Construing contexts: Problems and prospects of George Kelly's personal construct psychology. *British Journal of Clinical Psychology, 34(1),* 1–16.

Boyatzis, R. (1998). *Transforming qualitative information: Thematic analysis and code development.* Thousand Oaks, CA: Sage.

Cantor, J., Ashman, T., Schwartz, M. E., Gordon, W. A., Hibbard, M. R., Brown, M., Spielman, L., Charatz, H. J., & Cheng, Z. (2005). The role of self-discrepancy theory in understanding post-traumatic brain injury affective disorders: A pilot study. *Journal of Head Trauma Rehabilitation, 20(6),* 527–543.

Dewar, B-K., & Gracey, F. (2007). "Am not was": Cognitive-behavioural therapy for adjustment and identity change following herpes simplex encephalitis. *Neuropsychological Rehabilitation, 17,* 602–620.

Elliot, R., Fischer, C. T. & Rennie, D. L. (1999). Evolving guidelines for publication of qualitative research studies in psychology and related fields. *British Journal of Clinical Psychology, 38,* 215–229

Ellis-Hill, C. S., & Horn, S. (2000). Change in identity and self-concept: A new theoretical aproach to recovery following a stroke. *Clinical Rehabilitation, 14,* 279–287.

Fordyce, D., & Roueche, J. R. (1986). Changes in perspectives of disability among patients, staff and relatives during rehabilitation of brain injury. *Rehabilitation Psychology, 31,* 217–229.

Fransella, F., Bell, R., & Bannister, D. (2004). *A manual for repertory grid analysis* (2nd Ed.). Chichester, UK: Wiley.

Gergen, K. J., & Davis, K. E. (Eds.). (1985). *The social construction of the person.* New York: Springer-Verlag.

Glaser, B., & Strauss, A. (1967). *The discovery of grounded theory.* Chicago: Aldine.

Goldstein, K. (1959). Notes on the development of my concepts. *Journal of Individual Psychology, 15,* 5–14.

Gutman, S. A., & Napier-Klemic, J. (1995). The experience of head injury on the impairment of gender identity and gender role. *American Journal of Occupational Therapy, 50(7),* 535–544.

Higgins, E. T. (1987). Self-discrepancy: A theory relating self and affect. *Psychological Review, 94,* 319–340.

Kelly, G. A. (1955). *The psychology of personal constructs* (Vol. 1 and 2). New York: Norton.

Lieberman, M. D. (2000). Social cognitive neuroscience: A review of core processes. *Annual Review of Psychology, 58,* 259–289.

McGrath, J., & King, N. (2004). Acquired brain injury. In J. Bennett-Levy, G. Butler, M. Fennell, A. Hackman, M. Mueller, & D. Westbrook (Eds.) *Oxford guide to behavioural experiments in cognitive therapy.* Oxford: Oxford University Press.

Nadell, J. (1991). Towards an existential psychotherapy with the traumatically brain-injured patient. *Cognitive Rehabilitation, 9,* 8–13.

Neimeyer, G. J., & Neimeyer, R. A. (1993). Defining the boundaries of constructivist assessment. In G. J. Neimeyer (Ed.), *Constructivist assessment.* London: Sage Publications.

Nevid, J. S. (2007). Kant, cognitive psychotherapy, and the hardening of the categories. *Psychology and Psychotherapy: Theory, Research and Practice, 80(4),* 605–615.

Nilsson, I., Jansson, L., & Norberg, A. (1997). To meet with a stroke: Patients' experiences and aspects seen through a screen of crises. *Journal of Advanced Nursing, 25(5)*, 953–963.

Nochi, M. (1998). "Loss of self" in the narratives of people with traumatic brain injury: A qualitative analysis. *Social Science and Medicine, 46(7)*, 869–878.

Nochi, M. (2000). Reconstructing self-narratives in coping with traumatic brain injury. *Social Science & Medicine, 51(12)*, 1795–1804.

Paterson, B., & Scott-Findlay, S. (2002). Critical issues in interviewing people with traumatic brain injury. *Qualitative Health Research, 12(3)*, 399–409.

Pidgeon, N., & Henwood, K. (1996). Grounded Theory: Practical implementation. In J. T. Richardson (Ed.), *Handbook of qualitative research methods for psychology and the social sciences*. Leicester, UK: BPS Books.

Prigatano, G. (2000). A brief overview of four principles of neuropsychological rehabilitation. In A.-L. Christiensen & B. Uzzell (Eds.), *International handbook of neuropsychological rehabilitation* (pp. 115–125). New York: Kluwer Academic/Plenum.

Rous, B., & Gracey, F. (2007). *Dimensions of subjective self-construal following brain injury: Possibilities for mapping intra and interpersonal adjustment processes*. Presentation given at NeuroPsychoanalysis Conference, Kings College, London; December 2007.

Schonberger, M., Humle, F., Zeeman, P., & Teasdale, T. (2006). Patient compliance in brain injury rehabilitation in relation to awareness and cognitive and physical improvement. *Neuropsychological Rehabilitation, 16*, 561–578.

Teasdale, J. D., & Barnard, P. J. (1993). *Affect, cognition and change: Remodelling depressive thought*. Hove, UK: Lawrence Erlbaum Associates.

Turner, J. C. (1982). Towards a cognitive redefinition of the social group. In H. Tajfel (Ed.), *Social identity and intergroup relations* (pp. 15–40). Cambridge: Cambridge University Press.

Tyerman, A., & Humphrey, M. (1984). Changes in self-concept following severe head injury. *International Journal of Rehabilitation Research, 7(1)*, 11–23.

Williams, W. H., Evans, J. J., & Fleminger, S. (2003). Neurorehabilitation and cognitive-behaviour therapy of anxiety disorders after brain injury: An overview and case illustration of obsessive-compulsive disorder. *Neuropsychological Rehabilitation, 13(1–2)*, 133–148.

Wilson, B. A. (2002). Towards a comprehensive model of cognitive rehabilitation. *Neuropsychological Rehabilitation, 12*, 97–110.

Winter, D. A. (1992). *Personal construct psychology in clinical practice: Theory, research and applications*. London: Routledge.

Yardley, L. (2000). Dilemmas in qualitative health research. *Psychology and Health, 15*, 215–228.

Yeates, G., Henwood, K., Gracey, F., & Evans, J. (2007). Awareness of disability after acquired brain injury (ABI) and the family context. *Neuropsychological Rehabilitation, 17(2)*, 151–173.

Ylvisaker, M., & Feeney, T. (2000). Construction of identity after traumatic brain injury. *Brain Impairment, 1*, 12–28.

APPENDIX

Example list of bi-polar constructs elicited from a group in sub-sample 2

Have lots of energy	vs	Get tired easily
Able to maintain interest	vs	Lose interest easily
A limited range of physical activities	vs	A range of physical activities
Knowing/understanding your limitations	vs	Not being aware of limitations
Getting used to (accepting) limitations	vs	Finding out what I have to get used to
Finding strategies to help with difficulties	vs	Not finding strategies
Saying the wrong thing at the wrong time	vs	Knowing when and what to say
Good social life	vs	Being lonely
Feeling understood and accepted by others	vs	Being criticised/not being understood
Having a plan for the future	vs	Being uncertain about the future
Feeling "flat"/under-reacting	vs	Feeling emotional, over-reacting
Get wound up easily	vs	Even tempered, not wound up easily, having a "short fuse"
Not aware of inappropriate behaviour	vs	Being aware of my behaviour
Go out a lot	vs	Stay in a lot
Feeling equal with my friends	vs	Feeling betrayed
Not having confidence with relationships	vs	Feeling confident, able to trust
Being able to look on the bright side	vs	Feeling low and down
Being thoughtful and considerate, easy to get on with	vs	Shouting, swearing, being obnoxious
Serious	vs	Comical, joking around
Physically able, feeling strong	vs	Not being able to do things
Serious	vs	Good sense of humour
Knowing myself	vs	Being unsure of myself
Feeling vulnerable to instability	vs	Constantly stable

Coding key themes and descriptions after final analysis and discussion (not including full detail of indicators, exclusions and examples)

General rule for coding: if 2 themes seem present in a construct, decide on (a) which theme is most explicit and (b) which theme is referred to in both poles of the construct.

Theme 1:
Label: Self in Relation to Self
Definition/Description: This code captures how people feel or talk about themselves. There is a reflective or metacognitive component to this code. An articulation of who participants feel they are, or of the processes they feel they are going through.

Theme 2
Label: Activity
Definition/Description: "Things that I do'". Describes change in activity. No reference is made to a feeling, judgement or meaning.

Theme 3
Label: Outlook/Coping
Definition/Description: "The way I cope with and see the world"
This code describes people's constructs around coping and how participants' general outlook, and their emotional response to this outlook has changed. These represent conscious or unconscious coping, which seem to fall into two different areas of:

- Emotional coping.

- Strategies.

Theme 4
Label: Emotion
Definition/Description: Changes in the experience of emotion. There are two main categories in this theme:

- Quality of emotion, which involves speed of the emotion, amount of emotion and the range of the emotion, or controllability and predictability of emotion.

- Type of emotion: Different kinds of emotions are also described, e.g., happiness, sadness, anger, etc.

Theme 5
Label: Experience of Self in the World
Definition/Description: "How I feel and act in the world"
This code describes how people feel about themselves in relation to others and the world around them – subjective experience needs to be evident in one or both poles of the construct, along with stated or implied reference to context. Five sub-categories are identified, covering social, interpersonal and activity contexts:

- Relating with others, belonging, assertiveness: these include reference to sense of self where social context is stated or implied.

- Active self, independence – this describes construal of self where an activity is stated or implied. To use this code there needs to be a statement of personal experience of skills, abilities, and/or capacity in the context of self in the world, e.g., "Engaged, doing things that reinforce who I am – loss of key activities, not doing personally important things" . Sub-category "independence" may also refer to social context as well as activity, e.g., "Capable, able, making a contribution – feel like a waste of space".

Theme 6
Label: Motivation
Definition/Description: "Feelings about doing things". This code describes constructs around interest/drive about things. It also includes lacking in energy and things being more effort, reference to the self is absent.

Theme 7
Label: Social relating
Definition/Description: Describes changes in the quality of social interactions, when reference to the experience of the self, and feelings of the self, are absent. (Competence in social interactions recoded under "Basic skills – social").

Theme 8
Label: Uncertainty
Definition/Description: This is a directly described or implied internal state of uncertainty. This can be identified through terms such as worry, concern, or unsettling feelings associated with these statements. Usually with a future focus or anticipation implied.

Theme 9
Label: Basic Skills and Capacities
Definition/Description: Skills, capacities or deficits people have noted about themselves. Four sub-categories are identified:

- Physical aspects, such as sleep, fatigue, pain, mobility.

- Sensory aspects: vision, hearing, touch.

- Cognitive aspects: prioritising, "organised, decisive", etc.

- Social skills: social Behaviour such as "rude/polite", "think of others/don't think of others".

NEUROPSYCHOLOGICAL REHABILITATION
2008, 18 (5/6), 651–670

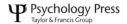

Traumatic brain injury and the construction of identity: A discursive approach

Karen Cloute[1], Annie Mitchell[2], and Phil Yates[3]

[1]*Somerset Partnership NHS and Social Care Trust, Yeovil, UK;* [2]*University of Plymouth, UK;* [3]*Mardon Neuro-Rehabilitation Centre, Exeter, University of Exeter, UK*

Using discourse analysis, this paper explores the co-construction of identity for individuals who have sustained a severe traumatic brain injury (TBI). An analysis of discourse, obtained through interviewing six adults with a TBI, each with one or two significant others, suggested four main interpretative repertoires which informed participants' co-construction of identity: "Medical model referencing", "dependence as intrinsic to TBI", "TBI as deficit" and "progression and productivity as key life-defining features". Medical model referencing is discussed in relation to the common, passive positioning of individuals with TBI, which often occurred in relation to memory loss. The construction of abandonment was also common, due to participants' dependence on the provision of specialist, expert services in the community. Clinical implications are discussed in terms of facilitating individuals in the co-constructing and re-authorship of more empowering and inclusive narratives and providing community services that promote meaningful social identities, separate from medical discourse.

INTRODUCTION

For individuals who have experienced a moderate to severe traumatic brain injury (TBI) (a nondegenerative, noncongenital insult to the brain from an external mechanical force, Dawodu, 2003), the neurological trauma results in an idiosyncratic mix of physical, cognitive and affective impairments.

Correspondence should be sent to Dr. Karen Cloute, The Balidon Centre, Summerlands Site, Preston Road, Yeovil BA20 2BX, UK. E-mail: Karen.Cloute@sompar.nhs.uk

---

DOI:10.1080/09602010701306989

Hidden disabilities are common, including problems with memory, concentration, emotional regulation, fatigue and sleep (Ponsford, 1995; Tate, 2002; Thaxton & Myers, 2002), and these can impact on family and marital relationships, employment and leisure activities (Kendall & Terry, 1996; Morton & Wehman, 1995). At 12 months post-TBI, it is the cognitive and behavioural consequences that appear most prevalent (Ponsford, 1995) with potentially devastating social implications for the survivor.

When considering the complexity of change described above, it is not surprising that individuals have reported "changing significantly 'as a person' as a result of their injury" (Tyerman & Humphrey, 1984, p. 16). Cantor et al. (2005) examined the utility of self-discrepancy theory (SDT) in explaining post-TBI depression and anxiety. The SDT model was expanded to include the discrepancy between the post-injury self and the pre-injury self. The findings suggest that further research is merited to investigate the impact of identity change in addressing issues of post-TBI depression and anxiety. While the literature acknowledges the role of neurological impairment in emotional and motivational disorders (Prigatano, 1992; Williams, 2003), the management of an individual's social identity is also felt to be critical, particularly in terms of psychosocial adjustment (Judd, 1999; Ylvisaker & Feeney, 2000).

Social identity is determined by identification with social reference groups (Vanbeselaere, 1991), yet social networks and contacts are known to be significantly disrupted post-brain injury (Morton & Wehman, 1995). In terms of service provision the UK, the Department of Health (2005) supports the crucial role of community-based rehabilitation and vocational rehabilitation services in promoting social inclusion and participation in meaningful life roles for people with long-term health conditions. Without such support it is accepted that social isolation and psychological problems can arise. The link between social role development and quality of life following brain injury has been established (Steadman-Pare, Colantonio, Ratcliff, Chase, & Vernich, 2001).

The formation and management of social identity is thus understood as an interpersonal process (Tajfel & Turner, 1979; Turner, Hogg, Oakes, Reicher, & Wetherell, 1987) and it is not uncommon to read accounts of individuals who describe a threatened sense of self by way of the labels they feel are imposed upon them (e.g., Nochi, 1998). Olney and Kim (2001) highlight the social stigma of being identified as "disabled" and the burden of explaining this to others and coping with their over-solicitous or invalidating responses, while simultaneously requiring the "label" to obtain needed support services. As such, "managing the perceptions of others" is seen as crucial to identity formation.

Through the use of ethnography, semi-structured interviews and documentary review, Krefting (1989) has provided some insight into the interactional component of identity formation for individuals with moderate head injuries. Three strategies of "concealment", "blind spots" and "redefinition" are described, by which individuals attempt to manage loss of self-identity. However it should be noted that seven out of eight excerpts presented in support of these strategies are comments from parents. Krefting's (1990) second paper, which subjects the same data to thematic and content analysis, outlines a "double bind" model of paradoxical communication. For example, an individual may receive direct messages from family members (as primary care givers) to be independent and responsible, while the contextual parameters identify them as adult dependents, reliant on them for financial, social and physical support.

It is clear that the literature highlights the importance of the interaction between the individual with the head injury and other parties in managing social identity. However, in terms of exploring the actual management *process*, the methodology and underlying epistemology has several limitations. Firstly, the literature base tends to privilege the voice of the carer or other. For example, the "users and carers" section within the Social Services Inspectorate report (1996) on TBI quotes only carers' and professionals' comments. Secondly, analyses tend to present excerpts from each party in isolation. Such research reflects the common positivist assumption that it is theoretically possible to obtain an objective perception of reality, which is accurately reflected by an individual's discourse. Thus, identity structures such as "dependence" are seen to assume a relatively stable and enduring ontological reality, which, although embodied or internalised within the individual, are accessible to inquiry through objective measure or subjective report.

Taking a social constructionist position, i.e., that knowledge is constructed between people in their everyday interactions with one another, avoids such assumptions (Burr, 1995; Gergen, 1985). In understanding the world through our interaction with it, phenomena traditionally thought of as "mental" are seen as being "intersubjectively constituted as the person speaks, writes, reminisces, talks to others and so on" (Potter & Wetherell, 1987, p. 178). In this respect, Widdicombe and Wooffitt (1995) assert that identity is "produced through, and embedded in, everyday forms of language use" (p. 66), rather than merely reflected by it. From this perspective, discourse can be understood as a form of "social action" in and of itself (Potter & Wetherell, 1995). Exploring the implicit negotiations that occur in conversational discourse (discursive negotiations) can therefore help us to understand the social action of identity formation.

In noting the impact of TBI on identity, as well as the importance of the interaction between individuals with a TBI and significant others in the process of identity management, this article explores identity formation using discourse analysis (DA). In interpreting discourse, in this case pieces of conversation, the presence and management of "interpretative repertoires" (IRs) are explored. IRs are understood as "broadly discernible clusters of terms, descriptions and figures of speech" (Potter & Wetherell, 1995, p. 89).

The following questions are asked: (1) What kind of IRs are used by individuals with a TBI and their significant others? and (2) How are they used in conversation to construct aspects of social identity? Finally, through the discussion, the function and consequences of such repertoires are explored at the wider socio-cultural level (Potter & Wetherell, 1987; Widdicombe & Wooffitt, 1995).

METHOD

Background

Interviewing individuals with a TBI with a significant other allows for more naturalistic conversation to occur between participants, increasing the likelihood of each challenging the other's accounts and thus, actively engaging in a process of identity construction. In emphasising the relational aspects of discourse within the text, this approach draws on discursive psychology (see Willig, 2003, for a review of approaches to DA). The work was guided by the principles of accountability and transparency in qualitative research (Elliot, Fischer, & Rennie, 1999) so as to allow readers to judge the trustworthiness of data collection (validity) and trustworthiness of data analysis (reliability) (Stiles, 1993).

Investigations of social meaning are liable to potential bias and therefore qualitative investigators must adopt a reflexive position by acknowledging and reflecting on their own interests in relation to the topic under investigation. All authors are non-disabled; the first and second authors (female) have no experience of neuropsychological rehabilitation of brain injury and were unknown to participants, while the third author (male) has professional experience in this the field. The first author has an interest in psychosocial adaptation to chronic illness and disability and the second author has a strong interest in empowering participants in the research process and functioned as a methodological adviser.

Participants

Discursive data were obtained by audiotaping six interviews conducted with an individual with a TBI (primary participant [PP]; age range 22–60 years; range of years since injury 4–20), together with one or two significant others of their choice (secondary participant [SP]; age range 40–69 years). All PPs had sustained a severe TBI (as defined by a length of coma of over six hours: Sohlberg & Mateer, 2001) as an adult and were now living in the community.

The PPs were first approached, on an opportunity basis, by the managers of Social Services' Adult Disability Teams in Devon (UK) and Headway, Devon (Brain Injury Association), of which they were either past or present users. They were then approached by letter, inviting them to take part. Two individuals approached declined to participate, stating they felt it would be too distressing. Five PPs were male, four with female SPs. In five interviews, SPs were family members and where they were living together, participants chose to be interviewed at home. Further demographics can be seen in Tables 1 and 2.

Data collection

A semi-structured interview schedule was used to elicit conversation around lived experience over time, from before the injury to future aspirations. The schedule and interview protocol were critiqued and refined with an individual from the population pool (Steel, 2004). To aid reflexivity, a research journal was kept and field notes written to reflect on the interview process, relationship dynamics, issues of identity and practical considerations.

The tapes were transcribed verbatim within a week of the interview and drafts checked against the tapes for accuracy. Notation was used for emphasis and delay, with additional observations from the tapes noted in the margins. An initial summary was made of each interview, which helped to highlight their broader action orientation, i.e., what it was *doing* in relation to the researcher, which was useful in interpreting the impact of the interview context.

TABLE 1
Demographic information for primary participants

Primary Participant (PP)	Age range	Years since injury	How injuries sustained	Length of coma	Employment status	
					Pre-injury	Time of interview
Roy	31–40	8	Assault	2 days	House husband	Unemployed
Colin	41–50	16	Assault	1 week	Full-time	Unemployed
James	21–30	7	Fall	Estimated 2–3 weeks	Full-time	Unemployed
Liz	51–60	20	Car accident	3 months	Full-time	Retired
Tom	21–30	4	Fall	3 months	University student	Unemployed
Dan	31–40	18	Car accident	9 days	Full-time	Unemployed

TABLE 2
Demographic information for secondary participants

Primary participant (PP)	Secondary participant 1 (SP1)	Age range	Relationship of SP1 to PP	Secondary participant 2 (SP2)	Age range	Relationship of SP2 to PP
Roy	Amy	31–40	Ex-partner	Linda	51–60	Mother
Colin	Janet	61–70	Mother			
James	Sarah	31–40	Service manager			
Tom	Dave	41–50	Father			
Liz	Harry	51–60	Husband			
Dan	Amanda	51-60	Mother			

Data analysis

The analysis involved cyclical periods of coding, reflecting and writing. To provide a helpful structure to compare interviews, participants' references to time frames were coded (a) pre-injury, (b) post-acute injury (hospital and rehabilitation stay and on return home), (c) intermediate time between "b" and "d" where (d) is current time and (e) is future time. Interpretive repertoires evident in each time frame for each interview were distinguished, compared and contrasted, while considering their potential "social action" in terms of identity construction, as well as issues of reflexivity.

To increase trustworthiness of data analysis, the analysis was reviewed with interested participants (Steel, 2004), as well as with colleagues working in the field of brain injury. Although the analysis presented is one of many possible readings, it is hoped that it provides interesting insights into the construction of identity and potential links to the literature base.

ANALYSIS

The analysis distinguished 29 interpretative repertoires (IRs) (see Table 3), which are conceptualised under four overarching interrelated IRs;

1. Medical model referencing.

2. Dependence as intrinsic to TBI.

3. TBI as deficit.

4. Progression and productivity as key life-defining features.

Common to all interviews, the PPs were often constructed as a passive party; in a sense absence, allowing little or no credibility in the telling of

TABLE 3
Interpretative repertoires for time frames across interviews

Broad repertoires	Specific repertoires by time frame				
	Pre-injury	Post-acute injury	Intermediate	Current	Future
Medical model referencing		TBI as pathology. PPs as not responsible for actions. TBI as requiring specialist health and social care services. Celebrated survivor.	TBI as requiring specialist health and social care services. Professionals as experts. PPs and SPs as abandoned by services.	TBI as pathology. TBI as requiring specialist health and social care services. PPs and SPs as abandoned by services.	PPs and SPs as abandoned by services.
Dependence as intrinsic to TBI		Significant other determination regarding recovery. Significant other guidance as permissible. Problematic care of PPs.	Caring as commitment and sacrifice. Change in traditional sex roles.	Significant other guidance as permissible. Caring as commitment and sacrifice.	Independence as key life-defining feature.
TBI as deficit	The idealised past. TBI as powerful force for change. Memory as indexing emotion.	Memory as indexing emotion. Amnesia as loss of legitimate voice. Memory as all or nothing. Memory as "truth". Memory as valued commodity.	PPs as physically impaired. PPs as victims/at risk.	Memory as power. PPs as socially deficient. PPs as functionally deficient.	Idealised lost potential future.
Progression and productivity as key life-defining features	Work as a primary identifying feature. "Getting on with it": Resilience as strength.	Plateaux as unacceptable. Achievement: Progression vs adaptation.	Progression and productivity indicative of worth. Achievement: Progression vs adaptation.	Progression and productivity indicative of worth.	Work as a primary identifying feature.

their story. This passive construction, or positioning, often occurred around the IRs of medical model referencing and the corresponding IRs of dependence and deficit. Referring to the PPs, the deficit experience of amnesia appeared key in the discursive negotiations around passive positioning.

In the following extract, TBI is co-constructed in terms of medical pathology, requiring intervention from specialist services. Roy (PP), Amy (SP1), his partner at that time, and mother Linda (SP2), emphasise that Roy's specialist needs were not met by general hospital services. With the implicit references to Roy's amnesia and explicit references to his "mental" state, he struggles to hold an active, validated position in the re-telling of the story. Transcription notation is adapted, in part, from Psathas (1995, pp. 70–78) where emphasis: italics; overlap: [; latching between talk: = ; pauses: (·) shortest (..), (...) longest; omitted sections of transcript: '...'; unclear speech: (unclear?); laughter: huhhuhhuh.

Amy:	... they put him on the ward which (.) really didn't specialise I think it was an orthopaedic [ward of some description (.) then he
Linda:	[umm
Amy:	(.) erm (.) had to do *occupational therapy* (.) and it (.) and he's (.) you could see he was (.) mental at the time you know he just (.) and they were *teachin'* 'im how to cook *sausages* and *potatoes* and I had to *sit* (..) and eat this [sausage and potatoes he had actually cooked =
Roy:	[yeah I remember *that* one
Linda:	= ummm =
Amy:	= and [you know and that's all the therapy he got
Roy:	[I remember that
Amy:	[whilst he was up
Linda:	[ummm
Amy:	there (.) an' we *walked* in one day (.) and they said oh we're discharging Roy this afternoon =
Linda:	= umm in that mean time he didn't know me from Adam
Interviewer:	right =
Linda:	= just didn't know me at all he thought I was some (..) a *couple* of times that happened he thought I'd come over from South Africa at one point
Interviewer:	right =
Roy:	= I was out of it yeah but I was totally in a mess

(Int.1, P3, L9–20)

It is argued that Amy and Linda increase the salience of Roy's traumatic injuries by providing emotive memories of events. Amy describes Roy using the arguably disparaging term "mental", indicating that the visible signs of this "pathology" were overlooked. Within her description, Amy communicates her irritation at the inappropriateness of Roy's "therapy". Roy then interrupts to acknowledge that he also remembers certain things, suggesting that there is much he does not remember. His interruption also suggests an urgency to be acknowledged as present at the event, as well as to hold agency in its recall. It is notable that he refrains from adding comment, in addition to factually stating his remembrance.

Roy's inability to offer an account of events positions him as somewhat absent and, therefore, he is unable to own the experience. Linda's description of Roy as not knowing who she was, adds to the sense of him being present in body, but not in mind. That Amy and Linda successfully co-construct Roy in terms of mental incapacity, strongly validates this position, making it difficult for Roy to disagree; "I was out of it, yeah." With its inherent threat to Roy's identity in terms of his sanity, he manages the positioning by stating what he does remember and justifying his behaviour; "But I was totally in a mess." This removes responsibility for his actions, although wavers his right to comment. The medical model of TBI also passively positions Amy, Roy, and Linda as dependent on the provision of more appropriate, expert services, for example Amy was unable to challenge Roy's therapy and discharge.

This pattern of the SP carrying the emotion of the trauma and the negotiations of passive positioning is also notable in Tom, Dan and Liz's interviews. Each of them attempts to manage the positioning and increase their agency in the re-telling of the story, through particular discursive strategies. For example, in the following excerpt, Liz (PP) discusses her time in coma as if an objective observer:

Liz:	. . . the *sister* came over to him (..) and Harry said *this* is the *only* time I *get* to have the *last* word
Interviewer:	humhum
Liz:	and I think the sister thought you *cold* bloody oaf
Interviewer:	humhum
Harry:	there was a time though Liz when (.) you were pretty pretty low (.) in state of coma
Liz:	um =
Harry:	= and they were quite concerned so I I whispered naughty things in your ear I I haha I ha watched the old needle huh suddenly huhhuh move very quickly [an' I knew you were there somewhere huhhuh
Interviewer:	[huff
Liz:	[um (.) and this nurse came rushing down from the *station*

Interviewer: [huhhuh
Harry: yeah but it is it is very peculiar to see one's wife (.) whose head's shaved *totally* inert (.) being you had *physio* every day when you were in coma (.) and then suddenly you'd be put on the tilt bed (. . .) er (.) it was quite surrealistic you know (.) it wasn't *you* it was you were viewing *somebody else*

(Int. 5, P38, L8-P39, L2)

The experience of coma signifies not just a threat to identity, but a significant threat to life. However, Liz's confident account of Harry's conversation with the nurse has the illusory function of positioning her as an objective observer, thus distancing her from the threat while allowing her agency in the conversation. During her narrative, she is able to portray emotion in the experience, for example in describing the urgency of the nurses rushing to the bedside. She also references motivational concerns, such as positioning Harry as a "cold bloody oaf". However, Harry's responses remind us that Liz was actually "pretty low in state of coma", thus emphasising her passivity and shattering the illusion. Although Liz attempts to re-establish some control in the storytelling, in her emotive description of the nurses rushing from their station, Harry reasserts his description of Liz as "*totally* inert", describing her physical manipulation by the physiotherapists. At this point, choosing to describe an account of whispering in Liz's ear, strengthens Harry's concerned and supportive, yet dominant position in the conversation.

Liz also used humour, as did Dan, as a way of remaining active in the joint process of story telling, thus mitigating the disempowerment arising from retelling the experience of coma. Below, Dan's mother Amanda (SP) gives an account of her first visit to Dan (PP) in coma.

Amanda: . . . *I* stayed
Interviewer: yeah
Amanda: slept on the floor in the hospital an (.) in the office (.) [in one of the offices
Interviewer: [really
Dan: that's what *she* said
Amanda: yeah that's what I said [(unclear ?)
Dan: [I reckon she threw me out of *my* bed
Amanda: *no I didn't*
Interviewer: huhhuh umm

(Int.6, P8, L8-12)

Amanda's account of her bedside vigil is highly emotive in its reference to the severity of Dan's condition and her commitment to him. Dan cannot objectively comment on the experience, however he uses humour to access the conversation, which requires and elicits a response from Amanda; *"No I didn't"*. This acknowledges Dan's comment but orientates back to the seriousness of the topic. However, the interviewer's socially appropriate (although perhaps somewhat untactful) laughter, irreversibly detracts from the gravity of the report and Dan's increased agency in the conversation becomes evident.

In contrast to the previous excerpts, the passive positioning in relation to medical model referencing in the following excerpt appears advantageous. James' service manager, Sarah (SP) has suggested that James (PP) feels unable to work.

James:	. . . the trouble is you know if I get a full-time job I'll be all right for a couple of days (..) and then the next two or three days (..) I might have a pounding headache and (.) I wont be going to work (.) so I've had that like I've *had* jobs (. . .) I've had too much time off and all that you know (.) I told my doctor about it an my doctor just told me to (.) *cease work* so
Sarah:	so it's because of your *headaches* and then your [*tiredness* that you
James:	[um yeah
Sarah:	get overtired and yeah and that's that's would you feel those are the two main =
James:	= it's like at the [place of work] when I used to go into work our boss used to say *"Oh oh you're here today then James (.) where have you been all week huhhuhhuhhuh"*

(Int.3, P12, L14-23)

In discussing the trouble of working full-time, James talks about the unpredictable nature of his physical complaints, which Sarah suggests is the primary reason for his unemployment. Although important, the medical co-construction of symptoms positions James as a passive subject at the mercy of his headaches, as opposed to, for example, the recognition of social barriers to successful employment, such as the provision of appropriately flexible working conditions.

The medical model of TBI is also referenced by James' reliance on his general practitioner, whose specialist knowledge affords him/her the right to legitimate James' status of unemployment. Thus, James is not held responsible and is identified as having a socially valued work ethic. This implicit passive positioning is accepted by James, possibly because his status avoids the potential ridicule and social stigma associated with being fired from an unsustainable position.

As opposed to James, Colin (PP), who lives alone, became very irritated in the interview at any attempt to construct a passive identity. Colin was interviewed with his mother, Janet (SP). However, Colin believed he would be interviewed alone. He was irritated at his mother's presence, which, it seems, he felt to be an insult to his independence.

> Colin: . . . I was 'oping it was gonna inter we was gonna-be interviewed separately (.) where Karen interviewed *you* and then *me* (.) *not together*
> Janet: *why was that?*
> Colin: (. . .) well cos (.) (tut) I don't know I mean I'm a big boy now mum I'm I'm
> Janet: *oh I know*
>
> (Int. 2, P2 L17-P3 L2)

For Colin, the dominant IR was progression and productivity as key life-defining features.

> Interviewer: so perhaps you could start by just telling me (.) something a bit about (.) your background erm and what life was like for you before (.) [your head injury
> Colin: [I'd say the same as it is now you've gotta *get on with it* it's no good *arsing* about is it (. . .) urm I'm I'm not a sit *sit round* (..) in a (.) in a hall (.) making papier-mâché *heads* an *so on* (.) I mean (.) these 'ead injuries I mean (.) you *get on* (.) doing by yourself (.) the system holds you back (.) they let you down.
>
> (Int. 2, P1 L1-6)

Colin constructs a sedentary identity for individuals with TBI, which he explicitly rejects, while at the same time implying he has also been "held back" and "let down".

In the following excerpt, Dave (SP) talks about his son Tom (PP) going to college. He despairs at the length of the course and what will happen after Tom has finished.

> Dave: . . . the course is only for 20 weeks (..) but what'll happen to him after that (.) will he just be put back on the scrap heap =
> Interviewer: = huf
> Dave: err because that's how he feels =
> Tom: = um

Dave: err obviously he feels as though and a lot of people and
                      even people we talk to it feels as though Tom has never
                      (.) he had the accident he got help for some time and
                      then all of a sudden boom he's just put aside
                                                        (Int.4, P14, L25-P15, L2)

Dave's questioning of whether or not Tom will be "put back on the scrap heap" implies the presence of an omnipotent third party, with Tom passively waiting for an acknowledgment of his worth. Although Tom acknowledges his father's description of his feelings, the imagery of "scrap heap" is powerfully emotive, possibly making it difficult to disagree. It is also markedly polarised, implying an all or nothing position: you are either on or you are off. It is notable that Tom's injuries are by far the most recent of all the PPs' and his provision of intensive inpatient services was described vividly and with much admiration. Dave talks clearly for Tom in recognising a sudden shift in the provision of help, which appears to contrast early acute services to his experience of living back in the community.

In discussing the college placement, it can be argued that Dave references the IR of progression and productivity as key life-defining features. In referencing this, while acknowledging the experience of being "put aside", a position of abandonment is constructed. It is notable that Tom is the youngest of the participants and his injuries occurred at a time when he was planning and preparing for his future, which may strengthen the position of current and future loss.

As well as Tom's father, Liz's husband and Dan's mother also raised concerns regarding services and/or work/college placements, themselves referencing the importance of progression and productivity and constructing a position of abandonment. As such, it would be interesting to consider how much of the concern around progression and productivity is actually held by significant others, who, living with the PP, is acutely aware of the PP's comparably more limited activities and have their own pressures of caring.

As a female trainee Clinical Psychologist and interviewer, I was constructed as an independent professional, interested in hearing, representing and disseminating the views of participants, which provided the contextual parameters for our conversation. Thus, it is likely I was understood as someone who could disseminate the implicit requests for additional support. In addition, I feel I was receptive to issues of social inequality and in presenting the analysis, I hoped to account for what I perceived to be their feelings of abandonment. In recognising my accountability to participants, I provided an opportunity for them to review and discuss the analysis, with the intention of disseminating their concerns via publication.

It should be noted that the interview context constructed the PP as the main focus; with the interviewer's discourse positioning them as "primary". Therefore, it is interesting that in recalling the time-frame of post-acute injury, the

SPs' discourse is privileged by passively positioning the PPs in relation to their experience of coma and amnesia. As such, this provided SPs with possibly a rare opportunity to validate their own experience of events and associated distress, which may indicate why it appeared to be carefully owned and guarded. Interestingly, emotional concerns are traditionally a female gendered topic. However Liz's husband and Tom's father clearly presented an emotive account of their experiences. It may have been that the presence of a female interviewer, whose job relies on an ability to empathise, implicitly socially validated the sharing of such emotive memories.

DISCUSSION

Overview and critique

The authors identified four overarching interpretative repertoires which informed participants' co-construction of identity: Medical model referencing; dependence as intrinsic to TBI; TBI as deficit; and progression and productivity as key life-defining features. In noting the self-selection of participants in terms of their agreement to the parameters of the research, it is likely that these do not represent all available IR and as such, care is required in discussing the implications of the analysis. However, with reference to quality standards in qualitative research (Elliot, Fischer, & Rennie, 1999), it is the hope that this paper provides a level of transparency that enables readers to judge the validity and reliability of the analysis for themselves and thus allow an informed critique of the impact and importance of the implications discussed here.

A strength of this method lies in the collection of conversational data between three or four individuals. This provided a more natural context than would have been achieved through dyadic interviewing, allowing individuals to challenge (implicitly and explicitly) each other's accounts (Bevan & Bevan, 1999). However, by positioning participants as either "primary" or "secondary", a context of inequality was inadvertently constructed, which requires acknowledgement.

Findings in relation to the literature

The analysis presented demonstrates a common pattern of passive positioning in relation to medical model referencing, with impaired memory appearing as a critical factor. Without clear recollection of events, PPs were less able to "own" their experience, constructing a position of disempowerment. The need to actively reconstruct missing narrative has been explored by Nochi (1997), who conceives of an individual's "void" in past memories as a barrier to self-understanding. Interestingly, Liz, who has had the longest time post-injury, was able to present a coherent narrative of her time in coma, although her active participation in the retelling was implicitly challenged in the discursive negotiations with her husband. Nochi's (2000) later paper, which explores the reconstruction of self-narratives in coping with TBI, acknowledges this interpersonal component. Thus, rather than advocating for professional intervention in terms of helping individuals to "fill in the blanks" (Nochi, 1997, p. 549), he goes on to suggest that any development of self-narrative needs to occur "in interaction with other people, society and culture" (Nochi, 2000, p. 1802).

Social constructionist accounts looking at the co-construction of meaning in health, illness and disability are presented in the literature (e.g., Corker, 2003; Fife, 1994; Scior, 2003; Yardley & Beech, 1998). However, these are often theoretical and/or do not explore interpersonal discursive negotiations. The consequences of referencing medical discourse in relation to subject positioning and identity formation has been discussed, whereby equating disability with illness positions individuals in the passive role of patient, requiring compliance to "expert" medical advice and intervention (Oliver, 1990). This pattern appeared evident here, whereby medical model referencing left participants seemingly dependent upon the active interventions of expert professionals and specialist services, thereby constructing a position of abandonment when referencing community life.

The medical model of disability, which has traditionally founded specialist acute in-patient services (Oliver, 1990), has been criticised for its pathologising nature and inability to support the provision of long-term community-based services (Willer & Corrigan, 1994). Although the social model of disability has gained in stature and respect (Oliver, 1990) and biopsychosocial models of rehabilitation are beginning to inform community provision (Yates, 2003), this study demonstrates that clients still reference medical model discourse, several years post-injury.

Clinical implications

In understanding identity as occurring in conversational discourse, the literature on narrative therapy may provide some useful clinical applications in terms of facilitating individuals in the co-constructing and re-authorship of more empowering and inclusive narratives (White & Epston, 1990). Harry suggested the use of diaries written by the family, not only for the injured party, but also for traumatised family members who may later have limited recall. Real-time diaries have been used in intensive care units to help individuals bridge their memory loss. However, careful assessment is needed to prevent re-traumatising the individual (Bennun, 2004, personal communication). In addition, Liz suggested that keeping newspapers from the time may also be helpful.

The development of specific models of identity construction for this population will be critical in developing and evaluating intervention. Although discourse analysis holds value in exploring how individuals resource prevailing discourse to construct notions of disability and how they are constructed by them (Chamberlain, Stephens, & Lyons, 1997), it has not as yet led to the development of "realist" clinical models. Rather, the knowledge gained can help practitioners to enhance the effectiveness of interventions based on realist models, as demonstrated for example in the expanding literature on "concordance" where application of qualitative understandings of patients' reasons for non-adherence with medical treatment has been shown to be associated with enhanced clinical control and medication use (Dowell, Jones, & Snadden, 2002)

At a service level, this research tentatively suggests that even many years after injury, families are frustrated by a lack of community-based support. The long-term adjustment of families has not traditionally concerned rehabilitation services, although it is now gaining some recognition (Ponsford, Olver, Ponsford, & Nelms, 2003). However, if referencing medical discourse creates the potential for dependency, agencies may need to consider how appropriate services can be provided while referencing more empowering repertoires, in order to facilitate the construction of positive identification. This would require professionals to undertake a process of self-reflection in order to "recognise and develop an awareness of the potential implications of the narratives/ discourses we adapt in our dealings with others" (Burr, 1995, p. 147) and in this way promote "positions in discourses which are less personally damaging" (p. 151). Such an approach has been formulated to assist professionals and clients with disabilities in sharing a philosophy and language to underpin services designed to empower individuals with disabilities towards role engagement and participation in the community (Fenton & Hughes, 1989). By shifting the power dynamics between professional and client towards collaboration and away from medical models, the language, roles and expectations of clients can shift from passivity to a more proactive empowered state.

Services are now recognising the need to help individuals develop meaningful social roles in the community (Yates, 2003) and outcome measures are beginning to reflect the importance placed on achieving personal life goals (Williams, Evans, & Wilson, 1999). McCluskey (2000) has highlighted the important and unexpected roles of paid attendant carers, who can become "protectors", "friends", "coaches" and "negotiators", promoting independence and mobility and increasing clients' social participation. In addition, Willer and Corrigan (1994) present a "whatever it takes" model of community-based services, which, in referencing "normalisation" and "social role valorisation", has maximum self-determination as its goal.

In addition, user involvement in service development could empower individuals through their identification of political activist, while user groups could provide the necessary power to inform and monitor developments, as well as provide means in themselves to help members manage threatened identities (Breakwell, 1986).

Limitations

The limitations of qualitative discursive methodology for those with more severe cognitive or language disorders following TBI are recognised. The methodology employed in this study may pose specific challenges in exploring identity construction for those with more severe impairments. There are also difficulties in utilising "case-focused" qualitative analyses because they compromise generalisation. A further limitation of this particular study was not being able to gain access to participant medical records to obtain clear information on Glasgow Coma Scale scores or length of post-traumatic amnesia in order accurately to determine severity of injury, although length of coma estimates were provided by secondary participants.

Future research

This study highlights the importance of deconstructing discursive negotiations in different socio-cultural settings, such as at home, with friends and with service providers. As Bevan and Bevan (1999) state, in this way, "these multiple contexts reflect, and individuals can reflect upon, the micro-political power present in them" (p. 26). Future research may benefit from exploring these multiple contexts prospectively, as individuals and their families move from hospital, through rehabilitation to the community, which may provide insights into ways of avoiding families' experiences of abandonment.

It is also notable that the empowerment of service users within the research process is rarely referenced in brain injury literature, which suggests this as an area for further development. By involving service users, i.e., clients as well as carers and relatives, we can ensure that the questions we ask are meaningful, that the process is respectful and that the findings are disseminated effectively. In this way, we can remain directly accountable to those individuals we hope to benefit (Blaxter, Thorne, & Mitchell, 2001).

Conclusions

It is hoped that it has been shown that discourse analysis provides a means by which we can begin to understand the dynamic process of identity construction for individuals with brain injuries. By exploring the interpretive repertoires evident in particular contexts, it is possible to consider how individuals are positioned and identified. This study demonstrates that passive positioning is a common occurrence for participants with TBI, particularly in reference to medical discourse. As professionals, by being aware of the impact of our own discourse, we can perhaps engage in conversation that promotes empowering identities for others, although the process by which this may occur requires further exploration. It is our hope that this article provides sufficient insight to stimulate further discussion and exploration into discursive means of understanding TBI and identity, as in the brain injury literature, social constructionist interpretations are rare. Traditionally, survivors of brain injury have been thought incapable of providing "accurate" descriptions of subjective experience (Sbordone, Seyranian & Ruff, 1998); in recognising the potential for co-construction of meaning, they are legitimated a voice.

REFERENCES

Bevan, S., & Bevan, K. (1999). Interviews: meaning in groups. In I. Parker & Bolton Discourse Network (Eds.), *Critical textwork. An introduction to varieties of discourse analysis.* Buckingham, UK: Open University Press.

Blaxter, L., Thorne, L., & Mitchell, A. (2001). *Small voices big noises: Lay involvement in health research. Lessons from other fields.* Exeter, UK: Washington Singer Press.

Breakwell, G. (1986). *Coping with threatened identities.* London, UK: Methuen.

Burr, V. (1995). *An introduction to social constructionism.* London, UK: Routledge.

Cantor, J. B., Ashman, T. A., Schwartz, M. E., Gordon, W. A., Hibbard, M. R., Brown, M., Spielman, L., Charatz, H. J., Cheng, Z. (2005). The role of self-discrepancy theory in understanding post-TBI affective disorders: A pilot study. *Journal of Head Trauma Rehabilitation, 20,* 527–543.

Chamberlain, K., Stephens, C., & Lyons, A. (1997). Encompassing experience: Meanings and methods in health psychology. *Psychology and Health, 12,* 691–709.

Corker, M. (2003). Deafness/Disability – problematising notions of identity, culture and structure. In S. Ridell & N. Watson (Eds.), *Disability, culture and identity.* London, UK: Pearson.

Dawodu, S. (2003). *Traumatic brain injury: Definition, epidemiology, pathophysiology,* Retrieved from: http://www.emedicine.com/pmr/topic212.htm.

Department of Health (2005). *National service framework for long-term conditions.* London UK: Department of Health.

Dowell, J., Jones, A. & Snadden, D. (2002). Exploring medication use to seek concordance with "non-adherent" patients: A qualitative study. *British Journal of General Practice, 52,* 24–32.

Elliot, R., Fischer, C., & Rennie, D. (1999). Evolving guidelines for publication of qualitative research studies in psychology and related fields. *British Journal of Clinical Psychology, 38,* 215–229.

Fenton, M., & Hughes, P. (1989). *Passivity to empowerment.* London, UK: Royal Association for Disability and Rehabilitation.

Fife, B. (1994). The conceptualisation of meaning in illness. *Social Science and Medicine, 38,* 309–316.

Gergen, K. (1985). The social constructionist movement in modern psychology. *American Psychologist, 40,* 266–275.

Judd, T. (1999). *Neuropsychotherapy and community integration, brain illness, emotions, and behavior.* London, UK: Kluwer Academic/Plenum Publishers.

Kendall, E., & Terry, D. (1996). Psychosocial adjustment following closed head injury: A model for understanding individual differences and predicting outcome. *Neuropsychological Rehabilitation, 6*, 101–132.

Krefting, L. (1989). Reintegration into the community after head injury: The results of an ethnographic study. *Occupational Therapy Journal of Research, 9*, 67–83.

Krefting, L. (1990). Double bind and disability: The case of traumatic head injury. *Social Science and Medicine, 30*, 859–865.

McCluskey, A. (2000). Paid attendant carers hold important and unexpected roles which contribute to the lives of people with brain injury. *Brain Injury, 14*, 943–957.

Morton, M., & Wehman, P. (1995). Psychosocial and emotional sequelae of individuals with traumatic brain injury: A literature review and recommendations. *Brain Injury, 9(1)*, 81–92.

Nochi, M. (1997). Dealing with the "void": Traumatic brain injury as a story. *Disability and Society, 12*, 533–555.

Nochi, M. (1998). "Loss of self" in the narratives of people with traumatic brain injuries: A qualitative analysis. *Social Science and Medicine, 46*, 869–878.

Nochi, M. (2000). Reconstructing self-narratives in coping with traumatic brain injury. *Social Science and Medicine, 51*, 1795–1804.

Oliver, M. (1990). *The politics of disablement.* Tavistock, UK: Macmillan.

Olney, M., & Kim, A. (2001). Beyond adjustment: Integration of cognitive disability into identity. *Disability and Society, 16*, 563–583.

Ponsford, J. (1995). *Traumatic brain injury: Rehabilitation for everyday adaptive living.* Hove, UK: Lawrence Erlbaum Associates.

Ponsford, J., Olver, J., Ponsford, M., & Nelms, R. (2003). Long-term adjustment of families following traumatic brain injury where comprehensive rehabilitation has been provided. *Brain Injury, 17*, 453–468.

Potter, J., & Wetherell, M. (1987). *Discourse and social psychology; Beyond attitudes and behaviour.* London, UK: Sage Publications.

Potter, J., & Wetherell, M. (1995). Discourse Analysis. In J. Smith, R. Harre, & L. Langernhove (Eds.), *Rethinking methods in psychology.* London, UK: Sage Publications.

Prigatano, G. (1992). Personality disturbances associated with traumatic brain injury. *Journal of Consulting and Clinical Psychology, 60*, 360–368.

Psathas, G. (1995). *Conversation analysis: The study of talk in interaction.* London, UK: Sage Publications.

Sbordone, R., Seyranian, G., & Ruff, R. (1998). Are the subjective complaints of traumatically brain injured patients reliable? *Brain Injury, 12*, 505–515.

Scior, K. (2003). Using discourse analysis to study the experiences of women with learning disabilities. *Disability and Society, 18*, 779–795.

Social Services Inspectorate (1996). *"A hidden disability": Report of the SSI traumatic brain injury rehabilitation project.* Wetherby, UK: Department of Health.

Sohlberg, M., & Mateer, C. (2001). *Cognitive rehabilitation: An integrative neuropsychological approach.* New York, USA: Guilford Press.

Steadman-Pare, D., Colantonio, A., Ratcliff, G., Chase, S., & Vernich, L. (2001). Factors associated with perceived quality of life many years after traumatic brain injury. *Journal of Head Trauma Rehabilitation, 16*, 330–342.

Steel, R. (Ed.) (2004). *Involving the public in NHS, public health, and social care research: Briefing notes for researchers* (2nd ed.). Eastleigh, UK: Involve Support Unit.

Stiles, W. B. (1993). Quality control in qualitative research. *Clinical Psychology Review, 13*, 593–618.

Tajfel, H., & Turner, J. C. (1979). An integrative theory of intergroup conflict. In W. Austin, S. Worchel (Eds.), *The social psychology of intergroup relations.* Monterey, CA: Brooks/Cole.

Tate, R. (2002). Emotional and social consequence of memory disorders. In A. Baddeley, M. Kopelman, & B. Wilson (Eds.), *The handbook of memory disorders*. New York: John Wiley & Sons.

Thaxton, L., & Myers, M. (2002). Sleep disturbances and their management in patients with brain injury. *Journal of Head Trauma Rehabilitation, 17*, 335–348.

Turner, J. C., Hogg, M. A., Oakes, P. J., Reicher, S. D., & Wetherell, M. S. (1987). *Rediscovering the social group: A self-categorisation theory*. Oxford, UK: Blackwell.

Tyerman, A., & Humphrey, M. (1984). Changes in self-concept following severe head injury. *International Journal of Rehabilitation Research, 7*, 11–23.

Vanbeselaere, N. (1991). The impact of in-group and out-group homogeneity/heterogeneity upon intergroup relations. *Basic and Applied Social Psychology, 12*, 291–301.

White, M., & Epston, D. (1990). *Narrative means to therapeutic ends*. New York: Norton.

Widdicombe, S., & Wooffitt, R. (1995). *The language of youth subcultures*. London: Harvester Wheatsheaf.

Willer, B., & Corrrigan, J. (1994). Whatever it takes: A model for community-based services. *Brain Injury, 8*, 647–659.

Williams, W. H. (2003). Rehabilitation of emotional disorders following acquired brain injury. In B. Wilson (Ed.), *Neuropsychological rehabilitation: Theory and practice*. Lisse: Swets & Zeitlinger.

Williams, W. H., Evans, J. J., & Wilson, B. A. (1999). Outcome measures for survivors of acquired brain injury in day and outpatient neurorehabilitation programmes. *Neuropsychological Rehabilitation, 9*, 421–436.

Willig, C. (2003). Discourse analysis. In J. Smith (Ed.), *Qualitative psychology; A practical guide to research methods*. London: Sage Publications.

Yardley, L., & Beech, S. (1998). "I'm not a doctor." Deconstructing the accounts of coping, causes and control of dizziness. *Journal of Health Psychology, 3*, 313–327.

Yates, P. (2003). Psychological adjustment, social enablement and community integration following acquired brain injury. In H. Williams & J. Evans (Eds.), *Biopsychosocial approaches in neurorehabilitation; Assessment and management of neuropsychiatric, mood and behavioural disorders*. Hove, UK: Psychology Press.

Ylvisaker, M., & Feeney, T. (2000). Reconstruction of identity after brain injury. *Brain Impairment, 1*, 12–28.

NEUROPSYCHOLOGICAL REHABILITATION
2008, 18 (5/6), 671–691

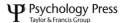

Maintaining group memberships: Social identity continuity predicts well-being after stroke

Catherine Haslam, Abigail Holme, S. Alexander Haslam,
Aarti Iyer, Jolanda Jetten, and W. Huw Williams

University of Exeter, Exeter, UK

A survey study of patients recovering from stroke ($N = 53$) examined the extent to which belonging to multiple groups prior to stroke and the maintenance of those group memberships (as measured by the Exeter Identity Transitions Scales, EXITS) predicted well-being after stroke. Results of correlation analysis showed that life satisfaction was associated both with multiple group memberships prior to stroke and with the maintenance of group memberships. Path analysis indicated that belonging to multiple groups was associated with maintained well-being because there was a greater likelihood that some of those memberships would be preserved after stroke-related life transition. Furthermore, it was found that cognitive failures compromised well-being in part because they made it hard for individuals to maintain group memberships post-stroke. These findings highlight the importance of social identity continuity in facilitating well-being following stroke and, more broadly, show the theoretical contribution that a social identity approach to mental health can make in the context of neuropsychological rehabilitation.

INTRODUCTION

A large body of research attests to the fact that many life transitions impact negatively on well-being, at least in the short-term (Sani, in press). This is

---

Correspondence should be addressed to Catherine Haslam, School of Psychology, University of Exeter, Exeter, Devon, EX4 4QG, UK. E-mail: C.Haslam@exeter.ac.uk

The research reported in this paper was supported by a grant from the Economic and Social Research Council (RES-062-23-0135).

---

because even positive transitions that are perceived to be "a change for the better" routinely bring with them upheaval, challenge and uncertainty. When people undergo negative life transitions (e.g., loss of job or home) the potential threat to well-being is all the more pronounced (e.g., Aneshensel, Botticello, & Yamamoto-Mitani, 2004; Dyson & Renk, 2006; Ethier & Deaux, 1994). This is particularly apparent where the transition itself entails some deterioration in intellectual ability — as is the case when individuals suffer from stroke. Such an unplanned transition requires significant adjustment and if not managed appropriately, can compromise well-being (e.g., Clarke & Black, 2005; Clarke, Marshall, Black, & Colantonio, 2002; Kim, Warren, Madill, & Hadley, 1999; King, 1996; Williams, Weinberger, Harris, & Biller, 1999; Wyller, Sveen, Sodring, Pettersen, & Bautz-Holter, 1997). The present paper investigates individuals' adjustment following stroke, and in particular considers the factors that predict their day-to-day work, life satisfaction and level of chronic stress. However, departing from the focus of previous research in this area, our emphasis is on the role that group memberships play in the adjustment process. This interest derives from evidence in the social psychological litera-ture that these memberships are central to the way people experience and respond to change because they furnish them with a sense of social identity (Tajfel, 1972; Turner, 1982).

Social identity and the importance of group memberships

According to social identity theory (Tajfel & Turner, 1979) and self-categorisation theory (Turner, 1982; Turner, Oakes, Haslam, & McGarty, 1994), group memberships are not external to a person's sense of self; rather they are often internalised and incorporated into a person's global sense of self (i.e., who they are, what they stand for, and what they do). As Turner suggests, group memberships form the basis of both our social and personal identities and hence are not always readily separable (e.g., Turner, Reynolds, Haslam, & Veenstra, 2006). Moreover, group memberships tend to have positive implications for well-being and play an important role in helping individuals adjust to the transitions they experience throughout life (Reicher & Haslam, 2006). A positive transition may involve moving to a higher-status group (e.g., a more prestigious organisation, a more desirable neighbourhood) and the positive implications of this for self-esteem can help counteract any adverse consequences of change itself. A corollary of this, though, is that negative life changes often involve loss of such member-ships or movement into less attractive groups — and this can accentuate pro-blems of uncertainty and challenge. In this context, people are often reluctant to forgo valued group memberships (Ellemers, 2003), and display consider-able resistance to new group memberships that are imposed upon them

(Jetten, O'Brien, & Trindall, 2002), especially if those group memberships are perceived to have lower status (Van Knippenberg, Van Knippenberg, Monden, & de Lima, 2002).

Consistent with this argument, many individuals who suffer from acquired brain injury, including stroke, find it necessary to give up professional identities (Bergmann, Kuthmann, Vonungernsternberg, & Weimann, 1991). They may be forced to leave recreational groups or to move out of the community and into care due to disability. Such changes constitute major social identity threats (Branscombe, Ellemers, Spears, & Doosje, 1999a; Breakwell, 1986), which may be critical to one's self-esteem and well-being. Rates of depression, for instance, are high in the stroke population (e.g., Brodaty, Withall, Altendorf, & Sachdev, 2007; Hackett, Yapa, Parag & Anderson, 2005; Kotila, Numminen, Waltimo, & Kaste, 1998; Robinson & Price, 1982; Robinson, Starr, Kubos, & Price, 1983; Robinson, Starr, & Price, 1984; Robinson, Bolduc, & Price, 1987) and yet they are typically attributed to neurophysiological (e.g., depletion of intra-cerebral neurotransmitters, Gainotti, Antonucci, Marra, & Paolucci, 2001; Wiart, 1997) and anatomical factors (e.g., location of lesion, MacHale, O'Rourke, Wardlaw, & Dennis, 1998; Torrecillas, Mendlewicz, & Lobo, 1997) rather than social factors.

There are many ways in which social identity can enhance well-being. In particular, a large body of evidence suggests that it provides the basis for individuals to receive and benefit from social support (Aspinwall & Taylor, 1997; Cohen & Wills, 1985; Underwood, 2000; for a detailed theoretical discussion see Haslam, 2004). Research has shown (a) that individuals are more likely to give and receive support from others with whom they perceive themselves to share a social identity (e.g., family members, colleagues; Haslam, O'Brien, Jetten, Vordemal, & Penna, 2005; Levine, Cassidy, Brazier, & Reicher, 2002; Levine, Prosser, Evans, & Reicher, 2005), and (b) that shared social identity is also a basis for any support to be interpreted positively (Haslam, Jetten, O'Brien, & Jacobs, 2004). When it is received, such social support also has the capacity to buffer people from the negative consequences of potentially stressful life events in a number of ways (Branscombe, Schmitt, & Harvey, 1999b; Cohen & Syme, 1985; House, 1981; Postmes & Branscombe, 2002). Specifically, it can provide people with (a) a sense of acceptance and self-worth (emotional support), (b) affiliation and contact with others (social companionship), (c) concrete aid, material resources, and financial assistance (instrumental support), and (d) information that is useful in understanding and coping with the challenges they face (informational support).

A number of epidemiological and longitudinal studies point to the importance of various forms of social support in predicting the long-term outcomes of patients with acquired brain injury (e.g., Beckley, 2006; Zencius & Wesolowski, 1999). For example in Beckley's (2006) research involving stroke sufferers, social support was found to moderate the relationship between functional limitation and the individuals' ability to participate in the community — where support was low, participation was predicted simply by functional competence, but where it was high, social support appeared to help individuals overcome their functional limitations. The importance of social support networks was also highlighted by Clarke et al. (2002) in research which found that satisfaction with these networks was associated with higher scores on several well-being indicators. Moreover, qualitative analyses of individuals recovering from stroke suggest that a person's subjective quality of life is determined as much (if not more) by their (re)engagement with the social world as by discrete physical function (Burton, 2000; Clarke & Black, 2005; Olofsson, Andersson, & Carlberg, 2005). These findings highlight the importance of addressing social processes and dynamics not only when considering community reintegration but at all stages of the rehabilitation process (e.g., Bendz, 2003; Pajalic, Karlsson, & Westergren, 2006).

The importance of multiple group memberships

The above analysis points to the fact that group memberships can make an important contribution to individuals' well-being. A question that follows is whether that contribution is moderated by the number of groups that a person belongs to. Although this issue has never (to our knowledge) been examined in the context of stroke recovery, it is one on which there are opposing views. On the one hand, role theorists have argued that having multiple roles or identities compromises well-being due the uncertainty and stress caused by role conflict and confusion (Marks, 1977; Seiber, 1974). In contrast, others have argued that — providing they are not inherently incompatible (Iyer, Jetten, Tsivrikos, Postmes, & Haslam, 2007) — access to multiple social identities increases "existential security" (Thoits, 1983, p. 175; see also Durkheim, 1951) and can thereby enhance mental health (Sarbin & Allen, 1968; Thoits, 1983).

This link between multiple identities and well-being is important for several reasons. First, having multiple identities can be seen to provide individuals with a source of social capital that buffers them from any negative consequences associated with identity change or identity loss (Bourdieu, 1979/1984; see also Bassuk, Glass, & Berkman, 1999; Burt, 1997; Hays & Oxley, 1986; Hirsch, 1981; Kawachi & Berkman, 2001; Puttnam, 2000). People who have only one source of social identity (e.g., their family, their work) are more vulnerable to the effects of change (e.g., the death of a family member, retirement) because their sense of self is invested exclusively in one group membership. Second, multiple identities provide people with more sources of support to draw on in times of difficulty and stress. When the ship of self encompasses more group memberships, it has more ports in which to find shelter if it is caught in a storm. Consistent with this idea Iyer et al. (2007, Study 2), found an association between the number of groups that first year university students were members of, and the amount of social support they reported receiving. Finally, the experience of managing multiple groups allows individuals to develop cognitive skills and flexibility that are useful intellectual resources in times of uncertainty and change. Support for this idea comes from research which indicates that individuals whose self-definition incorporates a greater number of independent self-schema (i.e., greater self-complexity; Linville, 1985) are better buffered against the negative effects of stressful life events than those whose self-complexity is lower (e.g., Steinberg, Pineles, Gardner, & Mineka, 2003; Woolfolk et al., 1999).

The importance of maintained group memberships

The existing evidence suggests that group memberships are a source of social psychological resources (or capital) that individuals can draw upon to enhance their well-being or protect themselves from threat. In reality, these resources are not static but are an ongoing source of self-definition and self-esteem (Iyer, Jetten, & Tsivrikos, in press; Sani, in press). Accordingly, the benefit of multiple group memberships may derive not (only) from the fact that these memberships enhance the resources available to the individual but (also) from the fact that where an individual is a member of multiple groups, there is a greater likelihood that he or she will be able to maintain at least some of these memberships following a life-changing event. Psychologically speaking, having one's eggs in multiple baskets enhances the likelihood of having some of those eggs intact after an accident.

This point is significant as there is growing evidence that, like social identity itself, social identity continuity (also known as collective continuity, cultural continuity) is an important determinant of a person's subjective well-being (Bluck & Alea, in press; Iyer et al., in press). Although there is little research examining the importance of social identity continuity in the general clinical population, it seems reasonable to assume that these factors would also contribute to their well-being. Anecdotal evidence is provided by Clarke and Black (2005) who studied the impact of maintained group membership on the well-being of a stroke survivor, Mrs NM, observing that her continued involvement in a tai chi class appeared to produce a significant improvement in quality of life. On the basis of these arguments, we would predict that well-being would be compromised to the extent that a stroke brings about changes that disrupt a person's connection with their past. However, a person's membership of multiple groups prior to the stroke may offer some protection by increasing the likelihood of maintained connection with the past (i.e., social identity continuity).

The present study

Although the arguments developed in the previous sections have received some support in the social psychological literature and in a range of non-clinical settings, they have not been tested in neurological populations. The present study attempted to address this gap by exploring the relationship between multiple and maintained group memberships and well-being in a clinical population comprised of stroke sufferers who were in contact with providers of community services.

Our predictions are represented schematically in Figure 1. First, we predict that the well-being of people recovering from stroke will be enhanced to the extent that they had belonged to multiple groups prior to the stroke (i.e., Hypothesis 1; H1). Second, well-being will be further enhanced to the extent that people are able to maintain membership of the groups that they belonged to prior to the stroke (i.e., H2). Related to this, we would expect that the relationship between multiple group membership and well-being will be mediated by continuity, or maintenance, of pre-stroke group memberships (i.e., H3). In addition, reports of cognitive impairment require consideration, given their impact on well-being following stroke (e.g., Clarke et al., 2002; Starchina et al., 2007) and their potential to hinder social identity continuity. Having more cognitive failures would tend to indicate that a person would be cognitively less well equipped to maintain group memberships. We address this in our final hypothesis and predict that the relationship between cognitive failures and well-being will be mediated by a person's inability to maintain group memberships after stroke (i.e., H4).

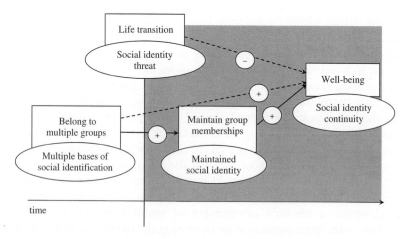

Figure 1. A schematic representation of relationships predicted under H1–H3.

METHOD

Participants

Participants were 53 recovering stroke patients in Cornwall, UK, over the age of 18 years, who were recruited on average 8.6 months ($SD = 5.1$ months) after their most recent stroke. Seven stroke care co-ordinators invited people on their caseloads to take part in the study and of the 66 people referred, three could not be contacted and 10 did not wish to take part. The sample comprised 34 men and 19 women whose ages ranged from 28 to 86 years ($M = 65.77$, $SD = 12.76$ years). Two-thirds of the participants ($N = 36$, 68%) were recovering from their first stroke, 10 (19%) were recovering from their second, and seven (13%) had experienced three or more strokes. No participant had (a) suffered any other form of brain injury (e.g., traumatic brain injury), (b) a previous psychiatric history (including clinical depression, psychosis or anxiety, personality or adjustment disorders), or (c) significant comprehension difficulties (as judged by stroke care co-ordinators) that would impact on understanding the questionnaires administered.

Procedure

After providing informed consent to take part in the study, participants were given a four-page questionnaire which they completed individually. They were then fully debriefed and thanked for their participation.

Measures

Group membership listings

Participants were asked to list the various groups that they considered themselves to be members of currently and to have been members of in the past. More specifically, the first question asked participants to list the groups they belonged to before their stroke and the second asked them to list the groups that they now belonged to after their stroke. Instructions stated that "These groups could take any form – for example, they could be work groups, professional groups, social groups, or sporting groups". Any grouping was permitted provided it was unique (i.e., so that it did not overlap with another listed)[1]. For purposes of analysis, the total number of unique groups that participants belonged to pre- and post-stroke was computed.

---

[1]Uniqueness was determined by one of the authors and only accepted if confirmed independently by another author.

Group affiliation ratings – EXITS

The questionnaire included a number of multiple-item measures designed to assess predictors of interest. Referred to as the Exeter Identity Transition Scales (EXITS), these were developed to examine group membership. Participants completed all items using seven-point scales (1 = do not agree at all, 7 = agree completely).

Multiple group memberships before stroke. Four items ($\alpha = .93$) assessed the extent to which participants had belonged to multiple groups before their stroke. These items were: "Before my stroke I belonged to lots of different groups", "Before my stroke, I joined in the activities of lots of different groups", "Before my stroke I had friends who were members of lots of different groups", and "Before my stroke I had strong ties with lots of different groups".

Maintenance of group memberships after stroke. Four items ($\alpha = .94$) were used to assess whether participants had maintained their pre-stroke group memberships after their most recent stroke. These items were: "After my stroke, I still belong to the same groups I was a member of before my stroke", "After my stroke, I still join in the same group activities as before my stroke", "After my stroke, I am friends with people in the same groups as I was before my stroke", and "After my stroke, I continue to have strong ties with the same groups as before my stroke".

New group memberships. Finally, four items ($\alpha = .85$) assessed whether participants had joined new groups after their most recent stroke, mirroring those for the previous scale. These items were, "After my stroke, I have joined one or more new groups", "After my stroke, I have joined the activities of new groups", "After my stroke, I am friends with people from one or more of these new groups", and "After my stroke, I have strong ties with one or more new groups".

Cognitive Failures Questionnaire (CFQ)

To assess their level of perceived cognitive function, participants were asked to complete the 25-item Cognitive Failures Questionnaire (Broadbent, Cooper, FitzGerald, & Parkes, 1982) for self-assessment. Items in this measure assessed the frequency of cognitive errors participants made in their daily lives over the previous six-month period. They did this by responding to questions such as "Do you fail to notice signposts on the road?" and "Do you fail to see what you want in a supermarket (although it's there)?" on five-point scales (0 = never, 4 = very often).

Dependent variables

Multiple-item measures were also used to assess two outcome variables of interest. Again, participants indicated their level of agreement with all items using seven-point response scales ($1 =$ do not agree at all, $7 =$ agree completely).

Life satisfaction.   Six items ($\alpha = .92$) assessed the extent to which participants were satisfied with their life after their stroke. These items related both to their life in general and to their daily work (e.g., chores and activities that they performed). These items were: "The conditions of my life are excellent", "My life is close to ideal", "I am satisfied with my life", "I enjoy my work", "I think the work I do is worth while", "My work is varied and interesting" (as used by Haslam et al., 2005).

Chronic stress.   Five items ($\alpha = .67$) assessed participants' feelings of chronic stress after their stroke. Items reflected the three core components of burnout (see Haslam, 2004; Haslam & Reicher, 2006): exhaustion ("I feel that I am working too hard" and "I feel energetic" [reverse-scored]), lack of accomplishment ("I feel I accomplish many worthwhile things in my life" [reverse-scored]), and callousness or depersonalisation ("I don't really care about what happens to my colleagues any more" and "I feel that I am becoming callous towards people").

RESULTS

Table 1 presents the descriptive statistics and inter-item correlations for all measures. Participants' listings of group memberships indicated that they belonged to an average of 1.74 groups (range: 0–9) before their stroke, and, after this, maintained an average of 1 (range: 0–5) old group membership. In general, they had not (yet) joined new groups after their most recent stroke ($M = 0.09$; range: 0–2).

Correlations

Relationships between group membership measures

As shown in Table 1, maintenance of pre-stroke group memberships after a stroke was correlated with having multiple group memberships before the stroke (group listings: $r = .75$, $p < .01$; group affiliation ratings: $r = .47$, $p < .01$). Gaining new group memberships after the stroke was associated with having multiple group memberships before the stroke (although his

TABLE 1
Descriptive statistics and bivariate correlations

Group	Mean (SD)	No. scale items	Scale α	Group affiliation listings		Neuro ψ ratings (EXITS)			Outcome predictor	Variables	
				No. old groups post-stroke	No. new groups post-stroke	Multiple groups pre-stroke	Old groups post-stroke	New groups post-stroke	CFQ	Life satisfaction	Chronic stress
Group listings											
No. groups pre-stroke	1.74 (2.23)			.75**	.06	.58**	.45**	.33*	.02	.27*	−.15
No. old groups post-stroke	1.01 (1.79)				.07	.60**	.60**	.34*	−.19	.40**	−.29*
No. new groups post-stroke	0.09 (0.35)					.19	.06	.54**	.00	−.11	−.10
Group affiliation ratings (EXITS)											
Belong to multiple group pre-stroke	2.94 (2.19)	4	.93				.47**	.37**	−.06	.27*	−.22
Belong to old groups post-stroke	3.94 (2.53)	4	.94					.18	−.30*	.47**	−.44**
Belong to new groups post-stroke	1.62 (1.22)	4	.85						.20	.01	.16
Neuropsychological predictor											
CFQ	36.96 (19.77)	25								−.36*	.26°
Outcome variables (DVs)											
Life satisfaction	3.89 (1.92)	6	.92								−.73**
Chronic stress	3.43 (1.31)	5	.67								

*p ≤ .05; **p ≤ .01; °p ≤ .10 (2-tailed). CFQ: Cognitive failures questionnaire.

pattern was only apparent for group affiliation ratings: $r = .37$, $p < .01$) but not with the maintenance of old group memberships.

Taken together, these patterns suggest that individuals who hold multiple group memberships prior to a stroke are more likely to maintain them after the stroke, and are also more likely to develop new group memberships. In addition, the development of new group memberships after a stroke is independent of the maintenance of old group memberships. In other words, the effort taken to maintain old group memberships does not seem to affect individuals' ability to join new groups.

Relationships between group memberships and well-being

Correlations between patterns of group membership and measures of well-being are also presented in Table 1. Consistent with H1, it is apparent that having multiple group memberships prior to the stroke (assessed through both group listings and group affiliation ratings) was associated with greater life satisfaction post-stroke, but was unrelated to chronic stress. Consistent with H2, the maintenance of old group memberships after the stroke (again assessed through both group listings and group affiliation ratings) was also correlated with both well-being measures—being positively correlated with life satisfaction and negatively correlated with stress. Participants' well-being was not associated with the number of new group memberships acquired post-stroke (which might reflect the low number of new groups individuals acquired).

Relationships between cognitive failures and well-being

As observed in previous research (e.g., Broadbent et al., 1982; Mahoney, Dalby, & King, 1998; Smith, Petersen, Ivnik, Malec, & Tangalos, 1996), there was a significant negative relationship between participants' reports of their cognitive failures and their well-being, such that the more cognitive failures people perceived themselves to have the more dissatisfied they reported being with their life and the more likely they were to experience chronic stress (although the latter effect was only marginally significant; $p = .06$). Interestingly too, the incidence of perceived cognitive failures was also negatively correlated with participants' reports of their ability to maintain pre-existing group memberships after their stroke.

Mediational analysis

In addition to the above hypotheses, H3 suggests that the positive effect of multiple group memberships on well-being should be explained by the maintenance of these group memberships in the context of changes resulting from stroke. To test this mediational hypothesis, separate path analyses were performed on both the group listings and group affiliation ratings data to examine the role that maintenance of group memberships played in mediating between membership of multiple groups prior to stroke and life satisfaction (the dependent measure with which it was correlated).

Following procedures outlined by Baron and Kenny (1986), these analyses involved (a) regressing the mediator (m, maintained group memberships) on the independent variable (i, multiple group memberships), (b) regressing the dependent variable (d; life satisfaction) on multiple group memberships, and (c) regressing the dependent variable on both multiple group memberships and maintained group memberships. For mediation to be present, there must be a significant relationship between the mediator and the independent variable (which there was for both group listings, $\beta = .75$, $p < .01$, and group affiliation ratings, $\beta = .47$, $p < .01$), but when the dependent variable is regressed on both the mediator and independent variable, a previously significant relationship between the independent and dependent variables should be significantly reduced or rendered non-significant.

As Figure 2 indicates, when life satisfaction was regressed on the listed number of maintained group memberships and the listed number of group memberships prior to stoke, the relationship between life satisfaction and number of group memberships became non-significant and was significantly reduced (applying Sobel's Test, Preacher & Leonardelli, 2001; $z = 2.37$, $p < .02$). Similarly, as Figure 3 indicates, when life satisfaction was regressed on group affiliation ratings of maintained group memberships and group affiliation ratings of multiple group memberships prior to stroke, the relationship between life satisfaction and multiple group memberships became non-significant and was significantly reduced ($z = 2.95$, $p < .01$). These analyses provide evidence of full mediation supporting the view that belonging to a larger number of groups prior to stroke predicts well-being post-stroke because individuals who belong to multiple groups are more likely to maintain these group memberships than are those who belong to fewer groups.

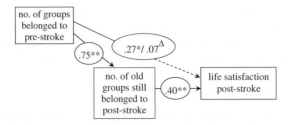

Figure 2. Mediation analysis for group membership listings.
Correlations: $^{**}p \leq .01$; $^{*}p \leq .05$; change: $^{\Delta}p \leq .05$; dotted lines indicate where a previously significant relationship is rendered non-significant.

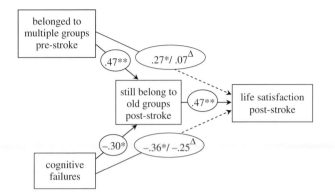

Figure 3. Mediation analysis for group affiliation ratings (EXITS).
Correlations: $**p \leq .01$; $*p \leq .05$; change: $^{\Delta}p \leq .05$, $^{\Delta}p \leq .10$; dotted lines indicate where a previously significant relationship is rendered non-significant.

The observed relationships between reports of cognitive failures and both life satisfaction and ratings of group membership maintenance also allowed mediational analysis to be conducted in order to test H4. As Figure 3 indicates, when life satisfaction was regressed on these two measures simultaneously, the relationship between cognitive failures and life satisfaction was reduced ($z = 1.78$, $p < .07$) and became non-significant. Although this reduction was only marginally significant, this pattern is consistent with the suggestion that one important reason why cognitive failures compromise stroke sufferers' well-being is that they interfere with their ability maintain valued group memberships.

DISCUSSION

The above findings reveal a pattern of relationships that is highly consistent with hypotheses derived from a social identity approach to clinical well-being that emphasises the importance of both social identities in general and social identity continuity in particular. In the first instance, as predicted under H1, there was evidence that individuals who had belonged to multiple groups prior to their strokes were more likely to report higher levels of well-being after their stroke. However, while this relationship was of moderate strength in the case of reported life satisfaction and apparent from both group listings group affiliation ratings, it was weaker (and non-significant) in the case of chronic stress. More pronounced, though, was the relationship, predicted under H2, between well-being and reports that pre-existing group memberships had been maintained after the stroke. This relationship was revealed with respect to both group listings and group affiliation ratings, and was apparent on measures of both stress and life satisfaction.

Furthermore, consistent with H3, path analysis provided evidence that support for H1 could largely be attributed to the relationship between maintained group memberships and life satisfaction. That is, there was evidence that the relationship between multiple group memberships and life satisfaction was fully mediated by maintained group memberships. This supports the view that multiple group memberships promoted well-being because there was a greater likelihood of these being preserved after a stroke than there was if participants had previously belonged to fewer groups.

Consistent with previous research (e.g., Clarke et al., 2002; Starchina et al., 2007), it was also apparent that stroke sufferers' perceptions of cognitive failures were generally predictive of their well-being—with a higher incidence of these failures being associated with reduced life satisfaction. A novel finding here, though, was that these perceived failures were also associated with participants' inability to maintain membership of groups to which they had belonged before their stroke. Other factors, such as mood, could have influenced perceptions of cognitive failure (e.g., see Farrin, Hull, Unwin, Wykes, & David, 2003; Merckelbach, Muris, Nijman & de Jong, 1996, for evidence of a relationship between depression and reports of cognitive problems), but in the absence of these data it is difficult to determine their impact. Nevertheless, consistent with H4, mediational analysis suggested that failure to achieve social identity continuity explained the impact of perceived cognitive failures on well-being. In other words, it appears that cognitive failures compromised stroke sufferers' well-being because these tended to interfere with their maintenance of valued group memberships.

Considered together, this pattern of results is highly consistent with the theoretical argument that group membership has an important role to play in clinical well-being (Haslam & Reicher, 2006; Iyer et al., 2007; Reicher & Haslam, 2006). In particular, the findings add to a growing body of research that points to the importance of social identity continuity as a predictor of mental health and adjustment to change (Chandler & Lalonde, 1998; Sani, in press). Where individuals have a strong sense of social identity and this can be preserved in the context of cognitive and social upheaval, this appears to increase the likelihood of their being able to cope with, and adjust to, change. Theoretically, this is predicted on the basis of evidence that shared social identities are a basis for individuals to derive positive self-esteem (Tajfel & Turner, 1979), to give and receive social support (Haslam et al., 2005; Levine et al., 2005), and to collaborate in endeavours both to resist the stresses of the present and to imagine and construct a path to a positive future (Haslam & Reicher, 2006).

An important contribution of the present paper is that it provides the first quantitative evidence of this trajectory within a clinical population. Although similar patterns have been reported in qualitative investigations (e.g., Burton, 2000) and studies of non-clinical populations (e.g., students adjusting to university life; Iyer et al., 2007), there was residual uncertainty about whether they would be revealed in a neurological population in need of rehabilitation. The fact that they were points to the importance of social factors in neuropsychological rehabilitation.

In terms of rehabilitation, the present findings suggest that interventions that aim to maintain and facilitate social identification may provide an additional solution to problems of community re-integration following acquired brain injury. This fits with previous recommendations about the importance of addressing issues of identity in clinical contexts (Folkman & Moskowitz, 2004; Ylvisaker & Feeney, 2000). Note, though, that the latter work has focused on issues of personal identity (i.e., a person's sense of themselves as an individual; Turner, 1982) and largely neglected issues of group membership and social identity. In signalling the importance of these latter dimensions of self, the present research thus points to important ways in which both theory and practice might be augmented.

Limitations and future research

Despite the support it provides for our hypotheses, it is clear that features of the present study's design place limits on our ability to derive conclusive support for our theoretical analysis. In this respect, several limitations need to be acknowledged. First, the reliance on correlational techniques means that it is impossible to draw inferences about the nature of the causal relationships between variables uncovered here (Haslam & McGarty, 2003). It is possible, for example, that post-stroke well-being encourages individuals to maintain pre-existing group memberships, or to report more positively on the strength of their maintenance. Against this, the fact that hypothesised patterns were apparent in both group listings and affiliation ratings reduces the likelihood that the observed patterns were a straightforward product of response bias. Path analysis also affords greater confidence in the nature of causal pathways than do simple bivariate correlations (Baron & Kenny, 1986).

Accordingly, alternative interpretations of the relationships we have observed are both possible and plausible. Indeed, along these lines, theoretical analysis suggests that group membership has the potential to create an "upward spiral" whereby identification with a group increases social support and psychological well-being, which in turn increase group membership identification (Haslam et al., 2005). To fully unravel the causal sequences here, there is a strong case for conducting both experimental and longitudinal research to explore the trajectory of group memberships and well-being over time and in response to particular interventions.

Another limiting feature of the present study is its lack of process measures. While our theoretical analysis asserts that group membership and social identity continuity are the key social psychological processes that underpin the relationships we have observed (after Tajfel & Turner, 1979), there is no direct evidence to support this assertion. Nevertheless, our confidence that these processes are implicated in the findings we have obtained is derived from previous research in which effects associated with maintained group membership have been shown to flow from underlying patterns of social identification (e.g., Iyer et al., 2007; Jetten et al., 2002; Van Knippenberg et al., 2002).

Due to the present study's relatively small sample size, little as yet can be said about the psychometric properties of the EXITS for neurological samples. While this limits interpretation of the data to some extent, it is important to acknowledge that these scales have proved to be both valid and reliable in previous social psychological research (e.g., Iyer et al., 2007). As in that research, the scales here also showed strong internal consistency, suggesting that items are capturing the same underlying constructs. Nevertheless, there is a clear need for future research to obtain further data about the clinical utility of these measures and to include more sophisticated measures of mental health and cognitive function in order to enhance confidence in the theoretical analysis upon which the present research is predicated.

Finally, the lack of clinical data on severity and location of insult raises questions about sample representativeness and clearly there is a need for more objective data for comparative purposes. In light of the fact that most of the participants in this study were men, there would also be value in confirming that the present demonstration of the importance of social identity continuity post-stroke is equally relevant to men and women.

Concluding comment

The above caveats notwithstanding, the present study extends our understanding of post-stroke rehabilitation by pointing to the significant role that group memberships play in this process. As such, it builds on a wealth of recent qualitative research (e.g., Bendz, 2003; Burton, 2000; Olofsson et al., 2005; Pajalic et al., 2006) which has emphasised the importance of social processes in recovery by providing, to our knowledge, the first quantitative support for this analysis. That said, more work needs to be done to explore the social and cognitive dimensions of the relationships revealed by the present research. As exploration of this form progresses, it is our conviction that social psychological approaches, and the social identity approach in particular, can make an important contribution to our understanding and management of well-being in the process of recovery from stroke and potentially other neurological conditions. Indeed, we feel this represents an important way forward for the field—encapsulating as it does an awareness of the fact that (neuro)psychology and social life are mutually interdependent (or "made for each other"). As the present data suggest, it is their implications for sustaining social life that make cognitive and physical damage particularly traumatic. Accordingly, the maintenance (and if necessary, repair) of that social life should be treated as a primary focus of attention and intervention, rather than as a matter of only secondary concern.

REFERENCES

Aneshensel, C. S., Botticello, A. L., & Yamamoto-Mitani, N. (2004). When caregiving ends: The course of depressive symptoms after bereavement. *Journal of Health and Social Behavior*, *45*, 422–440.

Aspinwall, L. G., & Taylor, S. E. (1997). A stitch in time: Self-regulation and proactive coping. *Psychological Bulletin*, *121*, 417–436.

Baron, R. M., & Kenny, D. A. (1986). The moderator–mediator variable distinction in social psychological research: Conceptual, strategic and statistical considerations. *Journal of Personality and Social Psychology*, *51*, 602–619.

Bassuk, S. S., Glass, T. A., & Berkman, L. F. (1999). Social disengagement and incident cognitive decline in community-dwelling elderly persons. *Annals of Internal Medicine*, *131*, 165–173.

Beckley, M. N. (2006). Community participation following cerebrovascular accident: Impact of the buffering model of social support. *American Journal of Occupational Therapy*, *60*, 129–135.

Bendz, M. (2003). The first year of rehabilitation after a stroke – from two perspectives. *Scandinavian Journal of Caring Sciences*, *17*, 215–222.

Bergmann, H., Kuthmann, M., Vonungernsternberg, A., & Weimann, V. G. (1991). Medical educational and functional determinants of employment after stroke. *Journal of Neural Transmission*, *33*, 157–161.

Bluck, S., & Alea, N. (in press). Remembering being me: The self-continuity function of autobiographical memory in younger and older adults. In F. Sani (Ed.) *Individual and collective self-continuity: Psychological perspectives*. Cambridge, UK: Cambridge University Press.

Bourdieu, P. (1979/1984). *Distinction: A social critique of the judgment of taste* (Trans: R. Nice). Cambridge, MA: Harvard.

Branscombe, N. R., Ellemers, N., Spears, R., & Doosje, B. (1999a). The context and content of social identity threat. In N. Ellemers, R. Spears, & B. Doosje (Eds.), *Social identity: Context, commitment, content* (pp. 35–58). Oxford: Blackwell.

Branscombe, N. R., Schmitt, M. T., & Harvey, R. D. (1999b). Perceiving pervasive discrimination among African-Americans: Implications for group identification and well-being. *Journal of Personality and Social Psychology*, *77*, 135–149.

Breakwell, G. M. (1986). *Coping with threatened identities*. London, UK: Methuen.

Broadbent, D. E., Cooper, P. F., FitzGerald, P., & Parkes, K. R. (1982). The Cognitive Failures Questionnaire (CFQ) and its correlates. *British Journal of Clinical Psychology*, *21*, 1–16.

Brodaty, H., Withall, A., Altendorf, A., & Sachdev, P. S. (2007). Rates of depression at 3 and 15 months poststroke and their relationship with cognitive decline: The Sydney Stroke Study. *American Journal of Geriatric Psychiatry*, *15*, 477–486.

Burt, R. S. (1997). The contingent value of social capital. *Administrative Science Quarterly*, *42*, 339–365.

Burton, C. R. (2000). Living with stroke: A phenomenological study. *Journal of Advanced Nursing*, 32, 301–309.

Chandler, M. J., & Lalonde, C. E. (1998). Cultural continuity as a hedge against suicide in Canada's first nations. *Transnational Psychiatry*, *35*, 191–219.

Clarke, P. J., & Black, S. E. (2005). Quality of life following stroke: Negotiating disability, identity and resources. *Journal of Applied Gerontology*, 24, 319–335.

Clarke, P. J., Marshall, V. W., Black, S. E., & Colantonio, A. (2002). Well-being following stroke in Canadian seniors: Findings from the Canadian study of health and aging. *Stroke*, 33, 1016–1021.

Cohen, S. & Syme, S. L. (1985). *Social support and health*. Orlando, FL: Academic Press.

Cohen, S., & Wills, T. A. (1985). Stress, social support and the buffering hypothesis. *Psychological Bulletin*, *98*, 310–357.

Durkheim, E. (1951). *Suicide*. London: Simon & Schuster.

Dyson, R., & Renk, K. (2006). Freshmen adaptation to university life: Depressive symptoms, stress, and coping. *Journal of Clinical Psychology*, *62*, 1231–1244.

Ellemers, N. (2003). Identity, culture, and change in organizations: A social identity analysis and three illustrative cases. In S. A. Haslam, D. van Knippenberg, M. J. Platow, & N. Ellemers (Eds.), *Social identity at work: Developing theory for organizational practice* (pp. 191–203). Philadelphia, PA: Psychology Press.

Ethier, K. A., & Deaux, K. (1994). Negotiating social identity when contexts change: Maintaining identification and responding to threat. *Journal of Personality and Social Psychology*, *67*, 243–251.

Farrin, L., Hull, L., Unwin, C., Wykes, T., & David, A. (2003). Effects of depressed mood on objective and subjective measures of attention. *Journal of Neuropsychiatry and Clinical Neuroscience*, *15*, 98–104.

Folkman, S., & Moskowitz, J. T. (2004). Coping: Pitfalls and promise. *Annual Review of Psychology*, *55*, 745–774.

Gainotti, G., Antonucci, G., Marra, C., & Paolucci, S. (2001). Relation between depression after stroke, antidepressant therapy, and functional recovery. *Journal of Neurology, Neurosurgery and Psychiatry*, *71*, 258–261.

Hackett, M. L., Yapa, C., Parag, V., & Anderson, C. L. (2005). Frequency of depression after stroke: A systematic review of observational studies. *Stroke*, *36*, 1330–1340.

Haslam, S. A. (2004). *Psychology in organizations: The social identity approach* (2nd ed.). London: Sage.

Haslam, S. A., Jetten, J., O'Brien, A., & Jacobs, E. (2004). Social identity, social influence, and reactions to potentially stressful tasks: Support for the self-categorization model of stress. *Stress and Health*, *20*, 3–9.

Haslam, S. A., & McGarty, C. (2003). Experimental design and causality in social psychological research. In C. Sanson, C. C. Morf, & A. T. Panter (Eds.), *Handbook of methods in social psychology* (pp. 235–264). Thousand Oaks, CA: Sage.

Haslam, S. A., O'Brien, A., Jetten, J., Vordemal, K., & Penna, S. (2005). Taking the strain: Social identity, social support and the experience of stress. *British Journal of Social Psychology*, *44*, 355–370.

Haslam, S. A., & Reicher, S. (2006). Stressing the group: Social identity and the unfolding dynamics of responses to stress. *Journal of Applied Psychology*, *91*, 1037–1052.

Hays, R. B., & Oxley, D. (1986). Social network development and functioning during a life transition. *Journal of Personality and Social Psychology*, *50*, 305–313.

Hirsch, B. (1981). Social network and the coping process: Creating personal communities. In B. Gottlieb (Ed.), *Social networks and social support* (pp. 149–170). Beverly Hills, CA: Sage.

House, J. S. (1981). *Work stress and social support*. Reading, MA: Addison-Wesley.

Iyer, A., Jetten, J., & Tsivrikos, D. (in press). Torn between identities: Predictors of adjustment to identity change. In F. Sani (Ed.), *Individual and collective self-continuity.* Mahwah, NJ: Lawrence Erlbaum Associates.

Iyer, A., Jetten, J., Tsivrikos, D., Postmes, T., & Haslam, S. A. (2007). *The more (and the more compatible) the merrier: Multiple social identities and identity compatibility as predictors of adjustment after life transitions.* Manuscript submitted for publication.

Jetten, J., O'Brien, A., & Trindall, N. (2002). Changing identity: Predicting adjustment to organisational restructure as a function of subgroup and superordinate identification. *British Journal of Social Psychology, 41,* 281–297.

Kawachi, I., & Berkman, L. F. (2001). Social ties and mental health. *Journal of Urban Health, 78,* 458–467.

Kim, P., Warren, S., Madill, H. & Hadley, M. (1999). Quality of life of stroke survivors. *Quality of Life, 8,* 293–301.

King, R. B. (1996). Quality of life after stroke. *Stroke, 27,* 1467–1472.

Kotila, M., Numminen, H., Waltimo, O., & Kaste, M. (1998) Depression after stroke: Results of the FINNSTROKE study. *Stroke, 29,* 368–372.

Kwok, T., Lo, R. S., Wong, E., Wai-Kwong, T., Mok, V., Kai-Sing, W., Kwok, T., Lo, R. S., Wong, E., Wai-Kwong, T., Mok, V., & Kai-Sing, W. (2006). Quality of life of stroke survivors: A one-year follow-up study. *Archives of Physical Medicine and Rehabilitation, 87,* 1177–1182.

Levine, R. M., Cassidy, C., Brazier, G., & Reicher, S. D. (2002). Self-categorization and bystander non-intervention: Two experimental studies. *Journal of Applied Social Psychology, 32,* 1452–1463.

Levine, R. M., Prosser, A., Evans, D., & Reicher, S. D., (2005). Identity and bystander intervention: How social group membership shapes helping behaviour. *Personality and Social Psychology Bulletin, 31,* 443–453.

Linville, P. W. (1985). Self-complexity and affective extremity: Don't put all your eggs in one cognitive basket. *Social Cognition, 3,* 94–120.

MacHale, S. M., O'Rourke, S. J., Wardlaw, J. M., & Dennis, M. S. (1998). Depression and its relation to lesion location after stroke. *Journal of Neurology, Neurosurgery and Psychiatry, 64,* 371–374.

Mahoney, A. M., Dalby, J. T., & King, M. C. (1998). Cognitive failures and stress *Psychological Reports, 821,* 432–434.

Marks, S. R. (1977). Multiple roles and role strain: Some notes on human energy, time and commitment. *American Sociological Review, 42,* 921–936.

Merckelbach, H., Muris, P., Nijman, H., & de Jong, P. J. (1996). Self-reported cognitive failures and neurotic symptomatology. *Personality and Individual Differences, 20,* 715–724.

Olofsson, A., Andersson, S. O., & Carlberg, B. (2005). 'If only I manage to get home I'll get better': Interviews with stroke patients after emergency stay in hospital on their experiences and needs. *Clinical Rehabilitation, 19,* 433–440.

Pajalic, Z., Karlsson, S., & Westergren, A. (2006). Functioning and subjective health among stroke survivors after discharge from hospital. *Journal of Advanced Nursing, 54,* 457–466.

Postmes, T., & Branscombe, N. R. (2002). Influence of long-term racial environmental composition on subjective well-being in African Americans. *Journal of Personality and Social Psychology, 83,* 735–751.

Preacher, K. J., & Leonardelli, G. J. (2001). *Calculation for the Sobel Test: An interactive calculation tool for mediation tests.* http://www.psych.ku.edu/preacher/sobel/sobel.htm

Puttnam, R. D. (2000). *Bowling alone: The collapse and revival of American community.* New York: Touchstone.

Reicher, S. D., & Haslam, S. A. (2006). Tyranny revisited: Groups, psychological well-being and the health of societies. *The Psychologist, 19,* 46–50.

Robinson, R. G., Bolduc, P. L., & Price, T. R. (1987). Two-year longitudinal study of poststroke mood disorders: Diagnosis and outcome at one and two years. *Stroke, 18*, 837–843.

Robinson, R. G., & Price, T. R. (1982). Post-stroke depressive disorders: A follow-up study of 103 patients. *Stroke, 13*, 635–641

Robinson, R. G., Starr L. B., Kubos, K. L., & Price, T. R. (1983). A two-year longitudinal study of post-stroke mood disorders: Findings during the initial evaluation. *Stroke, 14*, 736–741.

Robinson, R. G., Starr L. B., & Price, T. R. (1984). A two-year longitudinal study of mood disorders following stroke. Prevalence and duration at six months follow-up. *British Journal of Psychiatry, 144*, 256–262.

Sani, F. (Ed.) (in press). *Individual and collective self-continuity.* Mahwah, NJ: Erlbaum.

Sarbin, T. R., & Allen, V. L. (1968). Increasing participation in a natural group setting: A preliminary report. *Psychological Record, 18*, 1–7.

Seiber, S. D. (1974). Towards a theory of role accumulation. *American Sociological Review, 39*, 567–578.

Smith, G. E., Petersen, R. C., Ivnik, R. J., Malec, J. F., & Tangalos, E. G. (1996). Subjective memory complaints, psychological distress and longitudinal change in objective memory performance. *Psychology and Aging, 11*, 272–279.

Starchina, Y., Parfenov, V., Chazova, I., Sinitsyn, V., Pustovitova, T., Kolos, I., & Ustyuzhanin, D. (2007) Cognitive function and the emotional state of stroke patients on antihypertensive therapy. *Neuroscience and Behavioral Physiology, 37*, 13–17.

Steinberg, J. A., Pineles, S. L., Gardner, W. L., & Mineka, S. (2003). Self-complexity as a potential cognitive buffer among abused women. *Journal of Social and Clinical Psychology, 22*, 560–579.

Tajfel, H. (1972). La catégorisation sociale (English trans.). In S. Moscovici (Ed.), *Introduction à la psychologie sociale.* Paris: Larouse.

Tajfel, H., & Turner J. C. (1979). An integrative theory of intergroup conflict. In W. G. Austin & S. Worchel (Eds.), *The social psychology of intergroup relations* (pp. 33–48). Monterey, CA: Brooks/Cole.

Thoits, P. A. (1983). Multiple identities and psychological well-being: A reformulation and test of the social isolation hypothesis. *American Sociological Review, 48*, 174–187.

Torrecillas, J. L. G., Mendlewicz, J., & Lobo, A. (1997). Analysis of intensity of post-stroke depression and its relationship with the cerebral lesion location. *Medicina Clinica, 109*, 241–244.

Turner, J. C. (1982). Towards a cognitive redefinition of the social group. In H. Tajfel (Ed.), *Social identity and intergroup relations* (pp. 15–40). Cambridge: Cambridge University Press.

Turner, J. C., Oakes, P. J., Haslam, S. A., & McGarty, C. A. (1994). Self and collective: Cognition and social context. *Personality and Social Psychology Bulletin, 20*, 454–463.

Turner, J. C., Reynolds, K. J., Haslam, S. A., & Veenstra, K. (2006). Reconceptualizing personality: Producing individuality through defining the personal self. In: T. Postmes & J. Jetten (Eds.), *Individuality and the group: Advances in social identity* (pp.11–36). London: Sage.

Underwood, P. W. (2000). Social support: The promise and reality. In B. H. Rice (Ed.), *Handbook of stress, coping and health* (pp. 367–391). Newbury Park, CA: Sage.

Van Knippenberg, D., Van Knippenberg, B., Monden, L., & de Lima, F. (2002). Organizational identification after a merger: A social identity perspective. *British Journal of Social Psychology, 41*, 233–252.

Wiart, L. (1997) Post-CVA depression. *Encephale-Revue de Psychiatrie Clinique Biologique et Therapeutique, 23*, 51–54.

Williams, L. S., Weinberger, M., Harris, L.E. & Biller, J. (1999). Measuring quality of life in a way that is meaningful to stroke patients. *Neurology, 10*, 1839–1843.

Woolfolk, R. L., Gara, M. A., Ambrose, T. K., Williams, J. E., Allen, L. A., Irvin, S. L., & Beaver, J. D. (1999). Self-complexity and the persistence of depression. *Journal of Nervous and Mental Disease, 187*, 393–399.

Wyller, T. B., Sveen, U., Sodring, K. M., Pettersen, A. M., & Bautz-Holter, E. (1997). Subjective well-being one year after stroke. *Clinical Rehabilitation, 11*, 139–145.

Ylvisaker, M., & Feeney, T. (2000). Reconstruction of identity after brain injury. *Brain Impairment, 1*, 12–28.

Zencius, A. H., & Wesolowski, M. D. (1999). Is the social network analysis necessary in the rehabilitation of individuals with head injury? *Brain Injury, 13*, 723–727.

NEUROPSYCHOLOGICAL REHABILITATION
2008, 18 (5/6), 692–712

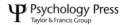
Ψ Psychology Press
Taylor & Francis Group

Participant perspectives on an individualised self-awareness intervention following stroke: A qualitative case study

Tamara L. Ownsworth[1], Merrill Turpin[2], Brooke Andrew[2], and Jennifer Fleming[2,3]

[1]School of Psychology and Applied Cognitive Neuroscience Research Centre, Griffith University, Mt Gravatt, Australia; [2]Division of Occupational Therapy, The University of Queensland, St Lucia, Australia; [3]Occupational Therapy Department, Princess Alexandra Hospital, Brisbane, Australia

Most research investigating the efficacy of neurorehabilitation has focused upon pre- versus post-intervention functioning, which is important for evidence-based practice but overlooks the therapeutic process. Therefore, this qualitative study aimed to investigate a participant's perspective of experiences in therapy throughout an awareness rehabilitation intervention. The participant (CP), a young male with awareness deficits following a right thalamic stroke, had repeatedly attempted to return to work and experienced recurrent periods of depression associated with his employment difficulties. Throughout a 12-session rehabilitation intervention, which targeted self-awareness and self-regulation skills, CP provided interview feedback concerning his experiences of different therapy exercises. The key themes emerging from the data regarding CP's perspectives included: understanding benchmarks and the value of feedback, learning through practical exercises, and individualising therapy. In collaboration with a disability employment support service, CP achieved paid durable employment. This study highlights the importance of

Correspondence should be addressed to Dr Tamara Ownsworth, School of Psychology, Griffith University, Mt Gravatt Campus, Nathan QLD 4111, Australia. E-mail: t.ownsworth@griffith.edu.au

A Public Health Fellowship from the National Health and Medical Research Council and a grant from the Centre of National Research on Disability and Rehabilitation Medicine jointly funded the present study.

http://www.psypress.com/neurorehab   DOI:10.1080/09602010701595136

considering participants' perspectives of the therapeutic process to assist in the design and evaluation of awareness rehabilitation interventions.

INTRODUCTION

Inaccurate self-appraisal following acquired brain injury (ABI) can pose a significant barrier to engaging clients in the rehabilitation process and achieving favourable outcomes (Toglia & Kirk, 2000). In a treatment context it can be challenging to determine how best to target the development of awareness of deficits while monitoring and supporting the emotional impact of this process (Ownsworth & Clare, 2006). Over the past two decades empirical evidence has emerged to support the efficacy of awareness interventions for improving self-awareness and everyday functioning (Fleming & Ownsworth, 2006). However, research is yet to examine participants' perspectives of the therapeutic process during sessions throughout rehabilitation. Thus, the main objective of this exploratory study was to identify participant perspectives of therapy during an intervention designed to enhance self-awareness and self-regulation skills.

Awareness of deficits: Key concepts

A review of conceptual models suggests that awareness of deficits following ABI refers to a broad range of interrelated metacognitive skills such as the capacity to: (a) accurately appraise changes to self and one's abilities, (b) understand the functional impact of these changes (e.g., the implications of deficits for independence or work), (c) set realistic goals, (d) recognise problems as they occur in day-to-day situations, and (e) anticipate that difficulties related to particular deficits will be experienced in the future (Crosson et al., 1989; Fleming, Strong, & Ashton, 1996). Toglia and Kirk (2000) made a distinction between *self-knowledge* of deficits that exists prior to task performance, and *on-line awareness*, involving the ability to recognise and anticipate errors in-situ or during performance. They proposed that these different aspects of awareness interact dynamically with personal characteristics (e.g., cognitive status, personality and coping style), the environment, and task demands. Awareness of deficits is a particularly pertinent issue in vocational rehabilitation.

Awareness of deficits and return to work

Awareness deficits are typically viewed as a barrier in the return to work process, which influence goals and expectations and the ability to benefit from feedback and develop compensatory strategies in the workplace (Ownsworth & Fleming, 2005). Ben-Yishay, Silver, Piasetsky, and Rattock (1987) found that the ability to set realistic goals was one of the key predictors of return to work outcomes following intensive holistic cognitive rehabilitation. Ezrachi, Ben-Yishay, Kay, Diller, and Rattock (1991) identified that individuals' acceptance of their injury during rehabilitation significantly predicted work outcomes six months after the programme. Greater acceptance of injury was associated with increased compliance with rehabilitation, active participation and willingness to disclose problems and follow therapists' recommendations. Such attributes in rehabilitation were viewed as important in achieving employment outcomes due to promoting realistic goals and expectations concerning work and the development of compensatory strategies.

Longitudinal studies have identified a significant association between awareness of deficits during rehabilitation and more favourable vocational outcomes (Ownsworth, Desbois, Grant, Fleming, & Strong, 2006; Sherer et al., 1998; 2003). Ownsworth et al. (2006) identified that individuals who achieved competitive employment between an initial assessment during rehabilitation and a 12-month follow-up experienced an associated increase in awareness of deficits while individuals who remained unemployed displayed little change in awareness. While the direction of this relationship was unclear, the findings emphasised the need to monitor developments in self-awareness as they occur during rehabilitation and the return to work process. It was further recommended that interventions target self-awareness and self-regulation skills while supporting the individual to cope with associated emotional reactions (Ownsworth et al., 2006). Techniques for enhancing awareness of deficits include psychoeducation, peer support and group therapy, role reversal, systematic feedback, performance predictions and guided self-evaluation of performance through participation on graded familiar tasks (Dirette, 2002; Fleming & Ownsworth, 2006; Toglia & Kirk, 2000). In general, multi-faceted approaches tailored according to an individual's characteristics are recommended in the context of a broader programme designed to achieve goals that are personally meaningful.

Participants' perspectives of rehabilitation

In a systematic review of evidence-based cognitive rehabilitation Cicerone and colleagues argued the need for future research to "move beyond the simple question of whether cognitive rehabilitation is effective, and examine the therapy factors and patient characteristics that optimise the clinical outcomes of cognitive rehabilitation" (2005, p. 1681). In terms of awareness interventions, most studies have focused on an evaluation of outcomes with only select studies investigating participants' perspectives of the process of developing awareness of deficits in the rehabilitation context.

Qualitative research by Kristensen (2004) examined changing goals and intentions during rehabilitation by interviewing participants before and after a 4-month programme. The findings suggested that before rehabilitation individuals generally strived to preserve "the former self" while after the programme individuals shifted towards self-autonomy, self-realisation and adjustment to their current situation. However, due to the pre- post-design, it is uncertain how this shift in self-presentation occurred. Further, Dirette (2002) interviewed three individuals with ABI who had "good awareness of cognitive deficits" and recently completed a day treatment programme. These individuals retrospectively recalled the slow process of developing awareness of deficits, which was triggered by critical events, and use of compensatory strategies. A recent qualitative study by O'Callaghan, Powell, and Oyebode (2006) conducted semi-structured interviews with 10 individuals receiving outpatient rehabilitation. Participants recalled that awareness of deficits developed through personal discovery and other people's reactions, typically outside of the rehabilitation setting, and was associated with fear, loss and grief. Rehabilitation assisted this process by explaining the effects of brain injury, normalising experiences and supporting individuals to accept their post-injury changes.

Overall, these studies reinforce the view that, from the participants' point of view, rehabilitation can be effective in increasing or supporting awareness of deficits. However, participants were required to recall and reflect upon their past experiences of rehabilitation. A further issue raised is whether individuals with awareness deficits and other cognitive deficits can comment insightfully on their experiences. However, as noted by Paterson and Scott-Findlay (2002), qualitative interviewing methods aim to capture the subjective accounts of reality for individuals despite their cognitive impairments. Rather than relying on retrospective accounts, however, it may be beneficial to seek participants' perspectives of their experiences of therapy on a session-by-session basis throughout rehabilitation. Seeking such timely and successive feedback may assist in the design and evaluation of awareness interventions.

Research rationale and objective

The main objective of this case study was to explore how an individual (CP) perceived and reacted to different components of an awareness intervention in the context of a return to work programme. To gain a sense of the experiential dimension of rehabilitation we sought feedback concerning CP's perspectives of different therapy exercises throughout the 12-session intervention.

METHOD

Research design

The present study employed case study methodology and use of multiple data sources to understand the phenomenon in depth (Yin, 2003). These sources included neuropsychological test findings, questionnaire data, field notes from observations by the research clinician and data from ongoing interviews with the participant about his experiences of the programme. CP was therefore a key informant in the research. According to Gilchrist and Williams (1999), key informants are "individuals who possess special knowledge, status, or communication skills, who are willing to share their knowledge and skills with the researcher, and who have access to perspectives or observations denied the researcher through other means" (p. 73).

Participant background

At the age of 33 CP experienced a stroke related to thrombosis in 2000. Prior to his injury CP had completed a university degree and worked in finance and administration positions. At the time of his injury he was single and undertaking further study. CP experienced a right thalamic infarction as a result of dissection of the right vertebral artery. He experienced a subsequent small left pontine infarct two days after the initial stroke. The thrombosis was treated with anti-coagulants.

Descriptive details of a neuropsychological assessment conducted nine months after the stroke indicated that CP's Verbal IQ was in the "high average to superior" range for his age with particular strengths noted on measures of immediate attention, abstract reasoning, arithmetic and general knowledge. His Performance IQ was described as "significantly lower than his Verbal IQ and relative to his age group". General difficulties were noted in the following areas: visuo-spatial construction, working memory, motor speed, speed of information processing, divided attention, verbal learning and coping with distractions or interference, mental flexibility and ability to monitor verbal responses. Visual memory abilities were at a lower level than verbal memory abilities. CP's pattern of deficits was noted to be "most certainly a consequence of his strokes" and consistent with right thalamic damage. The neuropsychological report also documented dysarthria, left-sided weakness, anosognosia, and emotional lability.

For several years after his injury CP worked as a volunteer in administration positions for charity organisations and received extensive return to work assistance from a specialised vocational rehabilitation service. He participated in work trials and applied for many positions in administration, often attending job interviews, but was unsuccessful. A work training evaluation indicated that despite CP's strong interpersonal skills, his speed and accuracy on clerical tasks was impaired and he required constant super-vision and checking of his work.

CP attempted to move out of home on a number of occasions with the support of his family and rehabilitation case manager. However, he would typically develop depression shortly after the move and return home to live with his parents. Various stressors and disappointments (e.g., not obtaining employment after a work trial or perceiving a lack of progress in his return-to-work plans) appeared to trigger depressive symptoms such as low mood, loss of motivation, lethargy and occasional suicidal ideation. In 2003 CP was prescribed antidepressant medication by his general practitioner and later began seeing a private neuropsychologist for counselling in 2004. The frequency of sessions varied from bi-weekly during periods of low mood to one session every 2–3 months. This intermittent psychological support continued throughout the present intervention. This treatment was generally based on a cognitive-behavioural model, particularly at times of crisis, and also included more general supportive psychotherapy.

Pre-intervention assessment findings

The findings of a neuropsychological review conducted just prior to the present intervention are presented in Table 1. Overall, the findings were con-sistent with the earlier assessment concerning CP's impairments in the areas of processing speed, visual perception, visual memory and visual attention (note: there was no evidence of unilateral neglect), although improvement was evident on measures of working memory and auditory attention.

Reports from CP's rehabilitation case manager of several years generally indicated that he had persisting awareness deficits concerning the effects of his stroke and unrealistic employment expectations. However, during periods of depression he would display a pessimistic view of his employment circumstances (i.e., stating that he may never return to work and that he was not "job-ready") and he occasionally expressed suicidal ideation. When CP's mood state improved he would restate unrealistic employment goals. His fluc-tuating mood state was observed at the start of one of the neuropsychological testing sessions, when he burst into tears, quickly composed himself, and then stated that he felt "brilliant".

CP completed standardised measures of awareness of deficits and emotion-al status six months before the intervention and again at two weeks prior to commencement. Six months prior to the intervention CP's scores on the Hospital Anxiety Depression Scale (HADS; Snaith & Zigmond, 1994) were in the "mild" range for depression (10/21) and the "normal" range for anxiety (5/21). However, he reported a "severe" level (16/20) of hopeless-ness on the Beck Hopelessness Scale (BHS; Beck, Weissman, Lester, &

TABLE 1
Neuropsychological assessment data at 5 years post-injury

Test	Raw score (Index or Standard Score)	Percentile (description)
NART-II	15 errors (estimated FSIQ = 112)	(High average)
WAIS-III		
VIQ	71 (111)	77 (High average)
PIQ	31 (76)	5 (Borderline)
FSIQ	102 (95)	37 (Average)
Processing Speed	8 (69)	2 (Extremely low)
Working Memory	37 (113)	81 (High average)
WMS-III		
Auditory Immediate	18 (94)	34 (Average)
Visual Immediate	7 (57)	<1 (Extremely low)
Immediate Memory	25 (73)	4 (Borderline)
Auditory Delayed	17 (92)	30 (Average)
Visual Delayed	10 (68)	2 (Extremely low)
Auditory Recognition	12 (110)	75 (High average)
General Memory	39 (84)	14 (Low average)
Memory		
RCFT Immediate	15 (T score = 42)	21 (Low average)
Delayed	10.5 (T score = 36)	8 (Borderline-low)
RAVLT-Total	35	7 (Borderline)
Attention		
Trails A	52 seconds, 0 errors	<1 (Extremely low)
TEA – Map Search I/II	32/58 (6/3)	<1–12 (Extremely low to low average)
Elevator Counting (EC)	7	Normal
EC with Distraction	10 (13)	80-88 (High average)
EC with Reversal	8 (11)	57-69 (Average)
Visual Elevator	9/3.7 (9)	31-43 (Average)
Executive Function		
Trails B	100 seconds, 1 error	<1 (Extremely low)
RCFT Copy	35	90 (High average)
FAS Test	29 words, 0 errors	15 (Low average)
Design Fluency	17 designs, 2 errors	>2 (Extremely low)
Haylings Brixton – A	0	75 (High average)
B – Speed	70	10 (Low average)
B – Accuracy	3	75 (High average)
Stroop Test: Color–Word	40	<2 (Extremely low)
Zoo Map Test	1	9 (Borderline–low)
Key Search Test	3	70 (Average)
Tinker Toy Test	5	15 (Low average)

NART-2 = National Adult Reading Test – Second Edition; RAVLT = Rey Auditory-Verbal Learning Test; RCFT = Rey Complex Figure Test; TEA = Test of Everyday Attention; WAIS-III = Wechsler Adult Intelligence Test–Third Edition; WMS-III = Wechsler Memory Scale–Third Edition. Source: Lezak, Howieson, and Loring (2004), Wilson, Alderman, Burgess, Emslie, and Evans (1996).

Trexler, 1974). On the Self-Awareness of Deficits Interview (Fleming et al., 1996) CP scored 5/9, which reflected some acknowledgment of post-injury changes (mainly activity restrictions such as driving) but suggested minimal recognition of cognitive deficits and largely unrealistic goals (e.g., anticipating full-time work in his previous field of finance). Interestingly, his goals were incongruent with his negative expectations and beliefs indicated on the BHS. On a measure of defensiveness and self-deception (Marlowe-Crowne Social Desirability Scale; Crowne & Marlowe, 1960) CP's score (18/33) was in the normal range.

Two weeks prior to the intervention CP's mood symptoms (HADS Depression = 8, Anxiety-1; BHS = 18/20), awareness of deficits (SADI = 4/9) and defensiveness (15/33) were largely consistent with the earlier assessment.

Opinion and rationale

The intervention was initially discussed with CP, his rehabilitation case manager and CP's parents. CP's rehabilitation case manager identified some concerns that due to CP's "fragile" psychological state he might become more distressed if he received feedback about his post-stroke deficits. While this was an important consideration, CP's frequent periods of depression and high level of hopelessness suggested that he was aware of negative circumstances following his stroke (e.g., lack of success in finding work, inability to drive, loss of independence), but could not identify the reasons for these limitations nor understand what he could do to improve his situation. CP's parents were keen to support an intervention that aimed to facilitate his personal goals to live independently and achieve paid work. CP was very motivated to commence the intervention and particularly valued the idea of providing the therapist with feedback concerning each therapy session.

A therapeutic intervention was designed to concurrently target the following: (a) development of awareness of deficits, (b) ability to self-monitor performance, (c) use of corrective or compensatory strategies, (d) self-efficacy and emotional adjustment; and (e) realistic goals and expectations. The awareness intervention was conducted independent of the long-term psychological support provided by the private neuropsychologist, although the objectives and components of the intervention were discussed with this therapist. The self-awareness intervention was considered to be complementary to the general therapeutic approach, in that both methods of intervention encouraged CP to identify evidence for both over and under-estimates of his performance; however, the psychological support focused more on his interpersonal interactions and self-worth while the rehabilitation intervention focused more on his functional competencies. Half way through the

TABLE 2
A summary of the intervention components and therapeutic focus of each session

Rehabilitation session	Therapeutic focus
Session 1	
(a) Psychoeducation regarding the brain and effects of brain injury	General knowledge of the brain and brain injury
(b) Specific questions about post-injury changes and their implications	Self-knowledge: Awareness of deficits and their everyday impact
Session 2	
(a) Self-ratings of personal strengths and limitations (ratings: High average, Average, Low, Very low)	Self-perception of physical, cognitive and behavioural abilities
(b) Feedback using a graph of self-ratings and objective performance indicators (neuropsychological test results and relative's ratings)	Self-evaluation of the discrepancy between self-ratings and CP's cognitive performance and relative's ratings
Session 3 – Role reversal	
(a) Therapist's prediction of her own cognitive performance on tasks with feedback from CP	(Task designed to increase CP's understanding of the function of self-predictions and feedback)
(b) CP's prediction of his cognitive performance on a different set of tasks and feedback from the therapist	Self-prediction prior to cognitive performance and self-evaluation of the accuracy of predictions
Session 4	
Performance predictions on functional tasks (e.g., paying rent, scheduling appointments, attending a work training course)	Self-prediction of functional performance on future activities (anticipatory awareness)
Session 5	
Adjustment counselling	Emotional support
Session 6	
Participation in a cooking task with prompts to self-monitor performance, followed by self-observation on video.	Pre-task predictions (anticipatory awareness) and self-monitoring (on-line awareness) and review of self-predictions
Session 7	
Practice on the cooking task with an initial review of performance on video	Identification of goals for improving performance and immediate practice of skills during cooking.
Session 8	
Participation in a group therapy session with 5 other individuals with ABI	Self-reflection on recovery and personal goals and sharing of experiences with peers
{Break from the intervention for 2 weeks to receive more intensive support from the private neuropsychologist}	
Session 9	
(a) A review of sessions to date	Exploring the impact of the intervention upon self-perceptions.
(b) Preparation for work experience in a bookshop and self-predictions of performance on a range of tasks	Performance predictions (anticipatory awareness) and planned use of compensatory strategies

(Table continued)

TABLE 2
Continued

Rehabilitation session	Therapeutic focus
Session 10	
Work sampling in a bookstore: training from a staff member on a range of tasks	Self-monitoring performance and self-evaluations according to prior predictions. Experience in receiving immediate feedback on-the-job
Session 11	
A follow-up session in the bookstore to assess the effects of previous training	Independent self-monitoring (without therapist prompts), self-correction and self-appraisal of performance
{A break of one month until CP obtained a work trial}	
Session 12	
Observation and application of self-monitoring procedures to a work environment (a large retail store) with a prospective employer and the job coach	Independent self-monitoring (without therapist prompts), self-correction and self-appraisal of performance

[a]Cognitive tasks included: line bisection, immediate recall of a number sequence, recall of a short story, copying a design, and constructing an object (speed and accuracy).

intervention CP was linked with a disability employment service to commence the job search, job placement and on-the-job support process. The latter sessions in the intervention were in part guided by the opportunities that developed to observe and provide training to CP in various work settings. An outline of the 12 sessions of the awareness intervention is provided in Table 2 with a summary of the therapeutic focus of each session. These therapy components are based upon the theoretical framework of Toglia and Kirk (2000); the efficacy of which has been supported by empirical research (see review by Fleming & Ownsworth, 2006).

Monitoring CP's reactions and feedback

Based on the principles of key informant interviewing (see Gilchrist & Williams, 1999), immediately after each therapy session an informal debriefing was conducted using a semi-structured interview format (10–15 minutes). Given the importance of established rapport, timely questions and the relevance of CP's feedback in tailoring the intervention to his needs the interviews were conducted by the therapist at the site of the session, which included CP's home, work experience site and the group therapy setting. General questions related to the content and process of the session and the therapeutic relationship. These included: "How did you find today's session?", "What, if anything, do you feel that you learnt?", "Was there anything particularly helpful or unhelpful?", and "How did today's session compare to previous sessions?" Specific questions inquired about particular aspects of the session. For example, "How did you feel when I gave you feedback that you had overestimated your performance on the memory task?" Memory prompts were used as needed during the interview. The therapy debriefing was audio taped and transcribed after each session. The therapist used a mental status examination format (Trzepac & Baker, 1993) to structure observations during the session. Observations were recorded as detailed low inference field notes.

Data analysis

The transcripts of the informal debriefing and field notes were analysed thematically with narrative data coded into categories. A researcher who was not involved with the intervention or data collection process conducted this analysis. The initial section of the results presents a description of CP's reactions and feedback throughout the 12-session intervention with selected illustrative quotes. The second section presents the major themes emerging from the analysis of interview transcripts.

RESULTS

CP's reactions and feedback throughout the intervention

Session 1(a) Psychoeducation about the brain and brain injury. CP observed that this was "very interesting. . .I had never been educated about different parts of the brain. . . . maybe you could tailor it more to the client and their background".

Session 1(b) Questions concerning the effects of CP's injury. CP found it difficult to answer specific questions about the effects of his injury and repeatedly stated that the therapist should ask his private neuropsychologist or rehabilitation case manager to obtain "an objective opinion". When prompted to consider the long-term effects of his stroke CP felt that acknowledging such problems would mean he was "a second class citizen". CP described this exercise as neither helpful nor unhelpful but "somewhere in between."

Session 2: Self-estimations of cognitive, physical and behavioural abilities. CP found it more difficult to rate his cognitive abilities (e.g., memory for conversations, ability to plan) than his physical and behavioural skills because he did not feel that there was a "benchmark" or "a standard" against which he could compare himself. When he received feedback that he rated his cognitive ability higher than his actual performance on the previous neuropsychological assessment he responded that it was an employer's or a therapist's responsibility to provide training for a person to improve. For example, he felt that someone with visuo-spatial impairments could receive training to become an air traffic controller or to learn to drive ("If a job requires it, you can work on it"). Thus, he did not view impairments as permanent nor a barrier to employment.

Session 3: Role reversal with predictions of cognitive ability and immediate feedback.   The therapist deliberately overestimated her performance on some cognitive tasks to enable CP to provide feedback. He commented: "Don't worry, everyone can make that mistake but at least now you know." When the roles were reversed and CP predicted his performance he received feedback that he had underestimated his skills in a particular area. He stated: "Wow, that is really good to know....it made me feel really good that I was better at something than I thought." After receiving feedback that he had overestimated his memory for a short story he commented: "Well, that is not as good....at least I know for next time." CP identified that receiving feedback immediately after performance is particularly important in a work setting, as follows: "I think it's important to get it [feedback] early because you've got to know how you are measuring up against their standard...but it needs to be accurate feedback."

Session 4: Self-prediction of functional performance on future activities.   CP predicted that many activities he had planned would go well over the next few weeks but also identified some for which he was less certain. He anticipated that his memory, visual attention and motor co-ordination skills might influence the outcome on some activities. CP's evaluation of this session was positive: "It's all about anticipation so that if anything crops up you have a plan. Planning the next couple of weeks of my life is just so important."

Session 5: Adjustment counselling.   CP became upset at the beginning of this session as he described a situation that had arisen during the week. The therapist focused the session on exploring these issues with him. CP felt concerned about people's expectations of him and that he did not know what the "benchmarks" were in a job. He identified that difficulty regulating his emotions might be problematic for job-readiness and living independently. CP explained: "Crying like this means that I am not normal, that I am still a second-class citizen." CP received psychological support from his private neuropsychologist and stayed with his parents for a few days.

Session 6: Self-predictions and self-evaluation of functional performance.   After completing the cooking task CP said that he had felt a bit nervous about being observed but liked the fact that "we were trying to make it more like a real life situation...like a work situation...and you are not always able to plan for things on the job" . He felt that this activity added to the previous sessions because: "Cooking is very hands on. . . . much more useful. That's another reason why we should do the work sampling... so you can get confidence and know exactly what the feedback is." CP wanted to watch the video of his cooking session and repeat the same meal during the next session to "Do it better. I think I could improve things and make changes...yeah."

Session 7: Practice on the cooking task. CP became distressed at the start of this session while discussing his perceived lack of progress with return to work plans. However, he was keen to commence the cooking task and identified several areas for improvement based upon the video self-observation. On completing the activity he identified: "The video was good because it was completely objective. So it wasn't just a person's opinion, it was what happened. And you could see that if there was something wrong you could fix it." When the therapist asked if there were other ways of obtaining feedback CP commented: "I suppose you could ask your boss or job officer to watch you and give you feedback." After a pause he added: "And, just think about what you did wrong and what you need to improve and how you can do it faster."

Session 8: Peer support and group therapy. Other group members offered their encouragement when CP became upset while discussing his work difficulties. CP seemed to take great interest in their perspectives. After the session CP noted: "I didn't realise that other people had been depressed after their injury too...it was good to hear that they could get on with their lives and get jobs and things." He also identified a limitation of the group session was that the suggestions were not specific to each individual.

Sessions 9, 10 and 11: Self-prediction and self-evaluation of work performance. In preparation for his work sampling in a bookshop CP made predictions about his performance on a range of tasks. In relation to one task he commented: "Actually, I think this could be a bit difficult because that needs a bit of fine motor." CP recognised that this prediction proved correct during performance and asked for advice so that he could adopt a strategy. During the debriefing CP identified: "It was really good and useful to, sort of, get me into the mould of work after a lapse" and that making predictions "helps because you know if you are going to find something easy or hard" .

During the second work sampling session CP predicted that he would take several attempts to complete particular tasks without prompts. However, CP completed these tasks correctly without any prompts and spontaneously applied strategies. He evaluated his performance as follows: "Well, I went better than I expected...but I wanted to give myself some leeway – expecting the worst and getting the best rather than expecting the best and getting the worst I suppose you could say." When the therapist raised the issue of job readiness CP commented: "Well, I guess it's something. Job readiness is something that is good now because you've done a couple of tasks, even if they're simple tasks...so this programme is a confidence building process."

Session 12: Observation at a work trial.   This session focused on the application of self-monitoring and feedback procedures in a prospective work environment (a large retail store) with staff and the job development officer. In the debriefing CP was asked to review the entire programme. He identified: "It's all about being more realistic isn't it? You have to find out what your strengths and downfalls are so that you can be realistic about the type of work you want to do." He additionally advised: "The comment I would make is to try and make things as close to the workplace and reality as possible."

During the post-intervention assessment on the SADI (score: 2/9) CP reported the following work goals: "Hopefully in six months time I'll be working 2–3 days a week, 6 hours per day – maybe at [place of work trial]. I'm not sure what will happen, but this is what I hope. I need to be realistic." On self-report measures of emotional status CP was in the "mild" range for anxiety and hopelessness and the "normal" range for depression.

Three weeks later CP was offered part-time paid work as a retail assistant (3 days per week, 5 hours per week) and had maintained this position at follow-ups conducted at 3, 6 and 9 months post-intervention.

Major themes

Understanding benchmarks and the value of feedback.   The main theme that pervaded the CP's responses over the 12 sessions referred to the concept of "benchmarks". At times he used this word and at other times he used different words and phrases, such as "yardstick", "standards" and "knowing what's expected", to convey this idea, depending on the focus of the session. His answers, particularly during the early sessions that involved direct questioning about his post-injury impairments, seemed to raise the question of who should evaluate his skills – him or someone else? CP often deferred to, or sought the opinions of others he considered to have more expertise. The issue of benchmarks and social standards appeared to place considerable pressure on CP, which affected his self-confidence and perception of work readiness.

In subsequent sessions throughout the programme, which entailed situation-specific feedback and skills practice, CP seemed to learn that he could better understand standards of performance by seeking feedback from various sources and that this needed to occur early or immediately after task performance for him to personally benefit. He discovered that while feedback could be obtained from therapists, employers and job development officers, he could also gain feedback from self-observations (e.g., on videotape) or by reflecting on his own performance.

Learning through practical experience.   The rehabilitation intervention utilised a range of different approaches to increasing CP's awareness of his skills and impairments. Both therapist observations and CP's comments demonstrated that he preferred and benefited most from learning through practical experience. In particular, following the cooking task, CP gave his evaluation that the practical session had been more helpful than the earlier ones because it was "hands on". However, he made the point that other sessions were useful when they involved making predictions about "real life".

Individualising therapy.   Throughout the 12 sessions, CP continually referred to the importance of individualising the task or exercise. In the group session he perceived a limitation that the suggestions were not specific to an individual. In CP's discussions about the sessions, he often made reference to his family background. As both of CP's parents worked in the scientific field and he previously worked in finance, he frequently made comments about the "scientific" perspective or "objectivity" being important to him. However, this reference was always placed in the context of understanding that the needs and experiences of others might be different to his. His answers to various questions related to his major goal of work, particularly in the field in which he was receiving training.

DISCUSSION

The present study investigated a participant's perspectives throughout a 12-week intervention designed to enhance self-awareness and self-regulation skills. His perceptions indicated that the therapy sessions promoted greater understanding of benchmarks and the value of feedback, and enabled learning through practical experience. Individualising or tailoring rehabilitation according to his background and personal goals also enhanced this process. CP's emotional reactions to the intervention were closely monitored and managed by the project clinician in collaboration with his private neuropsychologist and supportive family. Of note, CP described the programme as "a confidence building process", thus reinforcing that awareness interventions can enhance emotional adjustment (O'Callaghan et al., 2006; Ownsworth, 2005). CP's awareness deficits and reactions can be considered in a biopsychosocial context.

In terms of neurocognitive factors, CP displayed marked impairments in visual perception, speed of information processing, psycho-motor speed, visual attention and visual memory, consistent with right hemisphere damage and thalamic strokes (Kumral, Kocaer, Ertübey, & Kumral, 1995; Myers, 1999). Models of awareness deficits (see McGlynn & Schachter, 1989; Morris & Hannesdottir, 2004) propose that conscious experience of post-injury changes requires an interaction between relevant functional domains (e.g., sensory, perceptual, motor and cognitive functions), comparator mechanisms within the central executive system to detect change, and the conscious or metacognitive awareness system. This feedback system relies upon updates regarding the experience of success and failure on tasks thus contributing to an individual's self-knowledge of personal abilities and impairment (Morris & Hannesdottir, 2004). This might occur from feedback from other people and structured opportunities to self-evaluate one's performance. Awareness deficits can arise from a disruption at various stages of processing within this integrated network. While the components of this network have not been specifically localised, thalamic lesions are found to produce diverse impairments in sensory, perceptual, motor and cognitive processes (Kumral et al., 1995), while disturbances in mood and self-awareness have previously been observed after right thalamic lesions (Liebson, 2000). Direct damage to the thalamus and/or disruption of connecting pathways to various regions of the cortex (e.g., fronto-thalamic pathways) may have contributed to CP's deficits in awareness and emotional regulation (Bogousslavsky, 1994).

Interestingly, once CP learnt about performance expectations in relevant situations, with training and practice on specific activities, he learnt to self-monitor his behaviour, identify errors and correct these during performance. CP did not display global executive dysfunction on testing, and thus his capacity to adopt metacognitive strategies most likely relied upon some intact higher-order cognitive abilities. CP's relative strengths in language expression enabled him to articulate the reason why he found it difficult to judge his own abilities, which related to a failure to understand benchmarks for performance, both in therapy and in work settings.

In terms of psychosocial factors influencing CP's awareness of deficits, he indicated that he preferred to receive feedback on his performance on practical tasks rather than direct questioning about his abilities. The concern about appearing a "second class citizen" emerged when CP was feeling uncertain of his abilities and suggested more deep-seated issues concerning acceptance of his disability and social stigma. Similar grief and loss issues have previously been observed following ABI (see O'Callaghan et al., 2006; Ownsworth,

2005; Ruddle & Coetzer, 2005). Ideally, these maladaptive beliefs would be explored and addressed through individual or group psychotherapy within a more holistic rehabilitation context. Overall, CP's motivation during the intervention was high, however, when he experienced heightened emotional distress his support needs were accommodated in the programme by breaks or modifying sessions. Engaging in practical activities such as cooking was found to improve CP's mood state and shift the focus of his self-appraisal from negative thoughts regarding his job readiness to personal achievement in other activities. CP appeared to benefit considerably from psychological support from the private neuropsychologist, particularly to cope with reactive depression in relation to ongoing stressors and life events.

The present study suggested that by developing more realistic expectations and modified goals CP was able to participate more actively in the job search and placement process. Ideally, this attitudinal and behavioural shift occurs during the pre-vocational rehabilitation stage prior to seeking employment (Ben-Yishay et al., 1987). It appears that some individuals may need to experience a lack of success with goals in order to develop a greater understanding of the impact of their deficits. However, such negative experiences may be overwhelming and lead to the development of heightened psychological distress (Langer & Padrone, 1992; Ownsworth & Oei, 1998). In general, a graduated return to work process with work sampling and early supportive feedback is recommended to prevent long-term psychological dysfunction.

Clinical implications

The present therapy intervention was designed to provide structured opportunities for CP to learn about the effects of his stroke and develop self-regulatory strategies (Toglia & Kirk, 2000). These experiences commenced with general exercises that are commonly used in brain injury awareness interventions, such as psychoeducation, feedback on assessment results, and a strengths and limitations self-assessment (see Fleming & Ownsworth, 2006; Toglia & Kirk, 2000), but subsequently the intervention became increasingly tailored according to CP's goals, incorporating participation on familiar and meaningful activities that CP requested feedback and support with. The approach is consistent with the "client partnership" approach advocated by McKenna and Tooth (2006), and other client-centred practices adopted in brain injury rehabilitation (see Wilson et al., 2000; Wressle, Eeg-Olofsson, Marcussen, & Henriksson, 2002).

However, the present intervention additionally demonstrated the value of establishing a bi-directional feedback process between the client and therapist at the commencement of an intervention, and structuring time for such communication within each therapy session. Therefore, while the focus of many sessions involved the therapist providing feedback to CP regarding his performance on tasks, CP additionally provided consistent feedback to the therapist regarding his experiences and the value of particular exercises throughout the programme (i.e., during the therapy debriefing). This mutual approach is likely to contribute to the therapeutic alliance, which previous research suggests is related to awareness of deficits (Schönberger, Humle, & Teasdale, 2006). The present study supports the value of therapy debriefing, particularly in the context of awareness interventions, to monitor individuals' perceptions and reactions to different components and assist in processing the meaning of these experiences.

Methodological considerations

The present case study was designed to identify a participant's perspective of his experiences throughout an intervention designed to improve self-awareness and self-regulation. Clearly, however, the findings regarding this process for one individual with particular clinical characteristics (i.e., persisting awareness deficits, fluctuating emotional state, and high motivation for treatment) cannot be broadly generalised to other individuals with ABI. The comprehensive data provided in relation to CP's neuropsychological and psychological functioning may assist in determining the relevance of the findings to other clinical contexts. Additionally, the detailed description of the intervention components may support the application of therapy techniques, in this relatively sparse area of rehabilitation practice.

While the present study was primarily concerned with CP's perspective of the therapeutic process, rather than evaluating an awareness intervention or return to work programme, it is important to acknowledge that CP was receiving concurrent psychological support from a private neuropsychologist and the disability employment service. Therefore, although feedback concerning CP's experiences was sought immediately after each session of the awareness intervention, the outcomes of the intervention need to be considered in this broader support context. The treating therapist in this study conducted the therapy debriefings with CP to obtain timely feedback and assist in the design of subsequent sessions. It is important to acknowledge, however, that CP's responses may have differed if the interview had been conducted by a professional independent of the intervention.

Given the exploratory nature of this study, further research into participants' perspectives of participating in rehabilitation is needed to assist in the design and evaluation of awareness interventions. By progressively monitoring clients' reactions to therapy sessions it may be possible to identify common experiences regarding the value of different exercises. Combined with an evaluation of rehabilitation efficacy (i.e., pre- and post-intervention outcomes), this type of investigation has the potential to identify not only who benefits from different interventions but also participants' own evaluation of their experiences and therapy outcome. Although there are pragmatic and methodological issues to consider when interviewing individuals with awareness deficits and cognitive impairment, due to their potential difficulty in reliably recalling and articulating experiences (see review by Paterson & Scott-Findlay, 2002), such methods can provide a valuable insight into personal accounts of rehabilitation which to date have largely been overlooked in the literature.

In conclusion, the findings of the present study suggested that from CP's perspective the awareness intervention promoted greater understanding of benchmarks and the value of feedback, and enabled learning through practical experience. The importance of tailoring rehabilitation according to his background and personal goals was also recognised. Future investigations of participants' perspectives in rehabilitation may assist in understanding how clients perceive the value of different therapy components, thus assisting in the design of interventions that are meaningful to individuals with awareness deficits.

REFERENCES

Beck, A. T., Weissman, A., Lester, D., & Trexler, L. (1974). The measurement of pessimism: The Hopelessness Scale. *Journal of Consulting and Clinical Psychology, 42*, 861–865.

Ben-Yishay, Y., Silver, S. M., Piasetsky, E., & Rattock, J. (1987). Relationship between employability and vocational outcome after intensive holistic cognitive rehabilitation. *Journal of Head Trauma Rehabilitation, 2*, 35–48.

Bogousslavsky, J. (1994). Frontal stroke syndromes. *European Neurology, 34*, 306–315.

Cicerone, K. D., Dahlberg, C., Malec, J., Langenbahn, D. M., Felicetti, T., Kneipp, S., et al. (2005). Evidence-based cognitive rehabilitation: Updated review of the literature from 1998 through 2002. *Archives of Physical Medicine and Rehabilitation, 86*, 1681–1692.

Crosson, B. C., Barco, P. P., Velozo, C. A., Bolseta, M. M., Werts, D., & Brobeck, T. (1989). Awareness and compensation in post-acute head injury rehabilitation. *Journal of Head Trauma Rehabilitation, 4*, 46–54.

Crowne, D. P., & Marlowe, D. (1960). A new scale of social desirability independent of psychopathology. *Journal of Consulting Psychology, 24*, 349–354.

Dirette, D. (2002). The development of awareness and the use of compensatory strategies for cognitive deficits. *Brain Injury, 16*, 861–871.

Ezrachi, O., Ben-Yishay, Y., Kay, T., Diller, L., & Rattock, J. (1991). Predicting employment in traumatic brain injury following neuropsychological rehabilitation. *Journal of Head Trauma Rehabilitation, 6*, 71–84.

Fleming, J., & Ownsworth, T. L. (2006). A review of awareness interventions in brain injury rehabilitation. *Neuropsychological Rehabilitation, 16*, 474–500.

Fleming, J. M., Strong, J., & Ashton, R. (1996). Self-awareness of deficits in adults with traumatic brain injury: How best to measure? *Brain Injury, 10*, 1–15.

Gilchrist, V. J., & Williams, R. L. (1999). Key informant interviews. In B. F. Crabtree and W. L. Miller (Eds). *Doing qualitative research*. (2nd ed.). Thousand Oaks: Sage.

Kristensen, O. S. (2004). Changing goals and intentions among participants in a neuropsychological rehabilitation programme: An exploratory case study evaluation. *Brain Injury, 18*, 1049–1062.

Kumral, E., Kocaer, T., Ertübey, N. O., & Kumral, K. (1995). Thalamic hemorrhage: A prospective study of 100 patients. *Stroke, 26*, 964–970.

Langer, K. G., & Padrone, F. J. (1992). Psychotherapeutic treatment of awareness in acute rehabilitation of traumatic brain injury. *Neuropsychological Rehabilitation, 2*, 59–70.

Lezak, M. D., Howieson, D. B., & Loring, D. W. (2004). *Neuropsychological Assessment* (4th ed.). New York: Oxford University Press.

Liebson, E. (2000). Anosognosia and mania associated with right thalamic damage. *Journal of Neurology, Neurosurgery and Psychiatry, 68*, 107–108.

McGlynn, S. M., & Schacter, D. L. (1989). Unawareness of deficits in neuropsychological syndromes. *Journal Clinical Experimental Neuropsychology, 11*, 143–205.

McKenna, K., & Tooth, L. J. (2006). Client education: An overview. In K. McKenna & L. Tooth (Eds.), *Client education: A partnership approach for health practitioners* (pp. 1–12). Sydney: University of New South Wales Press.

Morris R. G., & Hannesdottir, K. (2004). Loss of 'Awareness' in Alzheimer's disease. In R. G. Morris & J. T. Becker (Eds.), *The cognitive neuropsychology of Alzheimer's disease* (pp. 275–296). Oxford: Oxford University Press.

Myers, P. (1999). *Right hemisphere damage: Disorders of communication and cognition.* San Diego: Singular Publishing Group.

O'Callaghan, C., Powell, T., & Oyebode, J. (2006). An exploration of the experience of gaining awareness of deficit in people who have suffered a traumatic brain injury. *Neuropsychological Rehabilitation, 16*, 579–593.

Ownsworth, T. (2005). The impact of defensive denial upon adjustment following traumatic brain injury. *Neuro-Psychoanalysis, 7*, 83–94.

Ownsworth, T., & Clare, L. (2006). The association between awareness deficits and rehabilitation outcome following acquired brain injury. *Clinical Psychology Review, 26*, 783–795.

Ownsworth, T. L., Desbois, J., Grant, E., Fleming, J., & Strong, J. (2006). The associations among self-awareness, emotional well-being and employment outcome following acquired brain injury: A 12-month longitudinal study. *Rehabilitation Psychology, 51*, 50–59.

Ownsworth, T., & Fleming, J. (2005). The relative importance of metacognitive skills, emotional status and executive functioning in psychosocial adjustment following acquired brain injury. *Journal of Head Trauma Rehabilitation, 20*, 315–332.

Ownsworth, T. L., & Oei, T. P. S. (1998). Depression after traumatic brain injury: Conceptualisation and treatment considerations. *Brain Injury, 12*, 735–751

Paterson, B., & Scott-Findlay, S. (2002). Critical issues in interviewing people with traumatic brain injury. *Qualitative Health Research, 12*, 399–409.

Ruddle, J. A., & Coetzer, R. (2005). The mourning after brain injury: Understanding loss and grief. *Journal of Cognitive Rehabilitation, 23*, 12–19.

Schönberger, M., Humle, F., & Teadale, T. W. (2006). The development of the therapeutic alliance, patients' awareness and their compliance during the process of brain injury rehabilitation. *Brain Injury, 20*, 445–454.

Sherer, M., Bergloff, R., Levin, E., High, W., Oden, K., & Nick, T. (1998). Impaired awareness and employment outcome after traumatic brain injury. *Journal of Head Trauma Rehabilitation, 13*, 52–61.

Sherer, M., Hart, T., Nick, T. G., Whyte, J., Thompson, R., & Yablon, S. (2003). Early impaired self-awareness after traumatic brain injury. *Archives of Physical Medicine and Rehabilitation, 84*, 168–176.

Snaith, R. P., & Zigmond, A. S. (1994). *The Hospital Anxiety and Depression Scale: Manual.* Windsor, UK: NFER-Nelson.

Toglia, J., & Kirk, U. (2000). Understanding awareness deficits following brain injury. *NeuroRehabilitation, 15*, 57–70.

Trzepac, P. T., & Baker, R. W. (1993). *Psychiatric Mental Status Examination*. New York: Oxford University Press.

Wilson, B. A., Alderman, N., Burgess, P. W., Emslie, H., & Evans, J. J. (1996). *Behavioural Assessment of the Dysexecutive Syndrome (BADS)*. Bury St. Edmunds, UK: Thames Valley Test Company.

Wilson, B. A., Evans, J., Brentnall, S., Bremner, S., Keohane, C., & Williams, H. (2000). The Oliver Zangwill Center for Neuropsychological Rehabilitation. In A. L. Christensen & B. P. Uzzell (Eds.), *International handbook of neuropsychological rehabilitation* (pp. 231–246). New York: Kluwer Academic/Plenum Publishers.

Wressle, E., Eeg-Olofsson, A., Marcussen, J., & Henriksson, C. (2002). Improved client participation in the rehabilitation process using a client-centred goal formulation structure. *Journal of Rehabilitation Medicine, 34*, 5–11.

Yin, R. K. (2003). *Case study research: Design and methods*. Thousand Oaks, CA: Sage Publications.

NEUROPSYCHOLOGICAL REHABILITATION
2008, 18 (5/6), 713–741

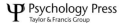

Metaphoric identity mapping: Facilitating goal setting and engagement in rehabilitation after traumatic brain injury

Mark Ylvisaker[1], Kathryn McPherson[2], Nicola Kayes[2], and Ellen Pellett[3]

[1]*College of Saint Rose, Albany, New York, USA;* [2]*Health and Rehabilitation Research Centre, AUT University, Auckland, New Zealand;* [3]*Pellett and Associates, Oakville, Ontario, Canada*

Difficulty re-establishing an organised and compelling sense of personal identity has increasingly been identified as a critical theme in outcome studies of individuals with severe traumatic brain injury (TBI) and a serious obstacle to active engagement in rehabilitation. There exists little empirical support for approaches to identity reconstruction that address common impairments associated with TBI. Similarly, there is as yet little empirical support for theoretically sound approaches to promoting engagement in goal setting for this population. This article has two purposes. First, theory and procedures associated with metaphoric identity mapping are discussed in relation to goal setting in TBI rehabilitation. Second, the results of a qualitative pilot study are presented. The study explored metaphoric identity mapping as a facilitator of personally meaningful goal setting with five individuals with significant disability many years after their injury. Drawing on principles of grounded theory, the investigators extracted data from semi-structured interviews with clients and clinicians, from focus groups with the clinicians, and from observation of client–clinician interaction. Analysis of the data yielded five general themes concerning the use of this approach: All clients and clinicians found identity mapping to be an acceptable process and also useful for deriving meaningful rehabilitation goals. Both clients and clinicians saw client-centred goals as important. Cognitive impairments posed obstacles to this goal-setting intervention and mandated creative compensations. And finally, identity-related goal

Correspondence should be sent to Mark Ylvisaker, 1171 Van Antwerp Road, Schenectady, New York 12309, USA. E-mail: ylvisakm@mail.strose.edu

© 2008 Psychology Press, an imprint of the Taylor & Francis Group, an Informa business
http://www.psypress.com/neurorehab   DOI:10.1080/09602010802201832

setting appeared to require a "mind shift" for some clinicians and demanded clinical skills not uniformly distributed among rehabilitation professionals.

Keywords: Traumatic brain injury; Rehabilitation; Identity; Goal setting; Self-regulation.

INTRODUCTION

After briefly reviewing the literature on identity and goal setting after traumatic brain injury (TBI), we describe the theoretical and procedural aspects of an approach to identity construction known as metaphoric identity mapping. This is followed by a report of a pilot study in which this approach was shown to be useful in enabling individuals with TBI to set meaningful rehabilitation goals.

IDENTITY AND GOAL SETTING AFTER BRAIN INJURY

As we use the term here, *identity* refers to the multiple ways individuals perceive themselves, including their values, goals, abilities, impulses, attitudes, action strategies, and the like, as well as their feelings associated with these representations of self (Rogers, 1974). As elaborated below, most people harbour multiple identities or "possible selves". In this broad sense, the concept of identity overlaps with but is not identical to the concept of *role* (Unruh, 2004; Unruh, Versnel, & Kerr, 2002). Roles include occupation (e.g., teacher, labourer), social relationships (e.g., husband, wife, friend), biological relationships (e.g., brother, sister), quasi-occupation (e.g., helper, volunteer), avocation (e.g., athlete, musician, collector), and affiliation (e.g., Catholic, club member). One and the same role, however, may be associated with dramatically different identities and fit into very different life narratives. For example, two mid-level managers may have the same occupational role, but differ substantially in the self-perceived "fit" of that role with other aspects of their life, such as their goals and level of ambition, and with the expectations of family and others. These areas of divergence may be clearer windows on their identity or "sense of self".

Identity or sense of self plays a variety of roles for individuals with or without disability. Identity enables one to have a sense of continuity in life, to experience the world through the lens of a "me" that remains relatively constant through the flow of events and changes in circumstances that define a life. Associated with this function is the established connection between sense of self and episodic memory (Levine, Freedman, Dawson, Black, & Stuss, 1999). In addition identity plays a fundamental role in motivation (Deci & Ryan, 2000; Markus & Wurf, 1987). Individuals often engage in difficult tasks not because of an anticipated pay-off, but rather simply because "that's something that a me sort of person does". Conversely, otherwise appealing activities might be avoided simply because "that's *not* something that a me sort of person does". This connection between identity and motivation is a central theme in the literature on self-regulation (see below).

The growing literature on identity after brain injury converges on two critical themes: (1) identity or sense of self is often shattered by the effects of the injury on the individual's abilities and roles, and (2) effective reconstruction of an organised, compelling, and reasonably realistic identity is central to the process of rehabilitation (Biderman, Daniels-Zide, Reyes, & Marks, 2006). Goals set by rehabilitation professionals for individuals with brain injury as well as strategies to achieve the goals may be rejected out of hand by the person simply on grounds that, "What you are proposing is *not me!*" In the absence of general congruence between the rehabilitation programme and the person's sense of personal identity, rehabilitation efforts, including vocational adaptations, are likely to be at best ineffective and at worst counter-productive by escalating the individual's negative reactions to disability, possibly including anger, resistance, and depression, and hardening negative attitudes to rehabilitation. Identity construction thus becomes central to rehabilitation (Klinger, 2005).

Johansson and Tham (2006) suggested that pursuit of identity after brain injury is associated with occupational role, but that its meaning may change, with work serving a social need and adding structure to life, but no longer the central feature of identity. Although return to work often serves as a motivator in rehabilitation, the construction of a positive sense of self independent of work identity is often critical to successful outcome.

Nochi (1998) identified three themes in loss-of-self narratives after brain injury. The individuals had difficulty developing a clear understanding of their abilities after the injury, they tended to compare current status with pre-injury status (thus emphasising their sense of loss), and they perceived the attitudes of others and labels used by others as exaggerating their losses. Comparisons of oneself to a "prior" self or to others without injury have also emerged as themes in studies of other populations with chronic and disabling conditions (McPherson, Brander, McNaughton, & Taylor, 2001, McPherson, Brander, Taylor, McNaughton, & Weatherall, 2004).

In a subsequent study, Nochi (2000) examined the self-narratives of 10 reasonably well-adjusted adults with TBI to identify patterns of successful identity reconstruction. Five categories of apparently effective self-narrative were identified: (1) The self as better than others (i.e., "Things could be much worse"); (2) The grown self (i.e., "The injury improved me in some way"); (3) The recovering self (i.e., "I continue to get better; I'm getting back to where I was before the injury"); (4) The self living here and now (i.e., "I won't compare myself with others or with myself before the injury; one day at a time"); (5) The protesting self (i.e., "The problem is with those who judge me, not with me; my job is to change society's attitudes"). The value of this study is that it illustrates the possibility of positive identity reconstruction after serious injury and underscores the individual variability in positive reconstruction. Other investigators have documented a strong relationship between a positive self-concept and general quality of life for this population. For example, Vickery, Gontkovsky, and Caroselli (2005) found that ratings of self-concept were correlated with perceived quality of life and, consistent with previous studies, that depressive symptoms were associated with lower quality of life ratings.

Goal setting and identity

Although goal setting is widely considered rehabilitation "best practice" (Siegert & Taylor, 2004), there is remarkably limited evidence for specific goal-setting procedures. Until recently, the only substantial (but non-systematic) review available concluded that evidence for the effectiveness of goal setting in rehabilitation was less robust than often assumed (Wade, 1998). Indeed, somewhat remarkably given its central place in rehabilitation, goal setting in clinical practice remains largely atheoretical and variable in both intended purpose and approach to intervening (Levack, Dean, McPherson, & Siegert, 2006a; Levack, Dean, Siegert, & McPherson, 2006b; Levack et al., 2006c). With this as background, there is growing acceptance of the need for a more carefully thought out conceptual approach to goal-setting practice and research, how it works and how it should be integrated into rehabilitation (Hart & Evans, 2006; Siegert, McPherson, & Taylor, 2004). Multiple theories have been proposed to underpin goal setting, most building upon research with healthy individuals (i.e., data collected from healthy psychology students and athletes). Motivation and engagement are common currency in the language of "non-rehabilitation" goal setting; however, the usefulness and application of findings from these fields is problematic for people with neurological deficit, given that many of the required skills and attributes, such as self-awareness and motivation, may be compromised (MacLean & Pound, 2000).

Siegert et al. (2004) and Hart and Evans (2006) are among those who have argued that self-regulation (SR) theory may yield procedures to assist individuals in developing the meta-cognitive skills needed for effective goal setting (e.g., awareness, motivation and goal-directed activity). Although alternative interpretations of SR exist (e.g., Carver & Scheier 1998; Locke & Latham, 1990), they tend to share the following five principles: (1) most of human behaviour is goal directed; (2) people typically strive toward multiple goals simultaneously; (3) progress or failure in goal attainment has affective or emotional consequences; (4) goal attainment, motivation and affect are closely related and interact; (5) success in achieving desired goals is determined in large part by individuals' skill at regulating their cognition, emotions and behaviour. Further, Emmons and Kaiser (1996) suggested that the most adaptive form of self-regulatory behaviour seems to require the ability to select concrete, manageable goals (lower order tasks) that are linked to personally meaningful (higher-order) representations of self. The educational psychology literature similarly highlights the critical connection between sense of self and goal setting (Boekaerts, 1998).

Arguably, people with TBI are at great risk of goal failure (and the consequences of self-regulatory failure) unless specific steps are undertaken to facilitate development of the skills associated with both lower order (task delineation) and higher order (identity exploration) issues involved in goal-related activity. Goal setting for individuals with TBI is often jeopardised by a natural but possibly unrealistic desire to return to pre-injury activities and levels of functioning. Therefore, there is often a conflict between the goals set by clinicians and those embraced by the individual (Levack et al., 2006a).

Identity construction after brain injury

Despite the growing literature documenting the importance of identity construction after TBI and repeated calls for clinicians to facilitate this process (Hill, 1999; Morris, 2004; Nochi, 1998, 2000), little research has been undertaken to identify and validate clinical procedures specifically designed to assist members of this clinical population with their identity reconstructive process. Indeed, the language used by many therapists, focusing almost exclusively on the individual's impairments, tends to contribute to a "self-as-damaged-goods" identity (Kovareky, Shaw, & Adingono-Smith, 2007). In this way therapists unintentionally contribute to a post-injury identity that is the opposite of that which holds the potential to support active engagement in the construction of a compelling new life.

Indeed, unawareness of deficits and psychoreactive denial can interfere with identity construction after brain injury and lead to poorer psychosocial outcomes (Yeates, Henwood, Gracey, & Evans, 2007). Therefore, helping individuals to understand their new profile of strengths and weaknesses is often a critical part of rehabilitation. Issues associated with unawareness and denial have a rich history in the research and clinical literatures (e.g., Prigatano & Schacter, 1991). Our experience suggests that unawareness or denial can be effectively addressed within the positive context of the identity construction procedures described in this article. For example, behavioural experiments and reality testing, identified as the most common strategy used by a sample of 21 UK psychologists in their psychotherapeutic work with individuals with TBI (Judd & Wilson, 2005), fit easily within the identity mapping process.

In addition to the emotional challenges associated with the need to construct a new sense of personal identity after a life-altering injury, the process is further complicated by the fact that those parts of the brain associated with construction and maintenance of an organised sense of self are themselves vulnerable in TBI. These include ventral prefrontal structures of the right hemisphere, proposed by Stuss and Alexander (1999) as a convergence zone for the neural processes that personalise experiences of self and represent awareness of that experience, and the hippocampus and amygdala, which contribute to the re-establishment of a stable identity because they are the substrates of integrated memories and emotional memories (Perna & Errico, 2004).

Theoretical underpinnings of metaphoric identity mapping

Theoretical support for metaphoric identity mapping as a set of clinical procedures is derived from a variety of sources, including (1) the theory of possible selves elaborated by Markus and Nurius (1986), (2) the cognitive processing theory of Barnard (Barnard, 1985; Teasdale & Barnard, 1993) within which a unique dimension of meaning is isolated as the connection between cognition, on the one hand, and affect and decision making on the other, (3) a neuropsychological theory of cognitive organisation and its associated clinical procedure, graphic organisers, and (4) theories of self-regulation cited in the previous section (Hart & Evans, 2006; Siegert et al., 2004).

Possible selves

In their now classic 1986 article, Markus and Nurius proposed that "possible selves" are individuals' complex mental representations of what they would like to become ("hoped-for selves") and what they are afraid of becoming ("feared selves"). Possible selves are the cognitive underpinnings of motivation in that they give form, meaning, organisation, and direction to "gut-level" hopes, fears, goals, and threats. For example, to be motivating, goals are not represented as an abstract end state (e.g., possession of a college degree). Rather they are embodied in a possible self, a cognitive and affective self-schema of *me* as possessing a college degree and the future this creates. With this as background, formulation of goals and engagement in goal-oriented rehabilitation efforts necessitate a focus on self or identity construction in rehabilitation.

Possible selves can arise from personal experiences, social and cultural forces, and the planned efforts of clinicians. Social and cultural influences are often largely negative for individuals with brain injury, focusing on impairments or the self as "unfixable damaged goods". However, the fact that possible selves can be and often are constructed in interaction with others underpins the positive therapeutic use of the concept in rehabilitation (Hermans, Kempen, & van Loon, 1992).

Possible selves are the context for evaluating one's current sense(s) of self. For example, if an individual's possible selves are largely negative, then a temporary setback will have a more profoundly negative impact than if the person primarily nurtures positive possible selves. In addition, possible selves serve as the basis for the active process of constructing one's own development. Furthermore, possible selves are necessarily associated with positive or negative emotions; thus feelings about oneself vary depending on which possible self is activated at any given time.

The psychological framework elaborated by Markus and Nurius serves as one of the theoretical pillars on which metaphoric identity mapping is built. It is also a framework for a variety of clinical approaches that have in common the coached development of a new life narrative after a life-altering injury (e.g., Heller, Mukherjee, Levin, & Reis, 2006). Narrative therapy has been supported by Bruner's work on narrative processing (2002) and by White and Epston's narrative approach to psychotherapy (1990).

Metaphor, meaning and motivation

In helping individuals with disability after brain injury construct an organised and compelling sense of personal identity, we also work with them to identify a personally meaningful metaphoric centre for that identity, possibly a heroic figure or some other meaningful symbol or image that can unify and give emotional valence to the characteristics and action strategies that comprise the identity schema. Positive metaphors are associated with positive, hoped-for identities and negative metaphors with negative, feared identities (if any). The premise for this search is that propositional thoughts by themselves do not drive choices or motivate behaviour, whereas the emotional meaning embodied by personally meaningful heroes, symbols, parables, and metaphors does.

Interacting cognitive subsystems (ICS) is a theory of information processing that offers an elegant theoretical framework for the metaphoric dimension of identity mapping. The ICS model (Barnard, 1985) includes nine cognitive subsystems (or qualitatively distinct codes) and their interrelationships. Teasdale and Barnard (1993) provided detailed descriptions of this cognitive architecture and illustrated its explanatory power in relation to both normal cognition and clinically significant phenomena.

From our perspective, the critical features of the theory are its distinction between propositional meaning (expressed by potentially true or false statements) and implicational meaning (conveyed by metaphor, symbol, narrative, and the like), its integration of emotion into theoretical accounts of information processing, and the central position accorded implicational meaning in the processing of information and regulation of emotions and behaviour (Teasdale & Barnard, 1993). Beliefs at the implicational level (e.g., "I am strong and heroic"; "I am a worthless victim") are not evaluated as true or false, but rather as motivating or disheartening, productive or stifling, inspiring or boring, calming or troubling, organised or diffuse, personally compelling or personally repugnant (Teasdale, 1997). Importantly, implicational meanings are bidirectionally tied to emotion, affect, and behaviour, whereas propositional meanings are not. For example, thinking of oneself as a person-in-control-of-my-destiny can elicit positive emotional states and positive behaviour. In contrast, worthless-self-as-victim thoughts can lead to negative emotions and lack of motivation. By tying identity descriptions to personally meaningful metaphors or symbols, those internalised descriptions can in this way play a role in motivation, decision making, and behaviour. Fitzsimons and Bargh (2004) summarised social psychology experiments showing that priming participants with thoughts about admired individuals can unconsciously activate goal states and induce superior performance on experimental tasks.

Metaphors also serve the purpose of collecting the multiple components of a complex cognitive schema, like sense of self, and making them accessible to memory with only one unit of thought – the metaphor. This contribution to efficient cognitive processing, "metaphoric compaction" (Ylvisaker & Feeney, 2000), is especially useful for individuals with impaired working memory or slow processing, both common after TBI. In a variety of publications, Lakoff and Johnson (1980, 1999) have illustrated the pervasive and largely subconscious impact of metaphors that are built into everyday language and influence emotions, thinking, and behaviour typically without being recognised as metaphors. Pinker's more recent treatment of the subject questions the universality and strength of the Lakoff and Johnson thesis, while at the same time affirming its core insight (Pinker, 2007).

Metaphor is often classified as an abstract use of language and therefore said to be difficult to comprehend for individuals who are concrete in their thinking. In contrast, metaphors that are very familiar or highly personal in their meaning may be easier to comprehend than a literal translation of the meaning expressed by the metaphor. Even young children are able to comprehend basic metaphors (Nippold, 1998). In our work with adolescents and adults with TBI, we have similarly found metaphor effective in exploring otherwise difficult-to-comprehend abstract or challenging concepts.

Because intrinsic motivation is critically related to a sense of competence (Deci & Ryan, 2000; Ryan & Deci, 2000), identity mapping should be accompanied by clinical efforts designed to enable the individual to experience success with meaningful tasks, using action strategies that are consistent with the newly constructed positive identity (Petrella, McColl, Krupa, & Johnston, 2005). For many people, vocational tasks or family responsibilities can serve this function. When work and family are not meaningful components of the person's life, contributory projects can be designed that enable the person to experience competence in playing a helping role. Project-oriented rehabilitation was discussed and illustrated by Ylvisaker, Feeney, and Capo (2007).

Cognitive organisation and graphic organisers

Grafman's theory of prefrontal function proposes that executive processes involve complex mental representations, "structured event complexes" or, at a higher level of generality, "managerial knowledge units" (Grafman, 2002). Injury to the frontal lobes creates inefficiency in self-regulation and all organisational activities, including organised and elaborated thinking, because of damage to these organising schemes. Sense of self is one of these potentially damaged or inaccessible managerial knowledge units, thereby creating a fragmented sense of self and difficulty creating a new and adequately organised sense of self after the injury. Studies in educational psychology and special education have yielded strong support for the use of external graphic organisers to enable students with organisational impairment to elaborate their thoughts, organise them, remember information more effectively, and express themselves in an organised manner (Bulgren & Schumaker, 2006). Our experience using identity maps as graphic organisers with adolescents and adults with TBI is consistent with this theory-based and empirically supported theme in educational psychology and special education.

Clinical uses and procedures: Metaphoric identity mapping

Metaphoric identity mapping may serve a variety of clinical purposes associated with the theoretical issues discussed in the earlier sections. Four specific purposes are outlined in Table 1. Figure 1 suggests that these purposes fall on a continuum of clinical activity that varies in complexity, intensity, and prerequisite counselling skill of the clinician. At the far left on that continuum, identity mapping can be used as a respectful "get to know you" procedure, with the goal of encouraging the individual to be open about values, goals, and associated feelings and action strategies (Mallinson, Kielhofner, & Mattingly, 1996). In this way a respectful therapeutic relationship is created. This process may lead naturally to other purposes listed to the right on Figure 1. Moving towards the middle of the continuum is the use of metaphoric identity mapping to enable the individual to set goals that are at the same time meaningful and realistic, and are associated with a sense of self that is coherent and adequately attractive.

Further to the right on the continuum, metaphoric identity mapping is used to enable the individual to overcome chronic resistance or other obstacles to important action strategies or to rehabilitation in general. This process may be

TABLE 1

Clinical uses and procedures of metaphoric identity mapping

Identification process	Action process	Rationale
A: Establishing a respectful therapeutic relationship with the individual		
• Organisation of at least one or more self-identity descriptions • Creation of "identity maps" based on these descriptions *Use B if the identification process is difficult*	• Identification of interests, goals, and values • Identification of obstacles to achieving goals • Identification of possible strategies and tactics *Connect to Level C Actions for ongoing work as required*	A process for understanding people as they understand themselves, thereby creating a therapeutic alliance, engaging them in rehabilitation, and ensuring that the rehabilitation process is informed by the individual's beliefs regarding what is important
B: Helping individuals to set meaningful goals for themselves and secondarily identify the action strategies/tactics needed to achieve the goals		
• Identification of a "general vision" of something that the person might like to do or be involved in • Identification of an admired person associated with that activity • Organisation of one or more identity descriptions • Creation of identity maps *Use C if the individuals can identify goals of importance they are struggling with.*	• Brainstorming about interests • Clarification of goals • Tying goals to a positive metaphor • Identification of obstacles • Identification of possible strategies and tactics *Connect to Level C Actions for ongoing work*	A process designed to facilitate the ability to determine what is important and achievable when either the level of impairment or emotional response to that impairment is hampering the process

C: Helping individuals to overcome chronic obstacles to achieving important goals and to become actively engaged in rehabilitation

- Identification of goals and related obstacles
- Identification of possible strategies and tactics
- Organisation of identity description(s). possibly including both hoped-for positive selves and feared negative selves
- Identification of positive images, heroes, or other metaphors to represent hoped-for selves; perhaps identification of negative metaphors to represent feared selves
- Creation of identity maps
  Use B if the identification process of C is difficult

- Supported practice using action strategies/tactics associated with the hoped-for self
- Modification of others' support behaviours so that the individual can achieve success
- Possibly engagement in a meaningful project to create a sense of accomplishment associated with a hoped-for self
  Development of scripts to support practice – changing over time as goals change

A process to connect existing goals with meaning and purpose, and to provide practical tools and supports for attainment of those goals

D: Facilitating "deep" changes in identity through a long-term psychotherapeutic process
This process may be required by certain individuals; however, it is not advocated as a tool for routine rehabilitation and referral to an appropriately trained clinician is required

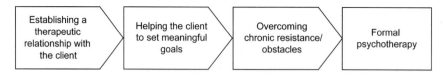

Figure 1. Points on a continuum of possible uses of metaphoric identity mapping in rehabilitation. Throughout the continuum, this clinical process is intended to foster motivation and engagement in rehabilitation. The movement from left to right corresponds to increasing intensity of the process and increasing counselling skill of the clinician.

a relatively straightforward framing of an important action strategy as the sort of action that is natural and admirable for the type of person represented by the metaphoric base of that sense of self. In other cases, identity mapping to overcome chronic obstacles is a more intensive and time-consuming clinical activity, as illustrated by the case described in the next section and by the cases described by Ylvisaker and Feeney (2000). In the study described below, identity mapping was used to help the individuals set meaningful goals and also to overcome difficulty engaging in rehabilitation activities, even the goal-setting process itself.

At the far right on the continuum is identity mapping as a procedure in formal psychotherapy. As such, the procedure is associated with more traditional approaches in psychotherapy, including cognitive-behaviour therapy (McMullin, 2000) and narrative therapy (White & Epston, 1990). Metaphoric identity mapping has been used clinically within a psychotherapeutic context for individuals with TBI, but that use is not the focus of this report. Appropriate training and credentials are required for all psychotherapeutic interventions. In our practice, we also encourage clinicians who lack training in clinical interviewing and counselling procedures to seek appropriate consultation support when using identity mapping toward the middle of the continuum of uses. When individuals with disability are served by more than one member of a multi-disciplinary team, identity metaphors and interventions should be coordinated within the team. In such cases, practitioners share responsibility for ensuring that identity metaphors and maps are consistent with psychotherapeutic interventions and with what is known about the individual's emotional vulnerabilities.

Figure 2 is an example of an identity map constructed collaboratively over the course of several therapy sessions with a young adult, John, who had a history of substance abuse and conflict with the authorities both before and after his brain injury. Initial conversations about his sense of self included his strong assertion that whatever else might be true about him, he had to consider himself an alpha male (his term). This was followed by extended conversations about different ways of being or appearing to be an alpha male. Some of the descriptors fit John's vision of a hoped-for self,

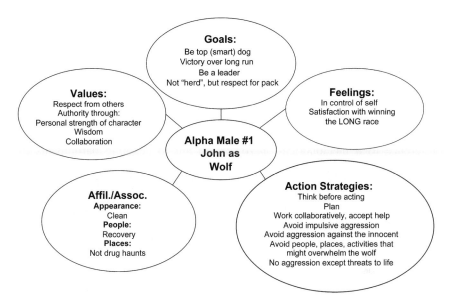

Figure 2. John's positive identity map, metaphorically representing himself as a "wolf" kind of person.

which came to be metaphorically represented as the Wolf. Other metaphors (and associated maps) fit his understanding of ways he had lived but no longer wanted to live (i.e., "feared selves"). In other cases, we have resisted constructing negative maps because dwelling on negative characteristics may lead to unwanted images of self that insidiously contribute to negative outcomes (Kelly, 2000).

In contrast to the expectations of some clinicians, John evidenced little reluctance to reflect on his various senses of self and participated actively in filling in the identity maps. Then with one positive and three negative maps in hand, he set about with the help of staff to implement the action strategies associated with the positive map and its associated metaphor. Other clients, including some of the participants in the current study, are more reluctant to participate in identity mapping or simply less capable of generating identity descriptors and action strategies. In such cases, client–clinician relationship building may be a necessary prerequisite. In addition, the clinician may need to suggest descriptors for the identity boxes, always seeking confirmation from the client before entering an item. Even in cases in which clients spontaneously offer descriptors or action strategies, they should repeatedly be asked to verify that these descriptions and strategies fit the possible self they wish to become or to avoid. In addition they should be invited to revise their descriptions or metaphors over time as they experience emotions associated with the action strategies they are helped to explore.

While clinical experience has been promising, studies are needed to validate targeted approaches to both goal setting and identity construction for individuals with TBI. As part of a larger study investigating novel interventions in goal setting, we undertook a pilot study of one approach drawing on previous work of Ylvisaker and Feeney (2000). The intervention, identity-oriented goal setting (IOG), used graphic organisational support and reference to a metaphorical "hero" as an aid to enabling participants to identify a meaningful, higher representation of what is important to them as a basis for deriving and pursuing rehabilitation goals. The objectives of this pilot study were to (1) explore the clinical application and utility of IOG as a goal-setting intervention for individuals with TBI, and (2) determine the acceptability of IOG to clients and their clinicians, and identify possible obstacles faced by community clinicians in applying IOG procedures.

METHOD

In keeping with recommendations from the UK Medical Research Council's *Framework for Trials in Complex Interventions* (2000), this pilot study was an exploratory trial incorporating qualitative methods, including observation, individual interviews, and focus groups. Ethical approval for the study was obtained from the Health and Disability Ethics Committee in New Zealand.

Participants

Two sets of participants were involved in the study: individuals with TBI and their primary clinicians. Participants were recruited from three inpatient or community rehabilitation services in the Auckland area in New Zealand. An initial information session was held with all key worker clinicians at each of the neuro-rehabiltation units to provide an overview of the study and its rationale, outline the intervention, indicate the time commitment required from clinicians, and discuss the recruitment protocol. Clinicians were then asked to consider if they would like to be involved in the intervention study and if so, which of their clients might be eligible to participate.

Individuals with TBI

Eligibility to participate in the study was based on the following inclusion criteria: (1) Potential participants had experienced moderate or severe TBI with disabling consequences defined as having a history of post-traumatic amnesia greater than one hour and moderate disability on the Extended

Glasgow Outcome Scale (Wilson, Pettigrew, & Teasdale, 1998). (2) They were receiving rehabilitation at one of the three neuro-rehabilitation units. (3) Their key clinician agreed to deliver IOG with the support of the researchers (NK and KM). Potential participants were excluded if (1) they were in a state of persistent unresponsiveness, scoring 8 or lower on the Glasgow Coma Scale (Teasdale & Jennett, 1974) when screened for the study; (2) cognitive deficits were so severe as to prevent participation in the study; (3) the individual was unable to communicate effectively with the researcher and/or clinician involved in the study; or (4) unstable medical conditions precluded participation in rehabilitation.

As part of the larger study into goal-setting approaches, 10 individuals who met all of the criteria and consented to participate were allocated to the identity-oriented approach (IOG). Of these 10, five completed the full intervention period. The results presented here are based on these five participants. The remaining five withdrew from the study, two immediately after allocation and three after receiving only one session of IOG. All but one of these withdrew for reasons unrelated to the intervention (discharge from the unit, referral for surgery, medical complication, commencement of a work trial). The remaining participant experienced anxiety during his first session. His keyworker believed this was due to co-existing mental health issues that needed to be addressed prior to engaging in IOG and therefore withdrew the client from the study. The five who withdrew from the study were also long-term post-injury and similar to the five who remained in age, gender, severity of injury, and ethnicity.

Characteristics of the five participants who completed the study are presented in Table 2. There were four males and one female, between the ages of 27 and 68. Three of the participants were in secondary school at the time of their injury. One was working as a physician and one was unemployed at the time of injury (highest educational qualification unknown). All were severely injured; however initial GCS scores are unavailable in three cases (3 and 7 in the other two cases). All were at least three years post-injury, with a range of three to 29 years.

TABLE 2
Characteristics of the participants with TBI

Participant	Age	Gender	Ethnicity	Pre-injury occupation	Time post injury (years)
P1	27	Male	Pacific Islander	Student	13
P2	45	Female	NZ European	Student	29
P3	28	Male	Maori	Unemployed	3
P4	30	Male	NZ European	Student	14
P5	68	Male	European (other)	Physician	20

Clinicians

Each neuro-rehabilitation service had an internal system whereby a key worker was identified for each client. Although this role varied among the three providers, the key worker tended to be the clinician who was predominantly working with that client and responsible for communicating with other members of the rehabilitation team and the client's family. Key workers of any profession were eligible to take part in this study if their client consented and they were able to meet with the client face to face at least once a week for 6–8 weeks during the intervention period.

The four key clinicians who worked with the five participants who completed the full IOG intervention included a physiotherapist, two occupational therapists, and a social worker. Although these professionals had practised for varying lengths of time (range 5–25 years), all had at least five years' experience in neurorehabilitation.

Intervention procedures

The intervention was delivered by the key workers with the support of the research team. Key workers met with their participants face to face and used the IOG strategy at least once a week for six weeks. To account for missed appointments, intervention delivery lasted up to eight weeks. This time frame was chosen to ensure standardisation of intervention (see below for more details) but also because the relatively brief intervention would test whether it would be deliverable in "real world" clinical practice. Actual duration of the sessions varied depending on the individual requirements of the participants, although sessions did not exceed two hours due to the fatigue often experienced by individuals with TBI.

A protocol for IOG intervention was developed in order to maintain a standardised delivery and thereby enable the investigators to draw conclusions about the clinical application, utility, and acceptability of the intervention. Identity maps (as described and illustrated in Figure 2 in the introduction and in Ylvisaker and Feeny, 2000) were developed for each participant using a scripted collaborative process (see Table 3). As discussed in the introduction, identity mapping is a collaborative process in which clinicians follow the client's lead while also facilitating the construction of a "possible self" that is compelling for the client and includes realistic goals and associated action tactics and strategies.

In contrast to the maps shown in Figure 2, the participants' maps included a box labelled "Facts" (i.e., what biographical facts would associate the participant with the metaphoric centre of the map?) and there was no box for "Values". Although possible selves are fluid, flexible, and variable within different contexts of individuals' lives, for purposes of standardisation, clinicians were advised to construct only one identity map (with associated goals)

TABLE 3
Collaborative procedures for constructing identity maps used in the study

Topic	Possible prompts
Talk with the client about desirable activities and identify someone highly admired by the client, possibly associated with such activities.	Tell me about activities in which you are interested, like sports, movies, family activities, music, church activities, and the like. And is there a person you especially admire in that world – a person whose goals and actions you might like to consider for yourself? (That person's name was then placed in the circle in the centre of the map.)
Discuss important *facts* of that person's life and possible associations with the client's life.	What roles does this person play? What does he or she do (e.g., for work and for fun)? What else do you know about this person? What are his or her struggles?
Talk with the client about relevant *associations* with being that kind of person.	Think of yourself as that kind of person (i.e., the admired person). Who would you associate with if you were acting as that type of person? What places would be important for you? What would you look like?
Talk with the client about *goals* associated with being that kind of person.	Thinking of yourself as that kind of person, what would your goals be? What would you like to accomplish for yourself?
Talk with the client about how he or she would *feel* if able to achieve those goals.	How would you feel about yourself if you were able to achieve one or more of those goals? Might there be feelings of satisfaction? control? mastery? accomplishment? contribution?
Talk with the client about various *actions and action strategies* that would be necessary or useful in attempting to achieve those goals.	What would you need to do to achieve those goals and therefore enjoy the feelings associated with achieving the goals? Let's try to think about specific actions or strategies that would help you to achieve those goals – even if the actions may be difficult.

during the intervention period. Clinicians were asked to discuss at some length each box in the map, remaining alert to the fact that an entry in one box might trigger a related entry in another box. In this way there was flexibility in completing the map.

Each of the clinicians had been working with their participating client for a period of time prior to the study. Therefore, they had established rapport and had some knowledge of the participant's background and the circumstances surrounding the injury. Nevertheless, the clinicians were advised to spend time in initial exploratory discussions, thereby enabling the clients to reveal aspects of themselves – or features of their vision for themselves – previously unknown to the clinician.

Clinician training

As mentioned previously, all key workers attended an initial information session providing an overview of the study and its rationale, including a summary of the literature on identity, goal setting, and self-regulation theory as well as the basic principles of the intervention. This was followed by two group sessions with those clinicians who volunteered for the study. The first of these sessions introduced the identity map and the clinician prompts. During the second session, the clinicians alternately role played client and clinician roles. At each of these sessions, clinicians were encouraged to consider the clients they had in mind for the study and to include in the role play barriers they may face in engaging that person in the process. This role playing helped to highlight potential pitfalls and enabled the research team to discuss strategies to overcome those difficulties.

In addition to these group sessions, clinicians were offered individual support by the research team, dependent on the individual needs of the clinicians. Support included some or all of the following: (1) Additional discussion of the intervention protocol prior to recommending clients for the study; (2) A specific meeting to prepare for the first session; (3) Ongoing support based on progress monitoring over the course of the study; (4) Investigator participation in a session (as observer or active participant) if requested by the clinician; this was followed by guidance for the clinician.

Data extraction and analysis

The primary aims of this pilot study were most appropriately addressed using qualitative methods to facilitate understanding of the experiences and views of the participants (Mays & Pope, 1996). Rather than make assumptions about the range of views that might be found, inherent in using standardised measures with a limited set of questions, the study drew on the principles of grounded theory (Strauss & Corbin, 1998) throughout each phase. Purposeful sampling (Denzin & Lincoln, 2000; Patton, 1990) was used to access a range of participants with TBI (in relation to severity of deficit, age, and gender) and a range of rehabilitation professions (in this case, physiotherapy, occupational therapy, and social work). Interviews (with clients and clinicians) and focus group discussions (with clinicians) used semi-structured prompts allowing both clients and clinicians to take part in a "guided conversation" about their experience of the intervention (Patton, 1990, 1999). Interviews were tape recorded and transcribed verbatim, with data coded and analysed manually to determine categories and themes that represented what was either a commonly or strongly expressed view or concern (Pope,

Ziebland, & Mays, 2000). These data were complemented by researcher records of sessions observed or participated in.

Rigour of data acquisition, analysis, and interpretation was tested using three strategies proposed by Mays and Pope (2000): Independent assessment of the interview material by two investigators to propose key categories and themes followed by discussion to reach consensus, systematic checking back with the interview transcripts to confirm the extent to which proposed categories and themes were reflected in or challenged by the data, and consideration of "expert" responses from a variety of health professionals, including members of the clinical teams involved in the project as well as other health professionals external to the project.

RESULTS

The findings presented here are a synthesis of the key categories and themes extracted from the data obtained from researcher observations and field notes in addition to transcripts of interviews (clients and clinicians) and focus groups (clinicians). Participants included the five clients and four clinicians who completed the IOG intervention period. Illustrative comments are included with each of the five themes, with some alteration of identifying information to preserve anonymity.

Theme 1: Both clients and clinicians found the identity mapping process to be acceptable

IOG was found to be acceptable to both clients and clinicians. Many clients reported a feeling of improved mood resulting from being involved in a meaningful activity (i.e., identity mapping) that yielded desirable rehabilitation goals. When asked what they liked about the process, participants often referred to a sense of achievement they felt when they achieved goals that they had set for themselves.

One client built his identity map around a favourite singer with whom he felt an affinity as the singer had come through "tough times", managing to overcome them. This participant found the experience of constructing the identity map a powerful one.

Client: "I remember that it was an emotional time thinking about how the Bronx singer, Kanye West, had had a similar experience and really made me think . . . the words of his music were healing and made me accept my disability and pushed me to do the very best . . . this has given me another opportunity to express feelings and emotions and move on with life."

The key worker for this client added to this:

Clinician: "... it actually helped him to see that someone he knew had actually made the journey and got there."
Researcher: "Do you think he enjoyed the process?"
Clinician: "He really did, he got a lot out of it."

Theme 2: IOG procedures were found to be useful for engaging participants in identifying meaningful goals

All of the clinicians acknowledged that although they believed goal setting to be a key component of their practice in rehabilitation, they had often found it difficult to engage clients with cognitive impairment in the goal-setting process. They found IOG provided a forum to discuss goals and formalised the process, helping to initiate collaborative goal setting with their client. Many clinicians found this was the case even in their clients with the most severe impairments.

Clinician: "I think it was good because they [clients] could still think globally; a lot of their cognitive functioning might have been a bit impaired or their memory, but they could often remember somebody they admired... even the ones who were quite severely affected did have the ability to come up with someone they did admire. So it was easier to find the starting point for it [i.e., goal setting]."

Clients appeared to find it easy to think about someone they admired around whom they could build their identity map. One client spoke about John F. Kennedy, whom he considered a very strong motivator.

Client: "I admired him because he was very persistent and he was a very powerful man and he was always positive and he managed the goals he had in his mind."

This client spoke about a JFK mantra which he would repeat to himself when he was working on his goals: "JFK was never defeated, never a failure – he was an achiever!"

Theme 3: Clients and clinicians recognised the value of setting client-centred goals

IOG seemed to be a particularly useful tool in helping clinicians to work in a collaborative way with the clients to establish a set of client-centred goals. Many of the clinicians admitted that previously they set their client's rehabilitation goals themselves in response to funder requirements rather than working with clients on developing their own goals.

Clinician: "We always had goals, but we never did sort of really collaborative goal setting; so it was quite a new concept using this sort of thing."

They reported that their failure to set client-centred goals is partly due to constraints that funding structures and processes place on them.

Clinician: "It's often something that the processes we work with in funding contracts don't allow us to really think about it... they don't encourage us to think in that way."

Often the identity mapping process led to clients nominating goals the clinician would never have thought the client would articulate. For example, one participant had only articulated one goal over the many years since his injury – to be able to walk again. Goal-setting sessions often left clinicians feeling frustrated because they did not believe that walking was a possibility, but they struggled to get him to consider other goals. The process of IOG enabled this participant to consider other aspects of who he wanted to be, which were just as meaningful and important to him as being able to walk again. For the first time he was able to articulate other goals, such as being able to make a contribution around the house and to improve his fitness. Indeed, he later expressed a sense of accomplishment in being able to achieve goals he set for himself for the first time since his injury.

Client: "You get a .... you get ... what do you call it ... from knowing that you've done it?"
Researcher: "... you get a bit of a buzz ....?"
Client: "Yeah"

For other participants, the IOG process enabled them to recognise aspects of themselves that they would like to change. For example, one participant found the metaphorical influence of his identity map useful in highlighting that his susceptibility to anger was a barrier to his engagement in rehabilitation. His clinician helped to articulate this.

Clinician: "It brought something very much to the fore in his consciousness ... think that it all added to ... where he is now and where he will be going because things like anger were a major issue ... I think it had a long-term benefit because it really made him start to think about himself."

Theme 4: Cognitive impairments posed a potential threat to the effectiveness of IOG procedures

When considering why some participants engaged better than others during the identity mapping process, the research team noted factors that appeared to be barriers to meaningful engagement, including weak generation of ideas and memory impairments. For example, some clinicians had difficulty helping their client move from the initial identification of their "hero" to thinking in more detail about the characteristics of that person or characteristics of themselves (their "possible self") as that kind of person.

Clinician: "What was difficult was trying to get out some of the characteristics of that person that they really admired and that's probably where the person delivering the intervention needed some quite good training and practice at doing it."

Clinician: "His brain injury wasn't as severe as some of the others, he could actually think a little bit more about perhaps individual features of someone, of their hero, when some of the other clients, it was really hard for them... they would perhaps be able to come across a person, but to actually crystallise it in their own mind and to be able to bring out what it was about them that they liked when they were cognitively impaired was actually really difficult."

Significant memory impairments also posed an obstacle for several participants. Although these participants were actively engaged in the face-to-face sessions with clinicians, they did not always recall their identity map and link it with their goals between sessions. In addition, clinicians needed to spend a significant proportion of each session reconstructing parts of the identity map before they could move on to the next stage of the process.

However, despite these setbacks, some positive observations were noted over the intervention period, even for those with the most significant memory impairments. For example, the process of reconstructing parts of the identity map at the beginning of each session became less and less necessary over the intervention period, with many participants ultimately needing only a small prompt to "spark" their memory of the previous session's content. Several strategies to help the participant remember the identity map and associated goals between sessions were useful, such as prompting from other rehabilitation team members and placing copies of the identity map or a picture of their metaphorical identity on their wall.

Missed appointments, not uncommon in brain injury rehabilitation, exaggerated problems for clients with memory impairments and were also problematic for others, particularly if the delay occurred early in the intervention process. Missed appointments required that considerable time be devoted to reviewing previous sessions for all clients, reducing the efficiency of the intervention. In addition, the delays reduced the ability of the clinician to establish a strong rapport with their client, which is essential to the success of IOG.

Theme 5: Identity-related goal setting requires a "mind shift" for many clinicians as well as clinical skills that not all rehabilitation clinicians possess

This theme was supported by focus group discussions, observation of clinicians delivering IOG, and specific expression of concern by some of the clinicians. Several participating clinicians found delivering IOG challenging and at odds with their normal practice. This was particularly so for the physiotherapist who expressed concern that she was funded to provide physiotherapy, rather than engage the client in dialogue. She was also concerned that clients would be unsatisfied if insufficient physical rehabilitation was provided during a session. More generally, all of the clinicians indicated that they face external pressures, including funder requirements and their own disciplinary commitments, to pursue priority goals that may be quite different from the goals set by clients. With these competing demands on their time, clinicians were often forced to decide which goals were most important. Even if the clinician perceived the clients' self-selected goals to be most important, more often than not the funder's goals took priority; failure to do so risked losing the client from the service.

Clinician: "There is often a reluctance to engage in this type of dialogue when we feel we should be doing some physical therapy at that time."

Clinician: "We are not used to planting the seed, nurturing it, weeding around it, and fertilising it. We plant it and expect it to grow."

In addition, more than one clinician expressed a lack of confidence in their ability to engage clients in the IOG process, perceiving the process as requiring training and skill in building relationships with people and bringing out their ideas.

Clinician: "Physios talk trivia with them [clients] while we are doing exercises, but we are not skilled in formulating dialogue that is used to facilitate thoughts and ideas from other people."

Clinician: "To be able to think on your feet at the same time as listening to someone and to generate ideas that are going to facilitate the person to say something. . .it was quite a challenge."

Whereas clinicians were positive about the initial phase of the goal-setting intervention (identifying a "hero"), they found it challenging to facilitate the process of identifying important aspects of that "hero" and constructing a positive, well-elaborated, and useful identity map, particularly if the clinician was unfamiliar with the client's metaphoric core. Indeed, some clinicians experienced internal tension, finding it hard to approve of the client's choice of a "hero" and fearing that the resulting identity map might be a negative influence.

Clinician: "It was good to start with, in that they could often pick the person – but that wasn't even the half of it. After that you had to really start thinking hard and trying to facilitate out of the person some of the "nitty gritty" and it was very hard trying to get that out and then translate that back into something that was going to be able to be done for the client."

Clinician: "It's a bit tricky if they come up with someone, particularly in the music world if I'm not familiar with their music. I don't know what culture goes behind that. . .. You want the person that they select to be socially acceptable or someone that's perhaps got characteristics that are going to help the person lead a good healthy life."

Internal tension was also experienced by some clinicians if they believed that the goals identified by the client as meaningful were outside of their scope of practice. Strangely these clinicians did not always engage other relevant team members in the goal-attainment process.

Clinician: "I mean, I am a physiotherapist and the things the client wanted to achieve were not within my discipline."

Despite these challenges, all of the clinicians were positive about IOG, and seemed eager to develop their skills.

Clinician: "It was a really good process to go through as a therapist . . . quite a big paradigm shift . . . I guess I almost felt a little bit embarrassed that I hadn't done things closer towards it in the past."

The IOG procedures were somewhat easier to implement for those clinicians with some background in person-centred services and counselling procedures. The social worker and both of the occupational therapists stated that IOG was consistent with their disciplinary commitments.

Achievement of goals

The focus of this study was engagement in meaningful goal setting, not achievement of goals. It is worth noting, however, that four of the five participants achieved their goals (two goals per person) at expected or higher levels on the Goal Attainment Scale (Kiresuk & Sherman, 1968).

The fifth participant set only one goal, which was achieved at a level below expected outcome. These results are suggestive of a positive impact of the study's clinical procedures; however additional studies using experimental methods are needed to establish this link.

DISCUSSION

The two main goals of this paper have been (1) to describe the theoretical underpinnings and clinical procedures associated with metaphoric identity mapping for individuals with TBI, and (2) to present a qualitative pilot study designed to explore the usefulness and acceptability (to clients and clinicians) of this approach when the clinical goal is to facilitate effective person-centred goal setting. In general both clients and clinicians found IOG to be procedurally acceptable and effective in yielding personally meaningful and achievable rehabilitation goals. In some cases, IOG enabled the client to overcome resistance to setting achievable goals and to experience for the first time since the injury the satisfaction associated with achieving self-set goals. Furthermore, IOG offers clinicians an organised and theoretically informed approach to goal setting that addresses specific TBI-related impairments that often interfere with effective goal setting. Based on this small sample, IOG appears to enable clinicians to facilitate meaningful engagement of their clients in the development of person-centred goals; this engagement has often been missing in traditional rehabilitation practice.

The investigators intended to include a wide variety of rehabilitation professionals as participants in the study. Because five of the original 10 IOG clients withdrew, the range of clinicians was limited to physiotherapy, occupational therapy, and social work. One of the themes that emerged from the data was a lack of preparation and subjective professional tensions experienced by some of the clinicians as they began to implement IOG procedures. In particular, the physiotherapist found it challenging, stating that it was difficult to facilitate well-elaborated identity descriptions. Despite excellent training in physical rehabilitation, some rehabilitation professionals have traditionally been less thoroughly trained in identity exploration and counselling procedures than other rehabilitation professionals. Those clinicians with training in person-centred services and counselling procedures experienced considerably less difficulty and discomfort, even though the specific procedures were new to them. Importantly, the physiotherapy participant judged IOG procedures to be acceptable and useful for her two clients, despite the novelty of the procedures.

All rehabilitation professionals must be competent in engaging clients in meaningful goal setting. If IOG or other quasi-counselling procedures are most effective in facilitating a goal-setting process that results in active client engagement in rehabilitation, then preservice or inservice training in all of the rehabilitation professions should be designed to ensure competence in implementing such interventions. In particular, clinicians should be competent in collaborating with their clients in constructing an organised, well-elaborated, and compelling description of a possible self capable of supporting the active pursuit of meaningful and achievable goals.

In addition, when clinicians work as members of intervention teams, those with less competence in delivering person-centred services and using psychologically oriented procedures should collaborate actively with team members with greater competence as they engage the client in identity exploration and reconstruction. This collaboration also addresses the concern of some professionals that metaphoric identity mapping may be outside of their scope of practice.

Because of the small number of participants and the non-experimental methods of this pilot study, its results can only be considered suggestive. Nevertheless these results are sufficiently strong to support additional investigations with larger numbers of participants, quantitative outcome measures, and control procedures in place. It may also be instructive to explore the usefulness of metaphoric identity mapping earlier in recovery. Comparison of alternative methods of goal setting may advance the field. Also welcome would be studies of the effectiveness of metaphoric identity mapping procedures as a component of counselling or psychotherapy after TBI. In a psychotherapeutic context, clinical procedures would be more complex and intensive than those used in this study, and require additional clinical expertise in their implementation. Finally, if more comprehensive studies support the conclusions suggested by this pilot study, then funders of rehabilitation must be systematically alerted to the importance of a more intensive and person-centred approach to goal setting than they may be accustomed to supporting.

REFERENCES

Barnard, P. (1985). Interacting cognitive subsystems: A psycholinguistic approach to short-term memory. In A. Ellis (Ed.), *Progress in the Psychology of Language* (Vol. 2, pp. 197–258). Hove, UK: Lawrence Erlbaum Associates Ltd.

Biderman, D., Daniels-Zide, E., Reyes, A., & Marks, B. (2006). Ego-identity: Can it be reconstituted after a brain injury? *International Journal of Psychology, 41*(5), 355–361.

Boekaerts, M. (1998). Boosting students' capacity to promote their own learning: A goal theory perspective. *Research Dialogue, 1*(1), 13–22.

Bruner, J. (2002). *Making Stories: Law, Literature, Life*. New York: Farrar, Straus, and Giroux.

Bulgren, J. A., & Schumaker, J. B. (2006). Teaching practices that optimize curriculum access. In D. D. Deshler & J. B. Schumaker (Eds.), *Teaching Adolescents with Disabilities: Accessing the General Curriculum* (pp. 79–120). Thousand Oaks, CA: Corwin Press.

Carver, C. S., & Scheier, M. F. (1998). *On the Self-regulation of Behavior*. Cambridge, UK: Cambridge University Press.

Deci, E. L., & Ryan, R. M. (2000). The "what" and "why" of goal pursuits: Human needs and the self-determination of behavior. *Psychological Inquiry, 11,* 227–268.

Denzin, N. K., & Lincoln, Y. S. (2000). *Handbook of Qualitative Research.* Thousand Oaks, CA: Sage Publications.

Emmons, R. A., & Kaiser, H. A. (1996). Goal orientation and emotional well-being: Linking goals and affect through the self. In L. Martin & A. Tessler (Eds.), *Striving and Feeling: Interactions Among Goals, Affect and Self-Regulation* (pp. 79–98). Hillsdale, N.J.: Lawrence Erlbaum Associates.

Fitzsimons, G. M., & Bargh, J. A. (2004). Automatic self-regulation. In R. F. Baumeister & K. D. Vohs (Eds.), *Handbook of Self-Regulation: Research, Theory and Applications* (pp. 151–170)). New York: Guilford Press.

Grafman, J. (2002). The structured event complex and the human prefrontal cortex. In D. T. Stuss & R. T. Knight (Eds.), *Principles of Frontal Lobe Function* (pp. 292–311). New York: Oxford University Press.

Hart, T., & Evans, J. (2006). Self-regulation and goal theories in brain injury rehabilitation. *Journal of Head Trauma Rehabilitation, 21*(2),142–155.

Heller, W., Mukherjee, D., Levin, R. L., & Reis, J. P. (2006). Characters in context: Identity and personality processes that influence individual and family adjustment to brain injury. *Journal of Rehabilitation, 72*(2), 44–49.

Hermans, H. L. M., Kempen, H. J. G., & van Loon, R. J. P. (1992). The dialogical self: Beyond individualism and rationalism. *American Psychologist, 47,* 23–33.

Hill, H. (1999). Traumatic brain injury: A view from the inside. *Brain Injury,* 13, 839–844.

Johansson, U., & Tham, K. (2006). The meaning of work after acquired brain injury. *American Journal of Occupational Therapy, 60*(1), 60–69.

Judd, D., & Wilson, S. L. (2005). Psychotherapy with brain injury survivors: An investigation of the challenges encountered by clinicians and their modifications to therapeutic practice. *Brain Injury, 19*(6), 437–449.

Kelly, A. E. (2000). Helping construct desirable identities: A self-presentational view of psychotherapy. *Psychological Bulletin, 126*(4), 475–494.

Kiresuk, T., & Sherman, R. (1968). Goal Attainment Scaling: A general method for evaluating community health programs. *Community Mental Health Journal,* 4, 443–453.

Klinger, L. (2005). Occupational adaptation: Perspectives of people with traumatic brain injury. *Journal of Occupational Science, 12*(1), 9–16.

Kovareky, D., Shaw, A., & Adingono-Smith, M. (2007). The construction of identity during group therapy among adults with traumatic brain injury. *Communication and Medicine,* 4(1), 53–66.

Lakoff, G., & Johnson, M. (1980). *Metaphors We Live By.* Chicago: University of Chicago Press.

Lakoff, G., & Johnson, M. (1999). *Philosophy in the Flesh: The Embodied Mind and Its Challenge to Western Thought.* New York: Basic Books.

Levack, W. S., Dean, S., McPherson, K. M., & Siegert, R. J. (2006a). How clinicians talk about the application of goal planning to rehabilitation for people with brain injury: Variable interpretations of value and purpose. *Brain Injury, 20*(13–14), 1439–1449.

Levack, W. S., Dean, S, Siegert, R. J., & McPherson, K. M. (2006b). Purposes and mechanisms of goal planning in rehabilitation: The need for a critical distinction. *Disability and Rehabilitation, 28*(12), 741–749.

Levack, W. S., Taylor, W. J., Siegert, R. J., Dean, S. G., McPherson, K. M., & Weatherall, M. (2006c). Is goal planning in rehabilitation effective? A systematic review. *Clinical Rehabilitation, 20*(9), 739–755.

Levine, B., Freedman, M., Dawson, D., Black, S., & Stuss, D. T. (1999). Ventral frontal contribution to self-regulation: Convergence of episodic memory and inhibition. *Neurocase,* 5, 263–275.

Locke, E. A., & Latham, G. P. (1990). *A Theory of Goal Setting and Task Performance*. Englewood Cliffs, NJ: Prentice-Hall, Inc.

Maclean, N., & Pound, P. (2000). A critical review of the concept of patient motivation in the literature on physical rehabilitation. *Social Science and Medicine, 50*(4), 495–506.

Mallinson, T., Kielhofner, G., & Mattingly, C. (1996). Metaphor and meaning in a clinical interview. *American Journal of Occupational Therapy, 50*(5), 338–346.

Markus, H., & Nurius, P. (1986). Possible selves. *American Psychologist, 41*, 954–969.

Markus, H., & Wurf, E. (1987). The dynamic self-concept: A social psychological perspective. *Annual Review of Psychology, 28*, 299–337.

Mays, N., & Pope, C. (1996). *Qualitative Research in Health Care* (1st ed.). London: BMJ Publishing.

Mays, N., & Pope, C. (2000). Qualitative research in health care: Assessing quality in qualitative research. *British Medical Journal, 320*, 50–52.

McMullin, R. E. (2000). *The New Handbook of Cognitive Therapy Techniques*. New York: W.W. Norton & Co.

McPherson, K. M., Brander, P. M., McNaugton, H., & Taylor, W. (2001). Living with arthritis: What is important? *Disability and Rehabilitation, 23*(16), 706–721.

McPherson, K. M., Brander, P., Taylor, W., McNaughton, H., & Weatherall, M. (2004). Consequences of stroke, arthritis and chronic pain: Are there important similarities? *Disability and Rehabilitation, 26*(16), 988–999.

Medical Research Council (2000). *A Framework for Development and Evaluation of RCTs for Complex Interventions to Improve Health*. London: Medical Research Council.

Morris, S. D. (2004). Rebuilding identity through narrative following traumatic brain injury. *Journal of Cognitive Rehabilitation, 22*(2), 15–21.

Nippold, M. (1998). *Later Language Development: The School-Age and Adolescent Years* (2nd ed.). Austin, TX: Pro-Ed.

Nochi, M. (1998). "Loss of self" in the narratives of people with traumatic brain injuries: A qualitative analysis. *Social Science and Medicine, 46*, 869–878.

Nochi, M. (2000). Reconstructing self-narratives in coping with traumatic brain injury. *Social Science & Medicine, 51*, 1795–1804.

Patton, M. Q. (1990). *Qualitative Evaluation and Research Methods*. Newbury Park, CA: Sage Publications.

Patton, M. Q. (1999). Enhancing the quality and credibility of qualitative analysis. *Health Services Research, 34*(5 Pt 2), 1189–1208.

Perna, R. B., & Errico, A. F. (2004). Neurological substrates of personal identity: Implications for neurorehabilitation. *Journal of Cognitive Rehabilitation, 22*(1), 10–12.

Petrella, L., McColl, M., Krupa, T., & Johnston, J. (2005). Returning to productive activities: Perspectives of individuals with long-standing acquired brain injuries. *Brain Injury, 19*(9), 643–655.

Pinker, S. (2007). *The Stuff of Thought: Language as a Window into Human Nature*. New York: Viking, Penguin Group.

Pope, C., Ziebland, S., & Mays, N. (2000). Qualitative research in health care: Analysing qualitative data. *British Medical Journal, 320*, 114–116.

Prigatano, G. P., & Schacter, D. L. (Eds.). (1991). *Awareness of Deficit after Brain Injury: Theoretical and Clinical Aspects*. New York: Oxford University Press.

Rogers, C. (1974). Some observations on the organization of personality. *American Psychologist, 2*, 358–368.

Ryan, R. M., & Deci, E. L. (2000). Self-determination theory and the facilitation of intrinsic motivation, social development, and well-being. *American Psychologist, 55*, 68–78.

Siegert, R. J., McPherson, K. M., & Taylor, W. J. (2004). Toward a cognitive-affective model of goal-setting in rehabilitation: Is self-regulation theory a key step? *Disability and Rehabilitation*, *26*(20), 1175–1183.

Siegert, R. J., & Taylor, W. J. (2004). Theoretical aspects of goal-setting and motivation in rehabilitation. *Disability and Rehabilitation*, *26*(1), 1–8.

Strauss, A. L., & Corbin, J. (1998). *Basics of Qualitative Research: Techniques and Procedures for Developing Grounded Theory* (2nd ed.). Thousand Oaks, CA: Sage Publications.

Stuss, D. T., & Alexander, M. P. (1999). Affectively burnt in: A proposed role of the right frontal lobe. In E. Tulving (Ed.). *Memory, Consciousness and the Brain: The Tallinn Conference* (pp. 215–227). Philadelphia: Psychology Press.

Teasdale. J. D. (1997). The transformation of meaning: The interacting cognitive subsystems approach. In M. Power & C. R. Brewin (Eds.), *The Transformation of Meaning in Psychological Therapies* (pp. 141–156). New York: John Wiley & Sons.

Teasdale, J. D., & Barnard, P. J. (1993). *Affect, Cognition, and Change: Re-Modelling Depressive Thought*. Hove, UK: Lawrence Erlbaum.

Teasdale, G., & Jennett, B. (1974). Assessment of coma and impaired consciousness. A practical scale. *Lancet*, *13*(2), 81–84.

Unruh, A. M. (2004). Reflections on: "So . . . what do you do?" Occupation and the construction of identity. *Canadian Journal of Occupational Therapy*, *71*(5), 290–295.

Unruh, A. M., Versnel, J., & Kerr, N. (2002). Spirituality unplugged: A review of commonalities and contentions, and a resolution. *Canadian Journal of Occupational Therapy*, *69*, 5–19.

Vickery, C. D., Gontkovsky, S. T., & Caroselli, J. S. (2005). Self-concept and quality of life following acquired brain injury: A pilot investigation. *Brain Injury*, *19*(9), 657–665.

Wade, D. T. (1998). Evidence relating to goal planning in rehabilitation. *Clinical Rehabilitation*, *12*, 273–275.

White, M., & Epston, D. (1990). *Narrative Means to Therapeutic Ends*. New York: W.W. Norton and Company.

Wilson, J. T. L., Pettigrew, L. E. L., & Teasdale, G. M. (1998). Structured interviews for the Glasgow Outcome Scale and the Extended Glasgow Outcome Scale: Guideliness for their use. *Journal of Neurotrauma*, *15*(8), 573–585.

Yeates, G., Henwood, K., Gracey, F., & Evans, J. (2007). Awareness of disability after acquired brain injury and the family context. *Neuropsychological Rehabilitation*, *17*(2), 151–173.

Ylvisaker, M., & Feeney, T. (2000). Construction of identity after traumatic brain injury. *Brain Impairment*, 1, 12–28.

Ylvisaker, M., Feeney, T., & Capo, M. (2007). Long-term community supports for individuals with co-occurring disabilities: Cost effectiveness and project-based intervention. *Brain Impairment*, *8*(2), 1–17.

NEUROPSYCHOLOGICAL REHABILITATION
2008, 18 (5/6), 742–765

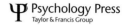

Psychology Press
Taylor & Francis Group

An exploratory case study of the impact of ambient biographical displays on identity in a patient with Alzheimer's disease

Michael Massimi[1], Emma Berry[2], Georgina Browne[2], Gavin Smyth[3], Peter Watson[4], and Ronald M. Baecker[5]

[1]*Department of Computer Science, University of Toronto, Canada;*
[2]*Neuropsychology Department, Clinical Neurosciences, Addenbrooke's Hospital, Cambridge, UK;* [3]*Microsoft Research Cambridge, UK;*
[4]*MRC-Cognition and Brain Sciences Unit, Cambridge, UK;* [5]*Knowledge Media Design Institute, University of Toronto, Canada*

One of the most troubling symptoms of Alzheimer's disease is the loss of the patient's sense of identity. This loss complicates relationships, increases apathy, and generally impedes quality of life for the patient. We describe a novel in-home ambient display called *Biography Theatre* that cycles through music, photographs, movies, and narratives drawn from the patient's past and current life. We conducted an exploratory case study with an 84-year-old male with moderate-stage Alzheimer's disease (Mr H). The study consisted of three phases: a baseline phase, a phase wherein autobiographical materials were collected and discussed, and a phase wherein the display was deployed in the home. The patient demonstrated improvement on standardised tests of apathy and positive self-identity, but did not improve on tests of autobiographical memory, anxiety, depression, and general cognition. We also report on caregiver reactions to the intervention and how the display helped them cope with and reinterpret their loved one's condition. This work suggests that interdisciplinary work involving "off the desktop" computing technologies may be a

Correspondence should be sent to Michael Massimi, Department of Computer Science, University of Toronto, 10 King's College Road, Toronto, Ontario, M5S 3G4, Canada. E-mail: mikem@dgp.toronto.edu

We would like to thank Steve Hodges and Ken Wood of Microsoft Research, Masashi Crete-Nishihata, Karen Louise-Smith, Thecla Damianakis, and especially Mr H and his family.

DOI:10.1080/09602010802130924

fruitful way to provide rehabilitative benefit for individuals with Alzheimer's disease.

Keywords: Identity; Alzheimer's disease; Ambient displays; Biography; Computing.

INTRODUCTION

The loss of identity is among the most devastating effects of Alzheimer's disease (AD). While it unclear how this "unbecoming" occurs (Kontos, 2005), it is possible that selfhood in AD degrades due to links to memory impairment (Downs, 1997). With this in mind, it is possible that sensitively designed technologies may help compensate for identity loss by acting as external memory or conversational aids. In this work, we describe an exploratory case study with a single participant wherein we examine how novel "off the desktop" technologies may help remediate identity through the provision of an external aid to memory and conversation.

Identity in Alzheimer's disease

Before examining how technology can help to remediate identity, it is necessary to break down the concept of identity further. The literature tells us that identity is commonly treated as a social process, whereby the individual defines him or herself as part of a group. Glover (1989) argues that we define our identities by responding to other people's actions towards us. These actions may be based on social structures such as gender, race, socio-economic status, or cultural upbringing, which also contribute to the way in which the individual understands his or her identity (Stryker & Burke, 2000).

Maintaining this sense of identity is important for people coping with AD. For instance, spouses of people affected by AD may attempt to affirm the patient's identity by maintaining gender roles despite the patient's inability to perform tasks culturally linked to gender (e.g., a husband caring for his wife may assume activities commonly considered "feminine" such as learning to cook and clean while at the same time helping her apply makeup) (Calasanti & Bowen, 2006).

Trends in person-centred care also share the belief that "people with dementia are ... people with unique biographies, personalities and life circumstances, all of which interact with the neurological impairment" (Downs, 1997, p. 598). These personalities and life circumstances may include changes in relationships with family members and environment as caregiving becomes more necessary.

Based on the notion that identity is created through both social and individual processes, we operationally define identity as a coherent internal, individualised self-concept that arises as a byproduct of intact autobiographical and personal semantic memory, in conjunction with understandings of one's relationship to others (Conway, 2005; Lundgren, 2004). This self-concept, in our study, is measured primarily through the participant's response to a formal test of identity for adults and through interview responses from his daughters and caregivers.

Approaches to rehabilitation of identity in Alzheimer's disease

In light of this movement towards acknowledging personhood in the care process, reminiscence therapy has become more popular (Woods, Spector, Jones, Orrell, & Davies, 2005). This therapy generally involves a caregiver sitting with the patient and using photos or keepsakes to motivate discussion. It is largely a conversational process. Lazarus, Cohler, and Lesser (1996) comment that "reminiscing reminds patients of a time when they felt more worthwhile, vital, and competent" (p. 256). Further, it reminds the family of the person they once knew. However, reminiscing can be time-consuming for family members already overburdened with other daily life activities. Patients may find the activity less satisfying when conducted with a hired care professional compared to a family member. In response to this, technological approaches may save caregivers time and effort and allow patients to reminisce on their own more easily.

There exists evidence that the decay of autobiographical and personal semantic memory is correlated with changes in identity for people with AD (Addis & Tippet, 2004). This supports current theories of identity, which posit that autobiographical and personal semantic memory systems play a role in formation of identity. In their study of 20 individuals with AD compared to 20 age-matched controls, Addis and Tippet found that impairment of memories from childhood and early adulthood were correlated with decreased strength and quality of identity as measured by the Twenty Statements Test and the Identity subscore of the Tennessee Self-Concept Scale. This finding supports current theories that memory plays a role in the formation of identity (Conway, 2005).

Other approaches to affirming or rehabilitating a sense of identity besides reminiscence therapy include validation therapy and reality-orientation therapy (Woods et al., 2005). Validation therapy suggests that caregivers simply listen to patients with AD and validate their concerns through creating a sense of shared understanding. It is not concerned explicitly with facts, but rather is about connecting at a more emotional level. Reality-orientation therapy, on the other hand, commonly involves discussing facts of which patients may not be aware (e.g., affirming the past) or asking patients to participate in activities designed to encourage information processing (Bennett, 2006). The movement towards personal or person-centred care emphasises identity and customised methods of treatment, although it is unclear how to treat identity in institutional settings: as a "thing" from the past that has broken, or as an ongoing process (Wellin & Jaffe, 2004).

Motivation for a technological approach

In this case study, we worked with a single patient to develop an in-home ambient display, called Biography Theatre, which displays digital life histories (DLHs) on an in-home touch-screen computer. We use the term "ambient display" to refer to an always-on, situated computer display which is not meant to be engaged as a foreground activity (as with traditional PCs), but is rather part of the background environment of the home. We consider this ambient display to belong to a class of emerging ubiquitous computing devices. This paradigm, thought by some computer scientists to be the "next wave" of computing, has the goal of enhancing human activity by embedding computational devices in the environment or making the devices mobile enough to be worn or carried (Weiser, 1993). The resulting interaction, it is believed, will be less focused on the mechanics of operating a computer, and more focused on engaging in an activity. In designing technology for reminiscence, it is critical that the focus remains on memories and social interaction rather than on operating technology. For this reason, we adopted a ubiquitous computing approach to designing the reminiscing technology and situated Biography Theatre in the participant's kitchen in a role similar to a picture frame.

In recent years, the use of technology to help rehabilitate mood and identity and communication in AD has been described in the literature. This study follows on from two previous influential projects that helped influence the design of the technology we describe. The main precursor for this work comes from Cohene, Baecker, Marziali, and Mindy (2006) and Baecker et al. (2007), wherein university students with little to no film-making experience worked with families of individuals with mild cognitive impairment and AD in order to produce "multimedia biographies" – 30–60 minute DVDs containing digitised photographs, music, videos, and narration drawn from the individual's life. Each DVD was organised into "acts" that revolved around a central theme such as "childhood", "marriage", or "my life in politics". Individuals were then asked to watch the DVDs on a regular basis, with qualitative results collected from video-taped observations of the individuals watching their autobiographies (often with family) at 6 month and 12 month follow-ups. Their findings indicated that the intervention stimulated enjoyable memories for the participants, that the families derived satisfaction from watching the DVDs with their loved ones, and that the biographies promoted conversation about past events. This work complements the previous study by providing additional evidence for the use of multimedia biography technology as a useful intervention for individuals with Alzheimer's disease.

The second source of inspiration comes from the CIRCA project at the University of Dundee (Gowans et al., 2004). In their project, researchers created an interactive storytelling device that contained public materials from the town of Dundee over the past several decades. These materials were presented on a touch screen interface and used in care facilities in order to stimulate conversation among residents. CIRCA differs from this work and the work by Baecker et al. (2007) in an important way; it contains public material rather than personalised materials. The rationale for this design decision was that public material would be less likely to elicit negative emotional responses (e.g., through seeing photos of a deceased spouse). Like Baecker et al. (2007), the CIRCA project prompted discussion and was viewed as a valuable piece of technology for the individuals with AD and their caregivers.

Hypotheses

In the current study, we examined the following hypotheses.

1. Participating in the collection process and display process would improve Mr H's autobiographical memory.

2. Mr H would report a stronger sense of identity after participating in the collection and display processes.

Our rationale for these hypotheses was as follows. For hypothesis 1, we predicted that exposure to materials from the past (e.g., photos) during the collection and display phases would cue Mr H's memory in ways that differ from cues he receives through everyday life. As a result, he would score higher on the Autobiographical Memory Interview (AMI) and be perceived to have higher cognitive functioning generally by his family as measured by the Informant Questionnaire of Cognitive Decline in the Elderly (IQCODE). We believed that because the topic of conversation would refer to Mr H's remote past, a period for which his long-term memory is still relatively intact, he would be able to participate in conversation more effectively compared to conversation about more current topics (hypothesis 2 above). This ability to engage in meaningful conversation and recall a time when he was a successful engineer and family man was expected to improve his sense of identity. As a result, his scores on the Self-Image Profile-Adult (SIP-AD) and the Twenty Statements Test (TST) were expected to improve. In response to these activities, it was considered possible that Mr H might experience a negative emotional response. For instance, reviewing his life history may highlight his current inabilities, prompting depression or anxiety. While the process was not expected to negatively impact Mr H's emotional status, we monitored levels of depression using the Geriatric Depression Scale–30 (GDS-30), levels of apathy using the Apathy Evaluation Scale–Informant (AES-I), and levels of anxiety using the Goldberg Anxiety Scale (GAS).

METHOD

In this single-subject case study, we specified three data collection points: (1) baseline, (2) after the collection of biographical material (interim), and (3) after the deployment of the Biography Theatre for a period of 2 weeks (final). At each time point, the participant underwent a neuropsychological battery containing eight standardised tests, one custom interview, and one custom questionnaire. At these points, we also collected informant data from three people: the participant's two adult daughters and his part-time daily caregiver.

PARTICIPANT AND CARE NETWORK

At the time of the study, Mr H was an 84-year-old right-handed British male. Before retiring, he worked and lived in over 10 countries around the world as an electrical engineer. He was diagnosed with Alzheimer's disease in 2005, and a standard assessment by a clinical neuropsychologist confirmed him to be in the moderate stages of the disease before the time of the study in 2007. His wife and brother both died in 2006. He lived at home during the course of the study, and was visited by caregivers and his daughters every day. He attended a bimonthly memory clinic at a local hospital and was referred to the study by a clinical neuropsychologist working at this hospital.

Mr H's care was overseen primarily by his daughters E and R. Both daughters had their own families and lived within 20 minutes of Mr H. They spoke to their father twice a day via the telephone, and picked him up for dinner on most nights. During weekdays, a hired caregiver L stayed with Mr H at his home and coordinated his schedule and daily activities. On nights that he did not have dinner with one of his daughters' families, an evening caregiver (D) stayed with him until bedtime. At the weekends, he usually stayed with one of his daughters. Together, these four individuals provided care during Mr H's waking hours. They coordinated their efforts through the use of a shared calendar and diary left in the kitchen.

Collection process (Phase I)

To develop a personalised biography of Mr H's life, it was important to involve him and his family in selecting materials to include. With the help of his daughters, we began by listing the major "chapters" of his life. Because Mr H and his wife and daughters lived in so many countries around the world, the chapters were often organised by the place where they lived (e.g., chapter titles included "Singapore" and "Egypt"). Additional chapters regarding his parents, childhood, marriage, children, and recent life also marked major life events.

A researcher then visited Mr H in his home approximately twice a week over the course of one month. At each visit, the researcher and Mr H would reminisce over old photos or memorabilia in an unstructured session lasting approximately 1 hour. At the end of each session, the photos were taken to the laboratory in order to be scanned and categorised into the appropriate life chapter. One session also focused on music, wherein the researcher asked Mr H to talk about his favorite musicians. Audio cassettes and CDs were similarly taken to the laboratory to be digitised into MP3 files. Each session was videotaped in order to collect Mr H's stories and narratives prompted by the materials under review.

In parallel, the researcher met with Mr H's daughters in sessions that helped us to obtain a richer story about his life. His daughters helped organise the DLH by providing appropriate chapters and stories. We also videotaped them as they told stories about their father relevant to each chapter. These stories were then included in the DLH and played alongside the photographs collected.

Digital life history viewing process (Phase II)

Previous work used DVDs in order to allow participants to watch their biographies (Baecker et al., 2007). However, we noted some technical limitations of these installations. Caregivers often had to be present in order to operate the DVD player and begin the biography. Subsequent interactions via the remote control could also be problematic, although replacing the remote control with a single large button partially helped to overcome this problem (Cohene et al., 2006). In addition, a DVD-based biography requires attention similar to watching a movie or television show, which may be prohibitive for some participants. We improved upon this process by creating a system called Biography Theatre.

Biography Theatre

Biography Theatre is an always-on permanent feature in Mr H's home which plays DLHs structured in a custom database (Figure 1). Biography Theatre sits in a "picture frame" on Mr H's kitchen table (actually a Sahara slate PC positioned on a stand). It consists of a menu which permits him or his caregivers to select a particular chapter of his life to review. If no chapter is selected within 5 minutes, the entire biography plays from the beginning until the end. At the end of the biography, the system returns to the main menu and repeats the biography after another 5 minutes. We originally programmed the system to dim the screen after 15 minutes of inactivity, but Mr H and his caregivers found this to be undesirable and so it was

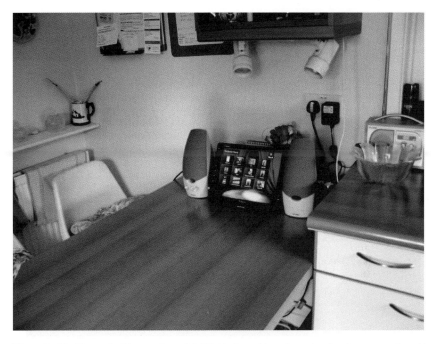

Figure 1. The Biography Theatre sits on Mr H's kitchen table and continually plays scenes from his past. The touch-screen interface allows users to select particular chapters, skip forwards and backwards through chapters, or pause the playback.

removed. The user can pause the chapter, skip to the previous chapter, skip to the next chapter, or return to a main menu of chapter listings by pressing simple buttons on the touch screen (Figure 2). The system is never turned off, and is connected to a pair of external speakers that can be used to turn off the volume if desired. All other operations are hidden from the user, as Biography Theatre runs in full-screen mode.

INSTRUMENTS

Two types of instruments were utilised during the study: formal psychometric tests and custom questionnaires and interviews specifically prepared for Mr H's family.

Psychometric tests

Psychometric instruments were chosen according to four major categories of measures in reminiscence therapy as set out by Woods et al. (2005). Below are the four major categories with the tests chosen for each category.

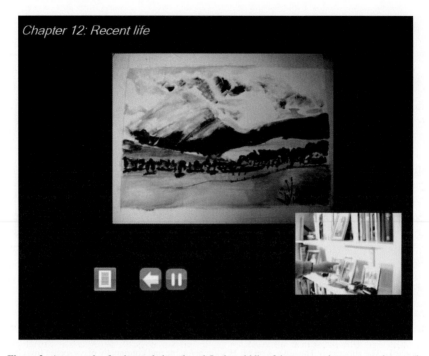

Figure 2. An example of a chapter being played. In the middle of the screen, photos pan and zoom (in this case, a watercolor painting Mr H recently completed). In the bottom right corner, video narratives (by Mr H or his daughters) accompany the photographs. Music plays in the background. The orange buttons allow the user to pause the chapter, to skip to adjacent chapters, or see a menu of all chapters.

1. Well-being: Depression, anxiety, identity, apathy, general mood.
   - Relevant instruments: Geriatric Depression Scale-30 (GDS-30), Goldberg Anxiety Scale (GAS), Apathy Evaluation Scale-Informant (AES-I), Self-Image Profile-Adult (SIP-AD), Twenty Statements Test (TST).
2. Communication and interaction: Conversation content, frequency, and initiation.
   - Relevant instruments: Custom interviews and questionnaires.
3. Cognition: Autobiographical memory, general cognitive functioning, memory.
   - Relevant instruments: Autobiographical Memory Interview (AMI), Mini-Mental State Exam (MMSE), Informant Questionnaire of Cognitive Decline in the Elderly (IQCODE).
4. Caregiver relationships: Caregiver strain, caregiver knowledge, emotional connection.
   - Relevant instruments: Modified Caregiver Strain Index (CSI), custom interviews and questionnaires.

Like Addis and Tippet (2004), we attempted to use the TST as a measure of identity on all three occasions. However, at each occasion, Mr H was unable to produce a single meaningful or unprompted statement about himself, even when the test was administered verbally. It is unclear whether he was unable to complete the test due to an actual diminishment of factors relating to self-identity or due to other non-identity related factors associated with the disease (e.g., language impairment).

Psychometric instruments included the MMSE in order to gauge global changes in cognition, and to ensure that changes on other tests were not the result of general disease progression. The AMI is a test wherein participants are asked to recall episodes from different eras of their life, and scored on the amount of detail produced. It was included to determine whether the collection process or DLH helped improve autobiographical memory through repeated exposure to reminiscence material. The IQCODE was administered to both daughters as a way to determine caregiver impressions of Mr H's cognitive ability. Given the suggestion from the CIRCA project that the use of personal items may cause depression or anxiety (Gowans et al., 2004), we administered the GDS-30 and the GAS. The GDS-30 involves responding to 30 Likert scale items regarding mood. The GAS is a short interview with up to nine questions which is intended to screen rapidly for the presence of anxiety. The AES-I was an informant questionnaire containing Likert items regarding how involved or withdrawn the patient was. It was included in order to determine if participating in the research helped Mr H feel more involved and active with his family. The SIP-AD is a questionnaire that asks participants to rate how strongly they feel particular characteristics apply to them (e.g., optimistic, hopeful, caring). It is organised into six subscores: Outlook, Consideration, Social, Physical, Competence, and Moral. Finally, the CSI was included to determine whether collecting biographical materials and using the DLH resulted in additional caregiver burden due to time spent collecting items or working with the computer.

Custom questionnaires and interviews

In order to ask more precise questions about the effect of the process and technology on Mr H and his family, we developed custom questionnaires and interviews to be administered to Mr H, his two daughters, and his daytime caregiver. These instruments included items regarding Mr H's ability to remember the past, frequency and types of conversation, emotional closeness to his family and community, and fulfilment with his life's work. The complete questionnaires and interview protocols can be found in Appendices 1 and 2.

RESULTS

We present the results of the formal psychological tests as quantitative results at each of the three assessments, supplemented by qualitative results provided by the participant and his family at those times.

Quantitative results

Overall, scores on the psychometric tests indicate an increase in self-identity and a decrease in apathy. However, due to the single-subject case study design and lack of appropriate norms for measuring identity in patients with Alzheimer's disease, we were unable to apply satisfactory inferential statistics. Of the norms that were available, none reported the central tendency or variance of change over time, making it difficult to draw reliable inferences regarding Mr H's progress. However, descriptive statistics and the most appropriate norms for the SIP-AD and AES-I are reported in Table 1.

Effect of collecting materials for a biography (Results from Interim Assessment)

After completing the collection process, we completed the interim psychological assessment battery with Mr H and his caregivers. Scores from the SIP-AD increased 13 points from 117 to 130, out of a maximum score of 180 (higher scores indicate more positive self-image). Informant measures from the AES-I indicated a decrease in apathy, dropping from 28 to 18 out of a maximum score of 54 (lower scores indicate less apathy). Depression and anxiety scores remained low. General cognition and autobiographical memory remained stable. One daughter reported a decrease in caregiver strain as measured by the CSI (from 100 to 87 on a scale of 160, higher numbers indicate higher strain). Reports from his daughters and caregivers indicated he "was more confident and had more self-esteem". There was no recorded change in conversation content or frequency.

Effects of viewing and interacting with a DLH (Results from Final Assessment)

After Mr H used the DLH for 4 weeks, we conducted the final assessment. Mr H continued to show improvement on the SIP-AD measure of identity, increasing from 130 to 148 (18 points higher than the interim assessment, and 31 points higher than baseline). His levels of apathy on the AES-I remained lower than baseline, but rose slightly compared to the interim. Depression, anxiety, and cognition maintained previous levels.

TABLE 1
Results of psychological assessments at baseline, interim and final stages

Test	Target construct	Baseline	Interim	Final
Mini-Mental State Examination (of 30) (Folstein, Folstein, & McHugh, 1975)	Cognition – global	23	24	22
Autobiography Memory Interview (Kopelman, Wilson, & Baddeley, 1989)	Cognition – autobiographical memory	35%	34%	21%
Informant Questionnaire of Cognitive Decline in the Elderly* (of 5) (Jorm, 2004)	Cognition – memory (general)	4.77	4.88	4.65
Geriatric Depression Scale–30 (of 30) (Yesavage et al., 1983)	Well-being – depression	2	1	0
Goldberg Anxiety Scale (of 9) (Goldberg, Bridges, Duncan-Jones, & Grayson, 1988)	Well-being – anxiety	0	0	0
Apathy Evaluation Scale–Informant* (of 54) (Marin, Biedrzycki, & Firinciogullari, 1991) (Norms: $M = 49.1$, $SD = 9.9$ for probable AD)	Well-being – apathy	28	18	20
Self Image Profile-Adult (of 180) (Butler & Gasson, 2004) (Norms: $M = 125.87$, $SD = 24.03$ for normal males aged 56–65)	Well-being – identity	117	130	148
Modified Caregiver Strain Index* (of 160) (Robinson, 1983)	Caregiver relationships – strain	100	87	124

*Tests with grey shading indicate informant measures completed by Mr H's daughters. Gains on the Self-Image Profile–Adult suggest the interventions improved identity, while a decrease in apathy was present on the Apathy Evaluation Scale–Informant.

The CSI score for Mr H's daughter rose to a high beyond the baseline (124, compared to baseline of 100), possibly because she took him along on a week-long holiday midway between the interim and final assessments. Autobiographical memory was seen to decrease from recalling 34% of discussed episodes to remembering 21%.

Feedback on the process of building the DLH

Overall, the experience of building the DLH was a positive one for the caregivers and Mr H. The family appreciated the opportunity to reminisce about the past with their father. However, the process was time-consuming, and required commitment from members of the family in order to make a high-quality account of Mr H's life possible. Mr H was, at times, fatigued by the process of reminiscing, and during some sessions, he would stand up and leave. This feedback suggests possible solutions in the form of automated technologies (e.g., a wearable camera such as SenseCam, Berry et al., 2007) or allowing for the DLH to be crafted over a period of months rather than a few weeks.

Feedback on keeping the DLH in the home

Keeping the DLH in the home was a very positive experience for Mr H and his caregivers and is, as of the time of writing, still in operation. During one telephone call with the family following the study, Daughter R reported that the entire family had gathered in the kitchen and was dancing and singing to the music from the ambient display. She further noted that Mr H had invited friends to come see the display, and had even shown off the system to the postman. It was additionally noted that the caregivers would like to have more control over the DLH – for example, they would like the ability to add and remove photos. In response, we are currently developing software called Biography Maker, which provides a user interface appropriate for care-givers to create DLHs without the assistance of a technologist.

DISCUSSION

Through the process of developing and using the DLH, we collected quanti-tative data from psychometric assessments in addition to qualitative data from interviews and observation. Overall, the use of an in-home display containing multimedia biographical materials implies improvement in the patient's sense of identity as measured by the SIP-AD. In addition, participating in the process appears to have reduced the patient's sense of apathy as measured by the informant version of the AES.

In some respects this work validates current theories that identity is depen-dent upon autobiographical and semantic personal memory (Conway, 2005). Just as external aids for prospective and semantic memory exist, it is possible that the DLH was an external aid for autobiographical and personal semantic memory. Correspondingly, Mr H scored higher on tests of identity.

Based on our observations in this exploratory case study, we explore how the DLH may have contributed to improvements in three ways. First, it may have acted as an external memory aid, permitting Mr H to engage in activities that rely on memory without actually improving memory itself. Second, it appears to have changed Mr H's relationships and communication. Because his friends and family viewed the DLH as well, they changed their behaviours and actions towards Mr H. Finally, Mr H's behaviour appears to have changed as a result of this new social emphasis on viewing his life and past as an achievement and an important topic for conversation.

Impact on memory

While the DLH by no means "restored" memory or improved cognition generally, it did change the way that memory factored into family life. Authoring and interacting with the DLH created an occasion to remember – an excuse, an opportunity, a "reminder" of the self, perhaps. In fact, family members often equated improvements in memory with improvements in communication:

> "[His memory] is much the same . . . Has it improved? Probably not. . . but he is remembering a lot about . . . [pause]. . . I guess I'm contradicting myself . . . he's *talking* a lot about what's on it. . . It's obviously made him more interested I think in the past. It's stimulated his interest in his memories, if you like."
>
> Daughter E

Mr H's daughter struggles to describe the concept that his memory has not improved, but he is *acting* in ways that imply it has. These were the actions that the family valued; the technology allowed them to bring the past to bear on the present – what Harper, Smyth, Evans, Heledd, and Moore (2007) describe as "memory-as-a-resource-for-action". It is one thing for Mr H to remember his holiday to Cyprus; it is quite another for him to laugh with his daughter about how much they drank at dinner on the first night. Our work demonstrates the value of situated technology that does not improve memory in a strict sense, but provides cues that bring memories to mind and is a tool to make *actions* that depend on memory like chatting and sharing possible.

Impact on relationships and communication

For family members caring for an individual with AD or mild cognitive impairment, the perceived person behaves differently from the person once known. The DLH worked to change this perception by providing a fuller, more encompassing depiction of who the person is and was. By changing the perception, the DLH changed the way that family members interacted with the participant.

> "[It] reminds us that he's not just an old man with a bad memory . . . he was clever and vibrant . . . This is a good way of reinforcing how he was."
>
> Daughter E

This quote illustrates the tendency for caregivers and family members to forget the role the individual played in the past, and instead see the individual primarily as a care recipient – in effect, a role transition or reversal (Stryker & Burke, 2000). In this case, as the disease progressed, the person's role changed from one of "parent" or "friend" to one of "old man". Creating and watching the DLH, however, worked to reverse these role changes – it gave Mr H a voice to assert his identity to others:

> "The fact that he's enjoyed seeing his past and remembered it, and he feels quite proud of what he's done. I think he feels he's got a sense of pride in the past, which he had forgotten before. He's reminded himself, in a way, of what he's achieved, I think."
>
> Daughter R

Also important is the ability to feel a connection to other people in the family despite being apart from them.

> "It has given him a sense of us being around even though we haven't been ... he phoned me up, he's often remarked 'I heard your voices! I heard you and [your sister] speaking!' He's obviously got up and heard it ... he has taken a lot of pleasure from it."
>
> Daughter E

According to interviews, conversation content changed greatly, with Mr H's daughters noting that he brings up items from the DLH in conversation more frequently than before.

The role of the biographer

One relationship that should not be overlooked is that between the participant and the biographer/researcher. By orchestrating a series of activities intended to "help" with the cognitive decline, we provided a social atmosphere that valued and affirmed the participant's prior role.

> "He's enjoyed the attention he is getting from everybody ... I think he's enjoying the process knowing that ... we're discussing his past more."
>
> Daughter R

Our relationship with the individual re-emphasised that the person was a human being and not "an old man with a bad memory" and may have even set an example for family members to follow. The introduction of the process and technology provided family members with an excuse to re-evaluate the way they saw their loved one.

Impact on behaviour

The activities undertaken in the two phases above appear to have altered Mr H's behaviour in important ways. For these results, we rely primarily on unprompted caregiver reports collected both during and after the two phases.

The first notable change in Mr H's behaviour is what appeared to be an increase in independent reminiscing between sessions. Perhaps prompted by the interest we expressed in his biographical material, he began to take more and more photos out of storage.

> "On Friday he kept going upstairs. I could hear a lot of thumping around. I said, 'Are you all right?' and he said, 'I'm just looking for some books and photos.' I haven't known him to do that, though. He came down with just a little album ... and wanted me to have a look at it. ... This particular day, we hadn't been talking about research or the past ... he did do that [on his own], nothing prompted it. That was quite odd, actually."
>
> Caregiver L

Once the DLH was installed in the home, Mr H exhibited a range of surprising behaviours which were not previously present. In the first week after installing the DLH, we phoned Mr H's caregivers. When Daughter R picked up the phone, we heard laughing and singing in the background. She explained that the entire family had gathered around the display and Mr H was "dancing around the kitchen, showing it off to everyone".

Mr H used the DLH to express himself to other people beyond his family members. Daughter R noted that he even invited the postman into the house to see his DLH. We find that the patient was able to assert his sense of self through sharing the display with others. Despite the inclusion of some potentially distressing memories (e.g., photos of his late wife), his scores on scales of depression and anxiety were uniformly low across all three data collection points.

Integrating our findings with current perspectives on person-centred care

This study has given some tentative support to the efficacy of interpersonal methods of rehabilitation, such as group reminiscence therapy, in which personal memories are stimulated by archive material. Like us, Head, Portnoy, and Woods (1990) found increased interaction in a group who were involved in reminiscent activities and Brooker and Duce (2000) noted higher levels of well-being during reminiscence groups which we also observed in our patient.

However our single case study, although preliminary, implies that sensitively developed technologies may encourage reminiscent activities which can potentially improve identity in people who may have difficulty articulating it otherwise and who may not respond well in a group situation. Interestingly, this study indicates that improvements to identity can be seen without necessarily improving autobiographical memory. That is to say, intact autobiographical memory does not appear to be a prerequisite for a positive sense of self, but may perhaps be only a contributing factor (Conway, 2005).

Furthermore, our preliminary findings may also indicate that identity is formed not solely through communicative and psychological processes, but also through interactions with the environment and its contents. Woods and Roth (2005) argue that traditional care environments for people with dementia do not support remaining skills and abilities, leading to underperformance and withdrawal from their environments, while Clare (2003) suggests that this loss of social and psychological function is commonplace following cognitive deterioration. There has therefore been a more recent shift to implement more positive, person-centred interventions for people with dementia and a growing evidence base to suggest that efforts to include and/or improve identity as a goal of rehabilitation may lead to improvements in treatment outcomes and to quality of life more generally. For example, one study found that including activities in a care home designed to correspond to a person's self-identity resulted in increased interest, pleasure, involvement in other activities, and orientation during the treatment period (Cohen-Mansfield, Parpura-Gill, & Golander, 2006a). A recent interpretive study found that people with dementia highly value being involved in meaningful activity, as defined by experiencing pleasure, sense of belonging, and retained sense of self-identity (Phinney, Chaudhury, & O'Connor, 2007). The authors further suggest that one way to create meaningful activity is through "creating a familiar social and physical environment that allows activity to happen in a way that is spontaneous and flexible" (Phinney et al., 2007, p. 391). The placement of Biography Theatre in our study promotes spontaneous conversation because it does not require set-up or demand to be the focus of attention. Its flexibility rests in the way it presents material, which can be incorporated into conversation or easily ignored.

Cohen-Mansfield, Parpura-Gill, and Golander (2006b) undertook an analysis of the importance of past identity roles to people with dementia. They identified four salient roles: professional, family, hobbies/leisure activities, and personal attributes and while they found that the importance of these roles decreased over the course of the illness, the family role was valued most. The group concluded that taking into account the past and present roles of a person with dementia was crucial for person-centred care and improving the individual experience. Our work provides a unique interdisciplinary way of bringing these roles to mind for both the patient and his caregivers.

This literature may in part explain the beneficial effect the Biography Theatre had for Mr H, as it appears that maintaining a sense of self is important for psychological and social well-being. Perhaps reviewing material that depicts self-defining experiences from the past is a powerful mechanism for maintaining identity, with secondary benefits to increased involvement in other activities.

Limitations of the approach

In this paper, we report on a single-subject case study which did not use a control condition – that is to say, the design was ABC rather than ABACA. Due to the small number and the lack of a control group, the results should not be generalised to other individuals or populations. As we continue to use this technology with more case study subjects, we intend to use experimental designs that are more sensitive to measuring the specific aspects of the multimedia biography that impact identity. However, due to the biographical and personalised nature of each DLH, it is impossible to apply the same treatment to each participant. This makes large-scale trials a difficult challenge. In addition, this process is time-consuming; developing the DLH took an experienced technologist approximately 30–40 hours of work over the course of a month. To combat this problem, we are presently developing software that may be used by caregivers to generate DLHs without the assistance of a technologist. Even so, the approach involves little to no risk and, as a byproduct, the family is left with a keepsake that can be passed down to future generations.

CONCLUSION

In this case study we have shown how an ambient display called Biography Theatre helped change memory and relationship-based behaviours and suggest that this display helped an individual with Alzheimer's disease improve his sense of identity. This work offers a proof of concept for inter-disciplinary efforts for rehabilitation of identity, combining the efforts and expertise of clinical neuropsychologists and computer scientists. While the results are not able to be generalised due to the case study method employed, we have contributed some evidence that this novel ubiquitous computing approach to remediating identity may be an effective intervention strategy.

REFERENCES

Addis, D. R., & Tippet, L. J. (2004). Memory of myself: Autobiographical memory and identity in Alzheimer's disease. *Memory, 12*, 56–74.

Baecker, R. M., Marziali, E., Chatland, S., Easley, K., Crete, M., &Yeung, M. (2007). Multi-media biographies for individuals with Alzheimer's disease and their families. *Proceedings of the 2nd International Conference on Technology and Aging.* June 16–19, 2007, Toronto, Ontario, Canada.

Bennett, P. (2006). *Abnormal and Clinical Psychology: An Introductory Textbook.* Maidenhead, UK: Open University Press.

Berry, E., Kapur, N., Williams, L., Hodges, S., Watson, P., Smyth, G., Srinivasan, J., Smith, R., Wilson, B., & Wood, K. (2007). The use of a wearable camera, SenseCam, as a pictorial diary to improve autobiographical memory in a patient with limbic encephalitis: A preliminary report. *Neuropsychological Rehabilitation, 17*(4/5), 582–601.

Brooker, D., & Duce, L. (2000). Wellbeing and activity in dementia: A comparison of group reminiscence therapy, structured goal-directed group activity and unstructured time. *Aging & Mental Health, 4*(4), 354.

Butler, R. J., & Gasson, S. L. (2004). *The Self Image Profile for Adults.* Oxford: Harcourt Assessment.

Calasanti, T., & Bowen, M. (2006). Spousal caregiving and crossing gender boundaries: Maintaining gendered identities. *Journal of Aging Studies, 20*, 253–263.

Clare, L. (2003). Neuropsychological rehabilitation for people with dementia. In B. A. Wilson (Ed.), *Neuropsychological Rehabilitation: Theory and Practice.* Lisse, The Netherlands: Swets and Zeitlinger.

Cohene, T., Baecker, R. M., Marziali, E., & Mindy, S. (2006). Memories of a life: A design case study for Alzheimer's disease. In J. Lazar (Ed.), *Universal Usability* (pp. 357–487) Chichester: John Wiley and Sons

Cohen-Mansfield, J., Parpura-Gill, A., & Golander, H. (2006a). Utilization of self-identity roles for designing interventions for persons with dementia. *Journals of Gerontology, Series B, Psychological Sciences and Social Sciences, 61*(4), 202–212.

Cohen-Mansfield, J., Parpura-Gill, A., & Golander, H. (2006b). Salience of self-identity roles in persons with dementia: Differences in perceptions among elderly persons, family members and caregivers. *Social Science and Medicine, 62*(3), 745–757.

Conway, M. (2005). Memory and the self. *Journal of Memory and Language, 53*, 594–628.

Downs, M. (1997). The emergence of the person in dementia research. *Ageing and Society, 17*, 597–607.

Folstein, M. F., Folstein, S. L., & McHugh, P. R. (1975). 'Mini-Mental State', practical methods for grading the cognitive state of patients for clinicians. *Journal of Psychiatry Research, 12*, 189–198.

Glover, J. (1989). *The Philosophy and Psychology of Personal Identity.* London: Penguin.

Goldberg, D., Bridges, K., Duncan-Jones, P., & Grayson, D. (1988). Detecting anxiety and depression in general medical settings. *British Medical Journal, 297*, 897–899.

Gowans, G., Campbell, J., Alm, N., Dye, R., Astell, A., & Ellis, M. (2004). Designing a multimedia conversation aid for reminiscence therapy in dementia care environments. *Extended Proceedings of the CHI 2004 Conference on Human Factors in Computing Systems*, 825–836.

Harper, R., Randall, D., Smyth, N., Evans, C., Heledd, L., & Moore, R. (2007). Thanks for the memory. *Proceedings of the British HCI 2007.* September 3–7, 2007, Lancaster, UK.

Head, D., Portnoy, S., & Woods, R. T. (1990). The impact of reminiscence groups two different settings. *International Journal of Geriatric Psychiatry, 5*, 295–302.

Jorm, A. F. (2004). The information questionnaire on cognitive decline in the elderly (IQCODE): A review. *International Psychogeriatrics, 16*(3), 1–19.

Kontos, P. (2005). Embodied selfhood in Alzheimer's disease. *Dementia, 4*(4), 553–570.

Kopelman, M. D., Wilson, B. A., & Baddeley, A. D. (1989). The Autobiographical Memory Interview: A new assessment of autobiographical and personal semantic memory in amnesic patients. *Journal of Clinical and Experimental Neuropsychology, 11*, 724–744.

Lazarus, L. W., Cohler, B. J., & Lesser, J. (1996). Self-psychology: Its application to understanding patients with Alzheimer's disease. *International Psychogeriatrics, 8*(3), 253–258.

Lundgren, D. C. (2004). Social feedback and self-appraisals: Current status of the Mead-Cooley hypothesis. *Symbolic Interaction, 27,* 267–286.

Marin, R. S., Biedrzycki, R. C., & Firinciogullari, S. (1991). Reliability and validity of the apathy evaluation scale. *Psychiatry Research, 38,* 143–162.

Phinney, A., Chaudhury, H., & O'Connor, D. L. (2007). Doing as much as I can do: The meaning of activity for people with dementia. *Aging and Mental Health, 11*(4), 384–393.

Robinson, B. (1983). Validation of a caregiver strain index. *Journal of Gerontology, 38*(3), 344–348.

Skaff, M. M., & Pearlin, L. I. (1992). Caregiving: Role engulfment and the loss of self. *The Gerontologist, 32*(5), 656–664.

Stryker, S., & Burke, P. J. (2000). The past, present, and future of an identity theory. *Social Psychology Quarterly, 63*(4), 284–297.

Weiser, M. (1993). Some computer science issues in ubiquitous computing. *Communications of the ACM, 36*(7), 75–83

Wellin, C., & Jaffe, D. J. (2004). In search of "personal care": Challenges to identity support in residential care for elders with cognitive illness. *Journal of Aging Studies, 18*(3), 275–295.

Woods, R., & Roth, A. (2005). Effectiveness of psychological interventions in older people. In A. Roth and P. Fonagy (Eds.), *What Works for Whom?* New York: The Guilford Press.

Woods, B., Spector, A., Jones, C., Orrell, M., & Davies, S. (2005). Reminiscence therapy for dementia. *Cochrane Database of Systematic Reviews* (2).

Yesavage, J., Brink, T. L., Rose, T. L., Lum, O., Huang, V., Adey, M., & Leirer, V. O. (1983). Development and validation of a geriatric depression scale: A preliminary report. *Journal of Psychiatric Research, 17,* 39–49.

APPENDIX 1: CUSTOM QUESTIONNAIRES

These questionnaires were administered to Mr H and his daughters. All items were presented in the style of question 1 below.

Questionnaire for participant

Please circle the number the best answer for each of the items below:

1. I can remember childhood events vividly.

1	2	3	4	5
Strongly disagree				*Strongly agree*

2. I have trouble remembering the specifics of important events in my life (e.g., who else was present, where it occurred).

3. Trying to remember events from long ago is frustrating.

4. I think about the past frequently.

5. Sometimes I daydream about things that happened to me long ago.

6. I worry about forgetting details of important events I attended.

7. I have trouble remembering events that happened in the past week.

8. I frequently bring up past events in conversation.

9. I like to have long, in-depth conversations with my friends and family.

10. I prefer to keep to myself about personal things.

11. When I meet someone new, I like to share my stories with them.

12. It's important for me to share my past with people in order to build a relationship.

13. I like to meet new people.

14. I like to chat with my family frequently.

15. I call my friends and family on the telephone frequently.

16. I'm not very good at keeping in touch with old friends.

17. I'm a talkative person.

18. I dislike it when my friends or family ask me personal questions.

19. I feel close to the members of my family.

20. I would consider myself a "family man".

21. I feel like my children don't understand the full story of my life.

22. There are things about my past I'd like to share with my children and grandchildren.

23. When I tell my family things about my past, I feel like I am boring them.

24. I have trouble keeping up with the goings-on of my family members.

25. My children and grandchildren understand me well.

26. I would like to spend more time with my family.

27. It's hard to start conversations about my past with my family.

28. I feel like I have lived a full life.

29. I feel connected to my family.

30. I feel connected to my community.

31. I feel connected to my friends and colleagues.

32. I feel spiritually fulfilled.

33. I am proud of my life's work.

34. I feel like I made a difference in the world.

35. I worry that people will forget me when I pass.

36. I am a nostalgic person.

37. I am grateful for the opportunities I have had.

38. I distress about mistakes I've made in the past.

39. I strongly defend what I believe in.

Questionnaire for caregivers and family members

1. [Participant] can take care of most everyday activities on his own.

2. [Participant]'s memory has gotten worse in the past 5 years.

3. [Participant] is able to follow instructions for simple appliances (like a television or DVD player).

4. [Participant] can be trusted to remember to complete important tasks.

5. [Participant] has difficulty remembering things from a long time ago.

6. [Participant] has trouble remembering events from the previous week.

7. [Participant] repeats himself frequently.

8. [Participant]'s memory seems to come and go depending on the day.

9. [Participant] reminisces about the past frequently.

10. [Participant] tells stories about his past a lot.

11. When it comes to personal things, [Participant] keeps to himself.

12. [Participant] likes to talk about the news and other current events.

13. [Participant] and I have long, in-depth conversations.

14. [Participant] and I talk often.

15. I usually initiate the conversation with [Participant].

16. I talk with [Participant] on the phone frequently.

17. I visit [Participant] frequently.

18. I like to check in on [Participant].

19. I think I know a lot about what [Participant]'s life was like when he was growing up.

20. I wish I knew more about [Participant]'s life.

21. It's important to understand my genealogy and family history.

22. I know what the most important events in [Participant]'s life are.

23. Sometimes I worry I won't get the chance to ask [Participant] something important about his life before he passes.

24. I feel awkward asking [Participant] to talk about his life with me.

25. When [Participant] and I talk, he usually seems enthusiastic.

26. I feel emotionally close to [Participant].

27. I wish I knew [Participant] better.

28. I feel like [Participant] and I have a lot in common.

29. On a day-to-day basis, [Participant] seems motivated and engaged.

30. [Participant] usually seems tired.

31. [Participant] seems proud of his life's accomplishments.

32. [Participant] seems proud of his children and grandchildren's accomplishments.

33. [Participant] seems worried or preoccupied.

34. [Participant] seems nostalgic.

APPENDIX B: INTERVIEW SCRIPTS

Interview with participant

1. How would you describe your ability to remember the past?

2. When you chat with people in your family, what topics do you generally discuss?

3. What kind of things do you talk about when you are out with friends?

4. How often do you chat with your family?

5. Who usually initiates the conversation? You or your family members?

6. Do you feel it is important for you to keep in touch with people from your past?

7. How would you describe your relationship with your children?

8. How would you describe your relationship with your grandchildren?

9. How would you describe your general well-being at this stage in your life?

10. Would you say you are a hopeful person?

Interview with caregivers and family

1. Could you please describe your perceptions of how [Participant]'s memory is?

2. What kinds of memory mistakes does [Participant] make?

3. When you and [Participant] have a conversation, what is it usually about?

4. What sorts of things does [Participant] usually like to talk about?

5. How often do you and [Participant] get a chance to talk?

6. When you and [Participant] talk, is it usually by phone, email, letter, or in person?

7. How would you describe your knowledge of [Participant]'s past?

8. How familiar are you with [Participant]'s life history?

9. How would you describe your relationship with [Participant]?

10. Who in your family would you say is the closest to [Participant]?

11. Does [Participant] seem generally happy with his life?

12. How would you describe [Participant]'s state of well-being?

NEUROPSYCHOLOGICAL REHABILITATION
2008, 18 (5/6), 766–783

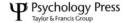

Holistic neuro-rehabilitation in the community: Is identity a key issue?

Rudi Coetzer

North Wales Brain Injury Service, Colwyn Bay, Wales, and Bangor University, Wales

Many people experience identity change after brain injury. Impaired self-awareness after acquired brain injury is also common and can, along with other factors, affect the identity change a person may experience. Holistic rehabilitation programmes attempt to address both cognitive and emotional difficulties and specifically problems of self-awareness after brain injury. Does identity change require longer-term rehabilitation interventions? This paper describes a community-based neuro-rehabilitation service that has incorporated some principles from more traditional holistic programmes with a view to providing long-term, low-intensity brain injury rehabilitation. Specific reference is made to problems of identity and how these may be addressed during long-term psychotherapeutic follow-up. The potential relevance of the total duration of rehabilitation input rather than simply the number of sessions when working with adjustment and identity change after brain injury in community settings is discussed. The service model is compared to more traditional holistic rehabilitation programmes. A case study and early outcome data are presented to illustrate some of these points and to provide more information about the nature of the programme.

Keywords: Identity; Brain injury; Psychotherapy; Holistic neuro-rehabilitation.

Correspondence should be sent to Rudi Coetzer, North Wales Brain Injury Service, Conwy and Denbighshire NHS Trust, Colwyn Bay Hospital, Hesketh Road, Colwyn Bay LL29 8AY, UK. E-mail: Rudi.Coetzer@cd-tr.wales.nhs.uk

The author would like to thank Lance Trexler and the other two reviewers for their thoughtful and helpful feedback on an earlier draft of this paper.

INTRODUCTION

Acquired brain injury can result in different combinations of cognitive, emotional, and behavioural impairments, contributing, with other factors, to significant disability in many cases. These impairments, directly or by default, can also result in a profound change of identity for the individual. Most practitioners would have been struck at some point by how difficult individuals find it to adjust to what is almost always a life-changing event. Hence, in addition to more traditional rehabilitation interventions, clinicians increasingly have to find ways to assist people with acquired brain injury to come to terms with the long-term effects of brain injury. In fact, Diller (2005) reminds us of the great importance of helping people to cease mourning, accept their limitations, and restore self-esteem during neuro-rehabilitation. Also, at a more strategic or policy level in the UK, to some extent the chronic nature of problems after brain injury is now recognised by the National Service Framework for Long-Term Neurological Conditions (Department of Health, 2005). It is hoped that this will shape how services are delivered over the next decade.

Acquired brain injury can, within a second, disrupt aspects of an individual's life. But what do we mean by a person's life? Perhaps looking beyond objective symptoms and signs associated with brain injury, can it be that one of the potentially most enduring changes after brain injury relates to the subjective experience of who someone is and is seen to be? As part of a person's development, identity is formed over many years and becomes more settled over time. For example, Erikson (1963) described eight stages of development, including the stage of identity formation during adolescence. Successful negotiation of this stage (Stage 5, Identity versus Confusion) results in the person having an integrated view of him or herself as a unique person (Erikson, 1963). However, it is unlikely that identity is formed during only one developmental stage of a person's life. Many of Erikson's (1963) other stages also impact on identity, for example the development of intimacy during early adulthood and the sense of fulfilment during older age. Many others have theorised about identity, sometimes using the term "self" as synonymous with "identity". For example, Hayes, Strosahl, and Wilson (2004) described the self as constituting a conceptualised self, ongoing self-awareness and an observing self. Myles (2004) applied this model to brain injury rehabilitation and suggested that the loss of sense of self after brain injury constituted a crisis in the conceptualised self (our historical view of ourselves). Within a cognitive-behavioural model, these would represent our thoughts about who we are. Clearly though, within Hayes, Strosahl, and Wilson's (2004) model, ongoing self-awareness also needs to be considered within the context of identity after brain injury.

One of the most perplexing symptoms after acquired brain injury is impaired self-awareness. Impaired self-awareness is recognised to negatively influence a person's engagement with rehabilitation interventions (Lam, McMahon, Priddy, & Gehered-Schultz, 1998) and employment outcome (Ownsworth, Desbois, Grant, Fleming, & Strong, 2006). Self-awareness has, in broad terms, been defined as the ability to consciously process information about the self in a way that reflects a relatively objective view, while maintaining a unique phenomenological experience or sense of self (Prigatano, 1997). Thus impaired self-awareness would represent the inability to perceive the self objectively, as others would, as well as a disturbance of personal identity. Hence besides the more obvious physical and cognitive impairments associated with acquired brain injury that can lead to significant changes in everyday life, impaired self-awareness can clearly further compli-cate the person's appraisal of his or her potentially changed identity. However, it is also worth noting that not all people suffer impaired self-awareness after brain injury and that we do not fully understand all the factors contributing to it.

Much has been written about the neurological basis of impaired self-awareness. Several specific anatomical regions have been postulated to be involved in self-awareness. However, keeping in mind the work of, for example, Bigler (2001), we are reminded of the importance of recognising the disruption of networks after brain injury as well as the not insignificant limitations of neuro-imaging. The finding of Sherer, Hart, Whyte, Nick, and Yablon (2005) that in their sample of sub-acute traumatically brain-injured adults impaired self-awareness was not associated with a lesion in a specific area of the brain but rather the actual number of lesions, is fascinat-ing. Sherer et al. (2005) concluded that the most likely explanation was that the disruption of widely distributed networks was more important to self-awareness than a single lesion in a specific region. Furthermore, Ownsworth, McFarland, and Young (2002) in their study of factors underpinning poor self-awareness concluded that one of the clinical implications was a need to assess both neuropsychological (cognitive) as well as psychological factors. Indeed, Giacino and Cicerone (1998) pointed out that problems of self-awareness could have multiple determinants. Furthermore, Anson and Ponsford (2006) found that there are interaction effects with self-awareness, for example, improved mood being associated with greater self-awareness after intervention, among other contributing variables. Clearly we have much to learn about not only the neuro-anatomical structures involved in self-awareness but also the psychological factors and rehabilitation.

Pragmatically, self-awareness can perhaps be seen as a fundamental cog-nitive building block underpinning a person's sense of identity. A change in sense of personal identity after acquired brain injury can take place in several areas. For example, employment or professional status, role in the family, parental role, friendships, and financial status are some of the more tangible areas of potential change after brain injury. But the individual as a person may also change as a result of cognitive impairment and behavioural and emotional changes. Impaired self-awareness may make it difficult for the individual to accurately process and, very importantly, come to terms with these changes. Nochi (1998) described how a loss of sense of self may take different forms, including loss of self-knowledge, loss of self by comparison, and loss of self in the views of others. Judd and Wilson (1999) pointed out that it is important to understand how people attribute meaning to their brain injury and impairment and how this process impacts on their understanding of themselves. Furthermore, a dislike of how the person views him or herself after brain injury may represent a mourning for their identity prior to injury (Judd & Wilson, 1999).

Focusing on rehabilitation in clinical practice, Gracey, Oldham, and Kritzinger (2007) provided a case report outlining the presentation of anxiety secondary to seizures after subarachnoid haemorrhage. This case report was about the efficacy of cognitive behavioural therapy (CBT) in managing anxiety symptoms and the difficulties related to using question-naires and disentangling neurological from psychological factors in the person's clinical presentation. Furthermore, this case report also illustrated how within a CBT model the patient's cognitions, or the way he saw himself, changed after his acquired brain injury—for example, never having been an anxious individual, not recognising anxiety after his brain injury and confusing anxiety symptoms for seizures. This case report helps practitioners to understand some of the links between change in identity, a person's cognitive appraisal of these changes, clinical presentation, and reha-bilitation strategies. At least some of the emotional difficulties (anxiety) in this case report appeared to stem from changes in who the person perceived himself to be after as compared to before sustaining his brain injury.

Does cross-fertilisation take place between rehabilitation in clinical prac-tice and development of theory and models of rehabilitation? Several theories and models of neuro-rehabilitation exist and Wilson (1997, 2002) provided comprehensive overviews of this complex topic. Broadly, these models encompass behavioural, cognitive, compensatory, and holistic approaches to rehabilitation (Wilson, 1997). Some models emphasise practice as the main factor responsible for improvement, while others use compensatory strategies to improve outcome. The person's need for adjustment and emotional re-integration are central to other models of neuro-rehabilitation, most notably holistic models. The holistic model of rehabilitation emphasises the need for developing self-awareness and identifies psychotherapy as part of the treatment package. However, in the individual case, it is unlikely that a single model or theory can always explain or guide treatment, and clinicians have to integrate different models and theories, as proposed by Wilson (2002). Of great importance also, of course, is how those who use our services experience rehabilitation. A pragmatic approach is perhaps that clinical practice (Wilson, 2005) is where models of rehabilitation can really be pushed forward. This historically appears to have been the case for holistic rehabilitation programmes.

Sarajuuri and Koskinen (2006) provided an overview of how holistic rehabilitation programmes were developed in the United States by Yehuda Ben-Yishay and George Prigatano during the late 1970s and early 1980s, respectively. These programmes subsequently underwent further development, for example, the use of a primary therapist for addressing some of the issues stemming from poor self-awareness (Trexler, Eberle, & Zappala, 2000). Further developments took place in several other countries of the world, for example, Finland (Sarajuuri & Koskinen, 2006) and Denmark (Caetano & Christensen, 2000). The Oliver Zangwill Centre (Wilson et al., 2000) played the leading role in developing a holistic neuro-rehabilitation centre of excellence in the UK. It is striking though that throughout the world, purely community-based services providing low-intensity long-term rehabilitation have not developed to the same extent. While there are many differences, for example, in length of time that input is provided and emphasis on types of interventions, in essence holistic neuro-rehabilitation programmes provide the following: individual and group interventions to address cognitive, behavioural, and emotional difficulties; increasing understanding or self-awareness; and providing work-trials or facilitation of return to education.

Rehabilitation strategies to address problems of self-awareness in holistic rehabilitation programmes include feedback, group therapy, videotaping, and psychotherapy (Prigatano, 2005). Fleming and Ownsworth (2006) provided a more detailed overview of interventions for problems of awareness. Holistic rehabilitation programmes traditionally have placed strategies to address problems of self-awareness at the centre of their treatment philosophy. Some have met with more success than others. In many holistic programmes, psychotherapy appears to play an important role in addressing problems of self-awareness. Prigatano (2005) asserted that psychotherapy could be an important strategy to work with problems of self-awareness, even where change was unlikely, because the therapeutic alliance can serve to help persons with brain injury make better decisions. Indeed several authors have advocated the role of psychotherapy in reconstructing the sense of self or identity after brain injury (Morris, 2004; Myles, 2004; Pollack, 2005; Prigatano, 1999). Reconstructing identity is central in the psychotherapeutic model described by Miller (1993), whereas Myles (2004) placed acceptance more centrally in the process.

The classic holistic rehabilitation programmes are perhaps not easy to replicate in the community, where high staff-to-patient ratios, therapeutic milieu, and intensity of interventions cannot be achieved for many reasons. And surely community-based rehabilitation should be seen as part of a wider spectrum of services rather than as a "one stop" type of service. Nevertheless there is an increasing desire to provide neuro-rehabilitation in the communities where people live. For example, recently the British Psychological Society Division of Neuropsychology (2005) produced a report outlining a proposed model of services for people with acquired brain injury, placing a strong emphasis on, for example, non-residential community brain injury rehabilitation centres. While there are limitations to what can be provided as regards neuropsychological rehabilitation in community settings, there are also good reasons to develop these services. For example, Trexler et al. (2000) described how their day treatment programme in the USA was designed to promote long-term community reintegration after inpatient rehabilitation has been completed. Community rehabilitation increasingly appears to be effective, even many years after injury (e.g., Powell, Heslin, & Greenwood, 2002). But is there perhaps a potentially overlooked reasoning behind developing holistic rehabilitation programmes in the community? The community is where people have to live their lives, and by implication with their identities. Even where good rehabilitation gains have been made prior to discharge into the community, it is here that people ultimately have to adjust and learn to live their new lives. Identity is, it can be argued, central to long-term rehabilitation and integration into the community.

HOLISTIC REHABILITATION IN THE COMMUNITY

There is evidence that intensive, community-based outpatient holistic rehabilitation can produce favourable outcomes (e.g., Cicerone, Mott, Azulay, & Friel, 2004). However, can limited, low-intensity holistic rehabilitation be provided on an outpatient basis? Such a programme has been developed in the UK (Coetzer et al., 2003) and is now described and compared to more traditional holistic brain injury rehabilitation programmes. The North Wales Brain Injury Service (NWBIS) is a multidisciplinary outpatient brain injury rehabilitation service with input from clinical neuropsychology, neurology, occupational therapy, social work, neuropsychiatry, physiotherapy, speech and language therapy, and rehabilitation assistants. The service is neuropsychology led and managed. The holistic model of brain injury rehabilitation provides both the theoretical foundations as well as the philosophical underpinnings of the programme. The clinical remit is to see individuals of most age groups with moderate to severe acquired (non-progressive) brain injuries. The majority of referrals have been in the severe category. While traumatic brain injury represents the largest proportion of referrals, the service accepts referrals of other non-progressive acquired neurological conditions including, for example, cerebrovascular accidents and brain infections.

Rehabilitation input is entirely individualised and based on the needs identified during the initial clinical assessment. The following characteristics of holistic neuro-rehabilitation programmes are embedded in the general model underpinning service delivery. Rehabilitation is provided individually and in groups. Members of the multidisciplinary team address cognitive, behavioural, physical, and emotional difficulties. Generally one clinician takes the lead in a patient's care. Increasing understanding or self-awareness is a central focus that permeates most of the clinical interventions. For example, the head injury education group aims to increase patients' understanding of brain injury as well as self-awareness. Another example is the way in which brain scan results are discussed in detail with patients to increase their understanding of the nature of their brain injury. Individual psychotherapy forms a core aspect of the programme for those who may benefit from it. One of the main aims of psychotherapy is to increase understanding and self-awareness, with a view to assisting patients over the long-term to come to terms with their lives after brain injury and re-form their identity. Re-integration to work or education is a major focus of occupational therapy interventions and involves close collaboration with local employers.

What then are the differences from other programmes? Perhaps the major operational differences from other holistic programmes, stemming to some extent from the individualised nature of the programme, is that patients are not discharged from the service, neither are they provided with a fixed number of sessions/length of time. Rather, long-term input is prioritised. This of course excludes delivering a predetermined, repeatable programme that is the same for everyone. Instead, based on their identified needs and rehabilitation goals, individuals can receive any combination of therapies for any period of time. Furthermore, the intensity (number of sessions per time period) is much lower than in other holistic programmes, peaking at approximately two sessions per week (about 2–3 hours), but usually less. By comparison, for example, Trexler (2000) reviewed several holistic programmes and found that intensity varied between 4 and 6 hours per day, whereas duration varied between approximately 4 and 7 months.

Another factor that makes it impractical within the NWBIS to deliver a circumscribed programme of interventions over a fixed period has to do with the large number of referrals and heterogeneity in clinical presentation. Not every person is suitable for all aspects of the programme. The programme has been designed specifically to reject as few referrals as possible. Hence the epochs of the programme vary and are determined more by factors such as time since injury and individuals' goals or needs. A general trend is for the number of consultations to be tapered over time, to facilitate generalisation and prevent long-term dependence on rehabilitation services. Groups are provided when there are enough suitable participants, rather than on a predetermined annual frequency. Clearly the programme has to cope with substantial heterogeneity of patients. How can we compare more systematically the characteristics of this programme with other holistic programmes? Trexler (2000) has described seven characteristics of holistic rehabilitation programmes. Table 1 follows Trexler's (2000) classification and provides a more systematic outline of the similarities and differences between the NWBIS programme and other holistic programmes.

What have we learnt from developing a community-based neuro-rehabilitation service incorporating some of the main principles from other holistic rehabilitation programmes? We have learnt that long-term change, especially as regards identity and adjustment, is slow, and hence careful titration of input over time may be more sensible in this setting. There is, undeniably, also the issue of geography. The NWBIS is located in a rural area and much time is inevitably spent driving from the unit to places in the community where input is provided, including people's homes. Interestingly, Ponsford, Harrington, Olver, and Roper (2006) also reported on this significant aspect of providing rehabilitation in the community. While this is a heavy price to pay, the benefit does appear to be significant opportunities for generalisation of therapeutic gains. And perhaps the fact that service users do come to the unit also provides a counterbalance for what can be a significant drain on valuable clinical resources.

What are the perceived strengths of this programme? Focusing therapies (including psychotherapy) to increase self-awareness and help people come to terms with the effects of brain injury in order to facilitate resolution of potential issues around identity has probably been a major strength of the programme. This is not an innovation, and in many holistic programmes psychotherapy, for example, has a central role. But allowing enough time for the lengthy process of facilitating adjustment for changed identity to take place is perhaps a luxury that a low intensity service can afford. Furthermore, the provision of groups is nothing new nor is the already mentioned interdisciplinary work, but co-ordinating this has been more difficult because of, for example, the amount of time spent travelling. One morning per week clinicians meet as a team to discuss new referrals and review existing cases. While this is cost-effective, it is recognised that it may risk mutual goals becoming vague or interventions unfocused. Correctly applying referral criteria has been invaluable and has certainly reduced inappropriate referrals. Medical colleagues in the service make a major contribution here and also contribute to helping people understand the physical factors contributing to their presentation, thus also facilitating self-awareness.

The greatest strength, operationally, of the service has probably been not discharging patients. While counter-intuitive to some extent, it has allowed patients to be followed up for much longer than would be the norm, albeit at a much lower intensity. In terms of facilitating the re-establishment of a patient's identity within a community setting, this seems a reasonable, if

TABLE 1
Holistic rehabilitation programme characteristics described by Trexler (2000): Application within the NWBIS

Programme characteristic	Degree to which provided	How provided	When provided and duration
Individualised goal setting	Moderate	Occupational therapists involve service users in individualised goal setting and review of goals. Type and intensity of therapies fully individualised.	At start of rehabilitation; during initial assessment following referral Initial assessment lasts approximately 1–4 sessions.
Holistic rehabilitation planning	Moderate	A lead clinician coordinates the patient's care within the service. Rehabilitation team meets once a week to discuss new referrals and existing patients. Regular informal discussion of patients' rehabilitation between clinicians involved. Fully integrated inter-disciplinary clinical notes.	Throughout the programme
Neuropsychological orientation	Extensive	The programme is neuropsychology led. Impairment of awareness addressed by different clinicians via feedback and psychotherapy. Provision of compensatory strategies for cognitive impairment. Psychotherapy provided to facilitate emotional adjustment.	After the early assessments by different clinicians have been completed, variation in duration depending on individualised needs identified during assessment. Individual psychotherapy can last from approximately 5 to >50 sessions.

(*Table continued*)

TABLE 1
Continued

Programme characteristic	Degree to which provided	How provided	When provided and duration
Therapeutic milieu	Limited	Limited provision of therapeutic milieu through groups, e.g., information group, problem solving group, employment group, occupational therapy groups. Feedback part of most clinicians' rehabilitation interventions.	Usually after individual therapies have started. Groups provided in parallel with individual therapies. Group psychotherapy not provided. Duration of education group approximately 8 sessions of 2 hours each (relatives in parallel group sessions).
Outcome-orientated rehabilitation planning	Extensive	Extensive provision of therapy away from the clinic setting. Long-term scheduled and unscheduled follow-up provided. Patients are not formally discharged from the service, as they can re-access services without a re-referral.	Throughout programme
Intensity of rehabilitation programme	Limited	Low intensity but lengthy duration of input to achieve meaningful psychological gains.	Throughout programme
Brain injury rehabilitation expertise	Moderate	Multi-professional staff, including medical, psychology, therapies and social work. No nursing staff. About half (9/16) of staff have at least 5 years or more direct experience of brain injury rehabilitation.	Varies very modestly as a result of staff turnover

not an essential approach to long-term rehabilitation. The community setting can perhaps be seen as a diffusion mechanism for shaping the application of some of the main characteristics of holistic rehabilitation, in as much as regards our resources, we can probably only really alter length of input or number of sessions. Hence in this service length of time was prioritised rather than intensity to alter and spread as widely as possible our limited resources, to help patients coming to terms with life and identity after brain injury and improve functional outcome while limiting reliance on social and health support where possible. Was this a wise decision? In an almost perverse way mirroring the aforementioned point, only time can tell. Next some initial outcome data and a case report are presented to further illustrate the characteristics of the programme.

OUTCOMES AND CASE DESCRIPTION

An important question remains to be explored. What clinical outcomes has this community programme achieved? Coetzer and Rushe (2005) retrospectively reviewed some early outcome data (European Brain Injury Questionnaire; Teasdale et al., 1997) of the NWBIS. Paired samples t-tests were performed between the first and repeated European Brain Injury Questionnaire (EBIQ) and effect sizes calculated. Significance was defined as $p <$ .05; effect sizes ranged from 0.25 to 0.54. The main finding was that this group of people with moderate to severe traumatic brain injury subjectively reported improved psychosocial outcome, including patients more than 2 years post-injury at the time the first EBIQ was administered. The data for this group ($N = 55$) revealed a significant reduction in EBIQ total scores for both patients (from an average of 119.6 to 107.1) and relatives (from an average of 122.7 to 116.3). A sub-group less than 2 years post-injury ($n = 23$) also showed a significant reduction in EBIQ scores for patients (from an average of 113.2 to 100.9) and relatives (from an average of 114.5 to 102.0). For a sub-group more than 2 years post-injury a significant reduction in EBIQ scores was found for patients (from an average of 126.8 to 114.1) but not for carers. These findings should of course be interpreted within context.

A strength of this outcome study was that the sample probably reflected the clinical population seen in many post-acute neuro-rehabilitation settings. Most were male (35 out of 55) and younger adults (mean age 38.9 years, $SD = 13.0$, range 19–75). A large proportion (47) sustained a severe traumatic brain injury (TBI), a small proportion (7) a moderate TBI, and only one person a mild TBI. Severity of TBI was determined by defining a moderate injury as a GCS score 9–12 or a loss of consciousness between 30 minutes and 24 hours; a severe injury as a GCS score 8 or lower or a loss of consciousness of more than 24 hours. There were several limitations that should be kept in mind when interpreting the findings, including small sample size and no non-treatment control group. Furthermore, it is important to be aware that it is difficult to use a single measure of outcome to chart the changes after holistic neuro-rehabilitation (Williams, Evans, & Wilson, 1999). Indeed, a significant limitation was the absence of data indicating "clinical significance", for example, employment outcome. While difficult to make direct comparisons, reassuringly these findings appear to be broadly similar to the findings from other holistic centres using similar questionnaires; for example, the EBIQ data reported by Bateman (2006). Furthermore, Svendsen, Teasdale, and Pinner (2004) also used the EBIQ as an outcome measure and concluded that their high intensity holistic neuro-rehabilitation programme can reduce symptoms in brain-injured patients, although the aim of restoring functioning to levels found in the non-brain-injured populations was not realistic.

Case study

The following case study provides more qualitative information to further illustrate the nature of the programme, especially the psychotherapeutic interventions. This case report has also been described elsewhere from within a general psychotherapeutic theoretical framework and applied to brain injury rehabilitation (Coetzer, 2007).

Ms C was in secondary school at the time she was injured in a road traffic collision. She suffered a severe traumatic brain injury. Her GCS score was 6/15 on admission to hospital. Computed tomography of the brain revealed a fracture of the occipital bone and generalised cerebral swelling, but no evidence of a focal mass effect or midline shift. No neuro-surgical intervention was required. Ms C was unconscious for about 36 hours, with post-traumatic amnesia for about 4 days in total. In the hospital notes it was recorded that by the 5th day after the accident she was able to communicate voluntarily and that by day 6 she was orientated. Ms C was discharged home to the care of her parents after a total length of stay of one week. She received no further rehabilitation at the time.

After a period at home, Ms C attempted to pass her A-level school exams. This, rather unexpectedly for her, was not successful. Ms C was generally considered to be confident and very able academically prior to the accident. After failing her A-levels, Ms C attempted to return to an undemanding part-time job as a cashier but could manage this for only one morning per week, mainly as a result of fatigue and poor initiation. These early failures contributed to feelings of despondency and worthlessness and were experienced as incongruous with her pre-injury identity. Three years after the injury her family doctor referred her for a neuropsychological opinion and asked for advice regarding her potential for further rehabilitation. Ms C was initially seen at her family doctor's practice. Clinically she presented with anxiety, depression, problems related to fatigue, irritability, and lack of motivation.

Initially Ms C was offered neuropsychology and occupational therapy input and later neurology review. The main proportion of her input consisted of psychotherapy. Ms C was provided with 62 individual sessions with a neuropsychologist. At the same time, occupational therapy input (10 sessions) was provided with a focus on return to work and higher education. Most sessions were at the unit, although many of the occupational therapy sessions were at home or elsewhere in the community. The neuropsychologist also provided two family sessions, and 48 individual sessions to one family member, who found it very difficult to come to terms with Ms C's brain injury. The sessions with the family member consisted of individual psychotherapy and some time allocated to regular review of Ms C's rehabilitation goals and achievement, the latter with Ms C present on many occasions.

The neuropsychologist and occupational therapist met regularly to discuss goals and progress and also jointly met with Ms C on a couple of occasions. Two neurology consultations were provided following a concern about possible seizures. Ms C had no physical impairments or difficulties of speech, hence no speech and language therapy or physiotherapy sessions were provided. Ms C did not attend any of the groups offered by the service, but later did become involved in a local voluntary sector advocacy group. It is important to plot the number of sessions against time. Ms C received input from the service for a total of 5 years, 6 months. Initially she and her family member were seen approximately every fortnight. After about 3 years the frequency had reduced to every 6 weeks, subsequently to 6-monthly reviews and finally two annual reviews. At this point Ms C reported having found her way or place in the community and appeared to have settled. She identified as her final goal to "go it alone", knowing that if needed she could directly re-access the service. Fourteen months after her last annual review Ms C let the service know that she was continuing to do well and that she had moved into more independent accommodation and was in virtually full-time employment.

While the total time under the care of the service was 5 years, 6 months, essentially Ms C received 3 years of relatively regular psychotherapy input. Early themes explored during psychotherapy included her understanding of what had happened to her and the nature of the associated changes. One of the main changes she reported was a change in identity. Ms C often attempted to understand this by comparing her identity after brain injury to that of individuals in her peer group. However, she found it difficult to explain these changes and for example reported that, "On the surface I seem to be fine, inside my head I am not." She experienced her change in identity as a major loss. Therefore, another theme during psychotherapy was to come to terms with her loss and attempt to make sense of who she now was. During this stage she expressed for the first time emotions congruent with loss. Subsequently Ms C focused less on her accident and injury. Psychotherapy then started to attempt to provide her with the skills to manage better some of the remaining difficulties, most notably anxiety, something she did not see as part of her identity prior to the accident. During this later stage CBT was provided to help her manage her anxiety. Increasingly, as part of CBT, more challenging functional goals were set.

Functional goals were regularly reviewed and as part of this the psychotherapy process was also intermittently reflected on. As regards more formal outcomes for Ms C, the first EBIQ was administered 69 months after her injury, some time after her community rehabilitation had started (as a newly developed service at the time, collection of outcome data lagged behind the early provision of rehabilitation). The EBIQ Self-Rating (total score) at baseline was 127, with a Relative-Rating (total score) of 123. Ten months later the corresponding EBIQ scores were Self 93, Relative 123. Interestingly, at this point her Awareness Questionnaire (Sherer et al., 1998) scores were 38 (Self), 33 (Relative) and 42 (Clinician), perhaps mirroring the EBIQ finding that her family member's perception was that Ms C difficulties were continuing. Finally, 97 months post-injury the EBIQ scores were Self 92 and Relative 84, now revealing a convergence between Ms C and her family member's perception of her functioning, perhaps also including perceived aspects of identity. As important perhaps, some of the functional improvements resulting from goals set in rehabilitation and subsequently achieved, included passing her driving test, finding local employment and resuming local and international travel.

There are some similarities between this case and the case described by Gracey, Oldham, and Kritzinger (2007). For example, Ms C's anxiety about seizures, having in the past never seen herself as an anxious person, hence finding her anxiety incongruous with her "remembered" identity. Furthermore, the use of CBT to manage some of the difficulties related to anxiety appears to have been effective in both cases. In addition, the importance of the family context (Yeates, Henwood, Gracey, & Evans, 2007) was also highly relevant in this case. There were of course also obvious differences, for example aetiology, and length and nature of the interventions provided. Perhaps these two cases again remind us about Wilson's (2002) point regarding combining different theories and models to rehabilitate individuals with acquired brain injury. While in Ms C's case rehabilitation started with community rehabilitation 3 years post-injury, perhaps negating to some extent at least spontaneous recovery as a confounding factor, it must be emphasised that for many people psychotherapeutic interventions are not indicated or even useful.

Finally we must keep in mind that there are also cases where, despite concerted rehabilitation input, improvement does not take place and conversely sometimes people make spectacular recoveries without any professional help.

CONCLUSIONS

This paper described how a community-based brain injury rehabilitation service has adapted and applied characteristics of holistic rehabilitation, trading off intensity for duration of input. Early outcome and other data for the NWBIS programme appear to be promising, but clearly need replication. Nevertheless, this type of programme is probably part of a continuum of services that can benefit persons with acquired brain injury. It is highly unlikely that it can provide all care on every occasion for every person with a brain injury. Community-based holistic programmes are more likely to be useful in augmenting other services, for example, inpatient and higher intensity early holistic rehabilitation services. High intensity holistic programmes potentially fit better in the brain injury care pathway as a "bridge" between acute and sub-acute rehabilitation and long-term community-based rehabilitation. Self-awareness, rehabilitation for cognitive impairments, and educational approaches are perhaps then better served by these intermediate services, while psychological difficulties related to identity and emotional adjustment can possibly be more effectively addressed in post-acute holistic rehabilitation services providing much longer-term input.

Ultimately, we also have to consider the role of the environment in the rehabilitation of people with acquired brain injury. While there are many difficulties associated with delivering low-intensity holistic neurorehabilitation programmes in community settings and we still have much to learn, there are also potentially moderating factors, such as a rural location (Farmer, Clark, & Sherman, 2003). Furthermore there are well-recognised opportunities for generalisation, tapping some of the strengths in close-knit communities and perhaps better social support structures. The change of identity that often follows brain injury may be central to many long-term brain injury rehabilitation interventions. Perhaps it is here that a community-based holistic programme that provides relatively low intensity intervention but of much greater duration may lead to desirable emotional outcomes within the environments where people live and their identities come to the fore on a daily basis. Hopefully this type of programme can augment other holistic programmes and further facilitate adjustment after brain injury, thus reducing the individual's long-term suffering as well as the collective burden on society.

REFERENCES

Anson, K., & Ponsford, J. (2006). Who benefits? Outcome following a coping skills group intervention for traumatically brain injured individuals. *Brain Injury*, *20*(1), 1–13.

Bateman, A. (2006). Conference presentation: *Oliver Zangwill Centre 10th Anniversary Outcomes*. 16–17 November 2006, Hinxton Hall, Cambridge, UK.

Bigler, E. D. (2001). The lesion(s) in traumatic brain injury: Implications for clinical neuropsychology. *Archives of Clinical Neuropsychology*, *16*, 95–131.

British Psychological Society Division of Neuropsychology (2005). *Clinical neuropsychology and rehabilitation services for adults with acquired brain injury*. Leicester, UK: British Psychological Society.

Caetano, C., & Christensen, A-L. (2000). The CRBI at the University of Copenhagen: A participant-therapist perspective. In A-L. Christensen & B. P. Uzzell (Eds.), *International handbook of neuropsychological rehabilitation* (pp. 259–271). Dordrecht: Kluwer Academic.

Cicerone, K. D., Mott, T., Azulay, J., & Friel, J. C. (2004). Community integration and satisfaction with functioning after intensive cognitive rehabilitation for traumatic brain injury. *Archives of Physical Medical Rehabilitation*, *85*(6), 943–950.

Coetzer, R. (2007). Psychotherapy following traumatic brain injury: Integrating theory and practice. *Journal of Head Trauma Rehabilitation*, *22*(1), 39–47.

Coetzer, B. R., & Rushe, R. (2005). Post-acute rehabilitation following traumatic brain injury: Are both early and later improved outcomes possible? *International Journal of Rehabilitation Research*, *28*(4), 361–363.

Coetzer, B. R., Vaughan, F. L., Roberts, C. B., & Rafal, R. (2003). The development of a holistic, community-based neurorehabilitation service in a rural area. *Journal of Cognitive Rehabilitation*, *21*(2), 4–8.

Department of Health (2005) *National service framework for long-term neurological conditions*. London: Department of Health.

Diller, L. (2005). Pushing the frames of reference in traumatic brain injury rehabilitation. *Archives of Physical Medicine & Rehabilitation*, *86*, 1075–1080.

Erikson, E. H. (1963). *Childhood and Society* (2nd ed.). New York: Norton.

Farmer, J. E., Clark, M. J., & Sherman, A. K. (2003). Rural versus urban social support seeking as a moderating variable in traumatic brain injury outcome. *Journal of Head Trauma Rehabilitation*, *18*(2), 116–127.

Fleming, J. M., & Ownsworth, T. (2006). A review of awareness interventions in brain injury rehabilitation. *Neuropsychological Rehabilitation*, *16*(4), 474–500.

Giacino, J. T., & Cicerone, K. D. (1998). Varieties of deficit unawareness after brain injury. *Journal of Head Trauma Rehabilitation*, *13*(5), 1–15.

Gracey, F., Oldham, P., & Kritzinger, R. (2007). Finding out if "The 'me' will shut down": Successful cognitive-behavioural therapy of seizure-related panic symptoms following subarachnoid haemorrhage: A single case report. *Neuropsychological Rehabilitation*, *17*(1), 106–119.

Hayes, S. C., Strosahl, K. D., & Wilson, K. G. (2004). *Acceptance and Commitment Therapy. An Experiential Approach to Behaviour Change*. New York: Guilford Press.

Judd, D. P., & Wilson, S. L. (1999). Brain injury and identity–the role of the counselling psychologist. *Counselling Psychology Review*, *14*, 4–16.

Lam, C. S., McMahon, B. T., Priddy, D. A., & Gehered-Schultz, A. (1998). Deficit awareness and treatment performance among traumatic head injury adults. *Brain Injury*, *2*(4), 235–242.

Miller, L. (1993). *Psychotherapy of the brain-injured patient: Reclaiming the shattered self*. New York: Norton.

Morris, S. D. (2004). Rebuilding identity through narrative following traumatic brain injury. *Journal of Cognitive Rehabilitation*, *22*(2), 15–21.

Myles, S. M. (2004). Understanding and treating loss of sense of self following brain injury: A behavior analytic approach. *International Journal of Psychology and Psychological Therapy*, *4*(3), 487–504.

Nochi, M. (1998). "Loss of self" in the narratives of people with traumatic brain injuries: A qualitative analysis. *Social Sciences Medicine*, *46*(7), 869–878.

Ownsworth, T., Desbois, J., Grant, E., Fleming, J., & Strong, J. (2006). The associations among self-awareness, emotional well-being, and employment outcome following acquired brain injury: A 12-month longitudinal study. *Rehabilitation Psychology*, *51*(1), 50–59.

Ownsworth, T. L., McFarland, K., & Young, R. M. (2002). The investigation of factors underlying deficits in self-awareness and self-regulation. *Brain Injury*, *16*(4), 291–309.

Pollack, I. W. (2005). Psychotherapy. In J. M. Silver, T. W. McAllister & S. C. Yudofsky (Eds.), *Textbook of traumatic brain injury* (pp. 641–654). Washington, DC: American Psychiatric Publishing, Inc.

Ponsford, J., Harrington, H., Olver, J., & Roper, M. (2006). Evaluation of a community-based model of rehabilitation following traumatic brain injury. *Neuropsychological Rehabilitation*, *16*(3), 315–328.

Powell, J., Heslin, J., & Greenwood, R. (2002). Community-based rehabilitation after severe traumatic brain injury: A randomised controlled trial. *Journal of Neurology Neurosurgery and Psychiatry*, *72*(2), 193–202.

Prigatano, G. P. (1997). The problem of impaired self-awareness in neuropsychological rehabilitation. In J. Leon-Carrion (Ed.), *Neuropsychological Rehabilitation. Fundamentals, Innovations and Directions* (pp. 301–311). Delray Beach, FL: St. Lucie Press.

Prigatano, G. P. (1999). *Principles of Neuropsychological Rehabilitation*. New York: Oxford University Press.

Prigatano, G. P. (2005). Disturbances of self-awareness and rehabilitation of patients with traumatic brain injury: A 20-year perspective. *Journal of Head Trauma Rehabilitation*, *20*(1), 19–29.

Sarajuuri, J. M., & Koskinen, S. K. (2006). Holistic neuropsychological rehabilitation in Finland: The INSURE program–a transcultural outgrowth of perspectives from Israel to Europe via the USA. *International Journal of Psychology*, *41*(5), 362–370.

Sherer, M., Bergloff, P., Levin, E., High, W. M., Oden, K., & Nick, T. G. (1998). The Awareness Questionnaire: Factor structure and internal consistency. *Brain Injury*, *12*, 63–68.

Sherer, M., Hart, T., Whyte, J., Nick, T. G., & Yablon, S. A. (2005). Neuroanatomic basis of impaired self-awareness after traumatic brain injury. *Journal of Head Trauma Rehabilitation*, *20*(4), 287–300.

Svendsen, H. A., Teasdale, T. W., & Pinner, M. (2004). Subjective experience in patients with brain injury and their close relatives before and after a rehabilitation programme. *Neuropsychological Rehabilitation*, *14*(5), 495–515.

Teasdale, T. W., Christensen, A-L., Willmes, K., Deloche, G., Braga, L., Stachowiak, F., Vendrell, J., Castro-Caldas, A., Laaksonen, R. K., & Leclercq, M. (1997). Subjective experience in brain-injured patients and their close relatives: A European Brain Injury Questionnaire study. *Brain Injury*, *11*(8), 543–563.

Trexler, L. E. (2000). Empirical support for neuropsychological rehabilitation. In A-L. Christensen & B. P. Uzzell (Eds.), *International handbook of neuropsychological rehabilitation* (pp. 137–150). Dordrecht: Kluwer Academic Publishers.

Trexler, L. E., Eberle, R., & Zappala, G. (2000). Models and programs of the Center for Neuropsychological Rehabilitation: Fifteen years experience. In A-L. Christensen & B. P. Uzzell (Eds.), *International handbook of neuropsychological rehabilitation* (pp. 215–229). Dordrecht: Kluwer Academic Publishers.

Williams, W. H., Evans, J. J., & Wilson, B. A. (1999). Outcome measures for survivors of acquired brain injury in day and outpatient neurorehabilitation programmes. *Neuropsychological Rehabilitation*, *9*(3–4), 421–436.

Wilson, B. A. (1997). Cognitive rehabilitation: How it is and how it might be. *Journal of the International Neuropsychological Society*, *3*, 487–496.

Wilson, B. A. (2002). Towards a comprehensive model of cognitive rehabilitation. *Neuropsychological Rehabilitation*, *12*(2), 97–110.

Wilson, B. A. (2005). The clinical neuropsychologist's dilemma. *Journal of the International Neuropsychological Society*, *11*(4), 488–493.

Wilson, B. A., Evans, J., Brentnall, S., Bremner, S., Keohane, C., & Williams, H. (2000). The Oliver Zangwill Center for Neuropsychological Rehabilitation: A partnership between health care and rehabilitation research. In A-L. Christensen & B. P. Uzzell (Eds.), *International handbook of neuropsychological rehabilitation* (pp. 231–246). Dordrecht: Kluwer Academic Publishers.

Yeates, G., Henwood, K., Gracey, F., & Evans, J. J. (2007). Awareness of disability after acquired brain injury and the family context. *Neuropsychological Rehabilitation*, *17*(2), 151–173.

NEUROPSYCHOLOGICAL REHABILITATION
2008, 18 (5/6), 785–790

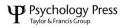

Subject Index